HEALTH, CULTURE
AND COMMUNITY

HEALTH, CULTURE AND COMMUNITY

*Case Studies of Public Reactions
to Health Programs*

Edited by
BENJAMIN D. PAUL

With the Collaboration of
WALTER B. MILLER

RUSSELL SAGE FOUNDATION
New York

STATEMENT CONCERNING PUBLICATIONS
OF RUSSELL SAGE FOUNDATION

© 1955
RUSSELL SAGE FOUNDATION
230 Park Avenue, New York, N.Y. 10017

Printed in the United States of America

Printed November, 1955	Reprinted April, 1972
Reprinted October, 1959	Reprinted December, 1973
Reprinted March, 1964	Reprinted February, 1975
Reprinted December, 1965	Reprinted March, 1976
Reprinted September, 1967	Reprinted May, 1978
Reprinted February, 1969	Reprinted June, 1978
Reprinted February, 1971	

Library of Congress Catalog Card Number: 55–10583
Standard Book Number: 87154–653–1

FOREWORD

Application of our available health knowledge is the weakest link in our chain of health protection. Vast stores of information about measures useful in solving health problems have been garnered through use of the scientific method of investigation. We have tremendously powerful tools with which to work: the laboratory, the epidemiological method coupled with statistical techniques for studying disease as it affects masses of people, our intricate and highly developed hospitals and other health facilities, the more than 150 types of health workers, and so on.

Nevertheless, experienced health workers know that it is not easy to persuade the public to make full use of the health information at hand, except when people are aroused by some obvious epidemic or other disaster. It is in the "public" part of public health that we are weak; the "health" aspects somehow seem simpler for us. It is not surprising that we come to this realization at the stage of development of western scientific medicine when community health measures which can usually be applied with only tacit acquiescence of the individual person, such as water purification and pasteurization of milk, are in general use in the more advanced countries. Much of our newer health work is with the individual. We must not only obtain his consent, but personal habits and ways of living must frequently be altered radically. If changes of this sort are to be brought about, we must apply what is known of human relations.

The behavioral or social scientists are also using the scientific method, and they can help in unraveling our human problems. Their concepts, tools, and methodology can be extremely useful in our efforts to understand the public with which we work. Many of these social scientists are eager to help us, even though they modestly tell us not to expect miracles. Accustomed as we are to the use of "miracle drugs," we wonder if they do not underestimate their potentialities! At the very least, it has been demonstrated again and again that they can help us remove the veil before our eyes which keeps us from seeing clearly the people we serve.

To aid health workers in understanding their human problems, the social scientist needs some experience of how the health worker thinks and of the kinds of problems he must face. In his teaching he needs examples which the health worker can easily understand, for social science terminology, like that in the health field, is not always easy for the neophyte.

Dr. Paul is one of the new group of social scientists who have taken the time to become familiar with health problems. He has a rare capacity to understand the health worker's aims and difficulties. His cases, collected from all over the world, represent actual health problems. In addition, however—and this is the significant point—the social scientist has been concerned in these particular situations and has contributed to understanding them. The cases illustrate numerous concepts from the behavioral sciences which are useful in health work.

Our experience in working with Dr. Paul at the Harvard School of Public Health has convinced us that these cases are most useful in demonstrating to health workers the kind of assistance they may expect from social scientists working with them as teammates. The cases will doubtless be equally valuable in bringing to the social scientist a clearer picture of health problems and of how he can be useful in seeking the right answers.

We are deeply grateful to Russell Sage Foundation for making this case collection possible, and for its vision in seeking to broaden and deepen the work of the health professions.

HUGH R. LEAVELL, M.D., DR. P.H.

Boston, Massachusetts

ACKNOWLEDGMENTS

This volume owes its existence to a happy conjunction of interest on the part of the faculty of the Harvard School of Public Health and the staff of Russell Sage Foundation. I am most grateful for their foresight and encouragement.

Preliminary versions of the case studies in this book have been tested in numerous staff and teaching seminars at the Harvard School of Public Health. I am much indebted to the many seminar participants for their reactions and criticisms, which helped materially to make the cases more instructive. I am equally indebted to the contributing authors for their patience and cooperation in meeting repeated requests for supplying new information and for rearranging portions of their material.

My particular thanks are due Dr. Walter B. Miller for his creative collaboration in the editorial task of aiding authors to maximize the effectiveness of their original contributions, and Mrs. Frances E. Martin for distinguished secretarial assistance in the preparation of manuscript.

BENJAMIN D. PAUL

CONTENTS

INTRODUCTION: Understanding the Community

A celebrated malariologist who worked on the Panama Canal project made a remark which lingers in the memory of his public health disciples. "If you wish to control mosquitoes," he said, "you must learn to think like a mosquito."[1] The cogency of this advice is evident. It applies, however, not only to mosquito populations one seeks to damage but also to human populations one hopes to benefit. If you wish to help a community improve its health, you must learn to think like the people of that community. Before asking a group of people to assume new health habits, it is wise to ascertain the existing habits, how these habits are linked to one another, what functions they perform, and what they mean to those who practice them.

When the aim is to bring mosquitoes under control, it may seem sufficient to understand the outlook of the insects and to ignore the outlook of the people they infect, on the assumption that the people will be pleased when their health improves as a result of the program, or, at worst, remain indifferent. This assumption may be valid in some cases, but can lead to unexpected trouble in others. In certain coastal zones of Peru, for example, technically successful DDT campaigns have resulted in public charges of incompetence and failure.

In one Peruvian zone the first year's campaign against malarial mosquitoes had a residual effect of six to nine months, but campaigns in succeeding years produced steadily shrinking effects as insects became more adapted to the mixture. Unprepared for this change, the villagers are now convinced that the spraying teams, originally conscientious, are becoming increasingly careless and that dishonest campaign officials are probably diverting the genuine DDT for some ulterior motive and substituting an inferior product in its place. Although the malaria rate has been reduced, the inhabitants do not associate this change with the spraying. Nor do they realize that the spray was aimed specifically at mosquitoes. To be sure, there are fewer mosquitoes and this is all to the good, but in their eyes mosquitoes have never been a

[1] Dr. Samuel Darling, as reported to the writer by Dr. Donald Augustine.

I

major insect pest, appearing only intermittently, unlike the perennial and bothersome housefly. According to popular assumption, the principal object of DDT spraying was to exterminate the fly, not the mosquito.

For several years this difference of interpretation did not matter; both mosquitoes and flies were cut down in substantial numbers. Malaria continues to be effectively controlled, but by now the flies have regained their lost ground. What campaign directors see as successful anti-anopheles work is seen by the local population as flagrantly unsuccessful anti-housefly work. Villagers say bitterly that the flies are worse than ever, appearing in great swarms a few weeks after communities have been sprayed.

Repercussions were more serious in another zone where anti-triatoma spraying actually brought Chagas' disease under control but was seen by the citizens as a fly-control fiasco. Aroused householders drew up a resolution, submitted it to the national Congress in Lima, and forced the health officer responsible for the campaign to answer charges of malfeasance. The officer was cleared but the episode did nothing to improve relations between health personnel and the population.

Evidently, then, we must reexamine the prevalent assumption that good results automatically carry conviction; dramatic effects in preventing or curing illness are not always self-validating. Facts do not speak for themselves; they are always cross-examined and given meaning in accordance with the assumptions of the examiner. We realize almost at once that the mosquito's image of the world must diverge sharply from our own. We realize less readily that different groups of humans, despite their constitutional similarities, can differ significantly and systematically in their perception of the same event. A given occurrence—an illness, an item of information, a DDT campaign—is really not the same event for all people. Observers located at different points in social space perceive the world from the perspective of their particular community or class or occupation.

Scope and Purpose of the Book

How does a human community accomplish its business? What keeps it on its course? How does it see and solve its problems? How does it perceive and receive efforts from the outside or the inside to improve its health? This volume provides case material for finding some of the answers. Each case deals with a concrete health situation or with a health program operating at the community level. All the cases are written by persons who were directly involved in the action or who lived in the community long enough to assess the situation at first hand through direct observation or interview.

Some of the cases appear as successes, others as failures. The case studies, however, have been selected not because they represent excellence of program or praiseworthy accomplishment but because they illuminate various facets of community process. In some instances these features are revealed most clearly when a program succeeds, in other instances when it fails. Some of the authors record the mistakes of others, a few bravely record their own. Virtue lies less in avoiding mistakes than in the capacity to recognize and explain them and thus to profit from experience.

Neither the cases nor the comments in this volume are intended to provide specific directives for action. The book reports what does happen, not what ought to happen. But clarifying by illustration what occurs in the community may help health workers make their own decisions and their own appraisal of results. George Rosen has written: "A knowledge of the community and its people . . . is just as important for successful public health work as is a knowledge of epidemiology or medicine. . . . The first principle in community organization is to start with people as they are and with the community as it is."[1]

A general book about social science and public health might dwell on the social antecedents of health conditions—the effects on health of increased productivity and rising standards of living; of urbanization, detribalization, and poverty; of social mobility and social strain; of new scientific knowledge and better medical techniques; of the growth of hospitals, nursing homes, and clinics. It might, on the other hand, dwell on the social consequences of medical developments such as the increase in human efficiency brought about by the reduction of debilitating illnesses, or the

[1] Rosen, George, "The Community and the Health Officer—A Working Team," *American Journal of Public Health*, vol. 44, January, 1954, pp. 14–16.

burdens of overcrowding and of an aging population. Some of these things inevitably become implicated in the case studies, but the book is not primarily concerned with the general social antecedents of health conditions or the long-range social consequences of medical developments. Its main concern is with the immediate situation where medicine and community meet.

Organization of the Cases

Each case study raises a problem, presents pertinent factual information, and draws attention to some of the larger issues illustrated by the data. Each study is complete in itself, and readers may select and compare specific cases as their tastes and interests direct. At the same time, the studies have been fitted into a larger framework, so that the total organization of the volume will add relevance and breadth to the individual reports. The 16 cases have been grouped into six sections, although some of the cases, because of their manifold implications, could fit equally well under several of the headings.

Reeducating the Community. In the long run the most efficient method of combating illness is to stop it at its source, to prevent its occurrence in the first place. The health sciences are discovering new means to promote sound health and prevent specific disabilities. The great challenge is to find ways of weaving the discoveries of science into the fabric of daily living. This is a task in community education, or more accurately, of reeducation.

It is a task in reeducation because every human community has developed an elaborate set of ideas, attitudes, and modes of behavior in response to the persisting problems of social living. Whether these are imparted to individuals through formal instruction or through the thousand diffuse ways in which cultural conditioning is effected, the adults of all communities are already educated. Whether or not one attends school, to grow up is to become educated. The content of this education varies with the cultural setting; knowledge of the digestive process imparted to a Zulu differs from that taught to a Peruvian peasant or a Canadian townsman.

Only in some communities do people venerate images or detect witches or conduct psychotherapy, but all have ways of coping with sickness and thinking about sickness. All peoples practice some form of preventive medicine, according to their own concepts of cause and prevention. People thus evaluate the acceptability of newly offered advice according to their own matrix of culturally conditioned understandings. New items of information must somehow be fitted into this matrix if they are to be received at all. The novel element must be reshaped to make it reasonably congruent with the existing framework of understanding, but in the process of assimilating new information, the framework itself is slightly transformed, like the growing organism that incorporates a bit of food. To enhance the likelihood of success, the educator must modify the form of his health message so that it makes sense to the particular audience for which it is intended. To do this well, he must be able to look at the world from the other person's frame of reference. The process of reeducation is thus two-sided, applying to the dispenser as well as the recipient of information. To teach, the health educator must be able to learn.

Reeducating the community was a primary aim in each of the first three cases. One study was written by a public health physician who played an active part in a comprehensive plan (first directed by Dr. Sidney Kark) to improve the health of South African people; heavy emphasis falls on reforming the diet. The author of another case is a social scientist who made a detailed assessment of one phase of a Peruvian health program initiated by Dr. John Hydrick, namely, the effort to convince housewives of the need to boil their drinking water. Another case is the joint product of a physician and a social scientist who conducted an intensive campaign to change popular conceptions about mental illness in a Canadian prairie town.

The three programs involved peoples with different languages and cultural traditions and used different methods to achieve varying degrees of success with different problems. Yet they teach similar lessons. What appears from the outside as irrational belief and behavior becomes intelligible when viewed from within. Perceiving the connections between items of belief and behavior as the people themselves perceive them enables us to make better sense of the seemingly capricious pattern of acceptance and rejection, of successful and unsuccessful educational efforts.

Why did the head of a Zulu family accept the verdict that several of his children were tubercular and should be hospitalized, yet vehemently reverse his stand when informed that his married daughter was the carrier? Why did Canadian citizens seem to tolerate a wider range of deviant behavior than those who were trying to educate them, yet refuse to accept the suggestion that there was a continuum rather than a hard line between personal normality and abnormality? Why did conservative Mrs. D in Los Molinos agree to boil her drinking water, while equally conservative Mrs. F scoffed at the idea of boiling hers? The cases give specific answers but they tell us something more general as well. They show in repeated detail that the culture pattern of a given people is made up of interwoven beliefs and dispositions, and why the pattern changes in some instances, but resists change in others.

Reaction to Crisis. Severe illness is always a psychological crisis for the individual and a social crisis for his family. All cultures anticipate such contingencies by furnishing criteria for weighing the severity of the crisis and specifying the steps to be taken when an event is identified as a crisis. Whether or not to call in a specialist, which type of specialist to summon, how to behave in his presence, how to utilize his advice, all depend on how the illness is classified. The category itself is determined as much by cultural definition as by the intrinsic nature of the ailment. Within any community the methods and assumptions of the specialist tend to be attuned to the beliefs of those who use his services since both parties are subject to the same system of expectation and the same cultural environment. To each, the behavior of the other is "natural."

But what seems natural in one social milieu often appears unnatural in another. A physician trained in one culture may experience confusion when he first faces a patient in another cultural setting; the patient, for his part, is frequently misled when the behavior of the alien physician diverges from his own expectations. Such cross-cultural encounters are potentially rich sources of insight into the social dimensions of sickness and therapy. Dr. Carstairs ably exploits these sources to give us a double view of his medical encounters in two communities of

India In a series of doctor-patient episodes, we see the situation both as he perceived it and as the patient and his family perceived it. The episodes make clear the divergence between our own and the rural Indian's conception of prognosis and healing, and demonstrate how powerfully these disparate expectations influence the process of transmitting health knowledge and medical care across cultural barriers.

Dr. Hsu's description of a severe outbreak of cholera in a Chinese town shows how pervasively the culture patterns of a community determine the people's response to an epidemic. Proceeding from different assumptions as to the ultimate causes of the crisis, the residents of the town and the agents of western medicine worked at cross-purposes, each side finding merit in its own method of protection and each failing to comprehend the logic behind the actions of the other.

The study by Dr. Hanks and his associates records a somewhat different situation. Spurred on by the death of a child they had tried to save, a social science research team alerted district health officials who arranged to have all the children of a threatened Thai community assemble for immunization against diphtheria. Many children appeared; even more did not. The authors investigated the reasons for the partial response. They wanted to know whether the evidence of an impending epidemic, as they saw it, was differently construed by most of the villagers or whether the information simply failed to reach them. What they found out about local culture and communication made it seem equally pertinent to ask why so many children actually appeared for immunization.

Sex Patterns and Population Problems. Although the concept of overpopulation is admittedly a relative one, certain areas such as Puerto Rico are commonly held to be seriously overcrowded. The advances of public health are partly responsible for this condition, and responsible health personnel are cooperating with experts in agriculture and industry to redress the balance between population and the means of support. The controversial issue of birth control rests on conflicting basic values and is thus not subject to scientific adjudication. Science cannot say what is preferable, but it is theoretically capable of saying what is possible, and a trained investigator can make a detached assessment of a going birth control program.

Dr. Stycos' study explains why Puerto Rico's numerous birth control clinics have made little impact on the high fertility rate. Local conceptions of virility, fidelity, and male authority are seen to be partly responsible.

On the Pacific Island of Yap, the pattern of relationship between the sexes differs markedly from the pattern in Puerto Rico. For years the population has been dwindling and although the elders want couples to have more children, women do what they can to remain childless until they are about thirty years old. Here again demographic problems hinge on culturally conditioned beliefs and practices surrounding sex and reproduction.

Effects of Social Segmentation. A community is more than a collection of individuals. Its members are part of a social system; they perform social roles and are bound to each other directly or indirectly by a network of rights and obligations. This system of interpersonal relationships, however, is seldom homogenous. It is usually divided into several distinguishable segments, each comprising its own subsystem of social roles. The segments are held together—tightly or loosely as the case may be—by certain cooperative or competitive arrangements. Characteristically, the segments of a social system differ in their respective activities, interests, and values. They often have different degrees of power, privilege, and prestige. In some instances the lines of cleavage are conspicuous; in others the magnitude or even the existence of cleavage depends on the purpose and standpoint of the observer.

Taking the standpoint of the Indian villager, Dr. Marriott recognizes three concentric social realms—the intimate realm of family and kinship, the familiar realm of village and caste, and the remote realm of the outside world. The author shows in detail why the western type of doctor, whether Indian or foreign, is perceived as a member of the outside world and is therefore distrusted in common with merchants and administrators. "Western medicine sits outside the door of the village, dependent upon governmental subsidy and foreign alms for its slim existence."

The Alabama town of Talladega is composed of three major social divisions: the elite white "community," the white workers, and the Negroes. Dr. Kimball's study shows how a self-survey which was intended to determine the health needs of the entire community was hampered by the separate values and organizational methods of each of these three social segments. In the author's words, "An overwhelming sentiment in favor of good health is no assurance that people will rush to support a program that promises health improvement. . . . With the organization and execution of Talladega's survey resting in the hands of its dominant powers, there was little likelihood that anything would be done to upset the existing system or threaten established interests."

The social segments which Dr. Naegele describes in his report on a mental health program in a Boston suburb are not divided by cultural and economic chasms as deep as those in Talladega. In this case the segments are three of Wellesley's social institutions: the school, the church, and the new Human Relations Service. All three are professionally concerned with individual character and social adjustment and therefore overlap in their aims and interests. But the organizational form and guiding principles of each institution differ significantly. These differences became manifest in joint meetings of the clergy and the staff of the Human Relations Service, as well as in the development of cooperative arrangements between the latter agency and the public schools.

Vehicles of Health Administration. Over the years, a number of organizational devices for bringing better health to the community have been evolved. These devices include, among others, the public health team, the community council, and the health cooperative. Three case studies deal directly with each of these organizational mechanisms.

The rationale for the team approach rests on the diversity of functions to be performed and the consequent need for combining the skills of several types of specialists. But in addition to this official and external task, every team faces the internal and unofficial task of sustaining itself as a going concern. A team is a small-scale social system and thus must maintain good communication between its members. The Chilean case by Dr. Simmons records the consequences of a decision to remove the nurses from a well-baby clinic in order to have them devote more time to health education in the home. This move led to a serious impairment of communication between doctor and patient in the clinic, throwing into relief the critical nature of the nurse's informal contribution to the functioning of the public health team.

Organizational devices that facilitate health action in one social setting may be obstructive in another, as shown by Dr. Oberg and Mr. Rios in their Brazilian case study. Apparently inspired by experiences in the United States, technical assistance experts set up a community council to enlist citizen participation in a village improvement project combining health, education, and agriculture. But in the context of local political realities, the community council proved to be more of a liability than an asset, and actually contributed to the premature termination of the demonstration project.

Professor Saunders and Dr. Samora present a comparable case of program failure caused in large part by an inappropriate organizational vehicle—in this instance, a cooperative health organization designed to provide better medical care for 7,500 Spanish-Americans in rural Colorado. Like the community council, the cooperative association proved to be a device that can operate successfully only where certain assumptions, values, and goals prevail. In attempts to profit from previous failure, new projects have recently been undertaken in Brazil and Colorado without a community council in the one instance or a cooperative organization in the other. Dr. Simmons' study warns against discarding effective organizational features; the Brazil and Colorado cases warn against clinging to organizational devices that prove ineffective.

Combining Service and Research. Public health workers continually seek better ways to apply proven medical techniques and disseminate known health information. But they are also eager to increase the store of scientific knowledge and develop new techniques for promoting health. Much research into the determinants of health and illness can be conducted in laboratories, but work with human populations is also necessary. Thus, to learn more about human growth and development it may be advantageous to use selected groups of children as subjects for nutritional experiments or psychological testing.

The Mexican case study by Dr. Lewis and the Guatemalan study by Dr. Adams are based on research projects involving school children. In the attempt to make such research acceptable to the public, both projects offered the community incidental services. The two cases raise the question as to whether the cause of research is enhanced or hindered by extending tangible services. In the Guatemalan case it was possible to dispel misunderstandings about blood sampling and the purpose of nutritional supplements. But community services, such as social nights and a community chicken coop, made no contribution toward winning good will for the research program; the medical clinic was poorly geared to the expectations of the villagers and proved a source of trouble. Once these extra services were withdrawn the nutrition experiment was able to proceed with less difficulty.

Residents of the large Mexican village studied by Dr. Lewis made it clear when he arrived that they needed a physician in their village. "Many people have come here to study us," they complained, "but not one of them has helped us." To meet their request and thus gain their cooperation for ethnological and psychological research, Dr. Lewis helped to organize a medical clinic. But this facility became entangled in a web of politics and was discredited indirectly by an attack on a more vulnerable part of the overall program, the psychological testing project.

Under some circumstances it can disturb community relations to undertake research as an adjunct to a program of service. This is generally recognized. It should also be realized that offering service as an adjunct to a research program can be equally inappropriate under some circumstances. Combining service and research is not always easy. This is attested in a number of the studies that follow. But the series of case studies taken as a whole also indicate that a combination of social action and social research can be mutually beneficial.

PART I

REEDUCATING THE COMMUNITY

Case 1

A COMPREHENSIVE HEALTH PROGRAM AMONG SOUTH AFRICAN ZULUS

by John Cassel

The habits and beliefs of people in a given community are not separate items in a series but elements of a cultural system. The elements are not all equally integrated, however; some are central to the system, others peripheral. Hence, some cultural elements can be altered or replaced with little effort, others only by applying great force. There are no ready rules for knowing in advance which items of health behavior and belief will yield readily under pressure from health education and which will offer tenacious resistance. But the reality of a sliding scale of resistance to change is well documented in Dr. Cassel's study. With more analyses of this kind from different communities, it may eventually be possible to derive workable principles about the relative mutability of different parts of a total culture.

Among the Zulus, cattle are intimately connected with veneration of ancestors and valued norms of human conduct. Witches violate these norms. Cattle and witchcraft thus symbolize good and evil; ideas and actions relating to these subjects are charged with strong emotions. Habits pertaining to the consumption of milk are hard to change; they partake of the emotional tone surrounding the subjects of cattle, ancestors, and proper behavior. It is even more difficult to alter conceptions about tuberculosis because the symptoms of this disease are seen as the effects of witchcraft, and the entire topic is surcharged with powerful feeling.

All this suggests that the most difficult task in health education is to change those cultural features which stand as symbols or indirect expressions of the fundamental moral code governing interpersonal conduct. In respect to these ultimate bases of resistance, the outcome of the mental health program reported in Case 2 by Dr. John and Dr. Elaine Cumming would seem to be directly comparable.—EDITOR

THE PROBLEM

Different Phases of a Program
Meet Varying Degrees of Resistance

Health conditions in a community of 16,000 Zulu tribesmen in southwestern Natal in the year 1940 were extremely poor. The infant mortality rate was 276 per 1,000 live births, the crude

15

mortality rate 38 per 1,000 population. Inadequacy of the diet was evident in the fact that more than 80 per cent of the people exhibited marked stigmata of nutritional failure and that malnutrition in the form of pellagra and kwashiorkor was rife. Frequent epidemics of typhoid, typhuş fever, and smallpox contributed to the high death rate; tuberculosis, venereal disease, and dysentery were major problems.

The Polela Health Centre, an enterprise based on a new approach to the pressing health problems of these Bantu-speaking peoples, was instituted in 1940. Operating on the principle that modern medical services could and should be brought directly to the people themselves, the Centre had at its disposal the most effective known techniques for the detection and treatment of disease.

Personnel of the Centre anticipated that it would be no easy task to implement their plans in a situation where health standards were so low and the culture of the people so different from their own. They could foresee in general that difficulties would arise, but they could not, at the outset of their program, know the specific kinds of conditions that did, in fact, serve to complicate their efforts. In their attempts to put into practice ameliorative health measures, they found that some of the obstacles encountered could be surmounted with a little ingenuity; others, more resistant, could be successfully circumvented; while still others appeared virtually insuperable.

For example, the people readily agreed to plant home vegetable gardens, thus adding important nutrients to their diet, once the proper incentive was discovered. On the other hand, no amount of demonstration of the nutritional importance of milk could convince the people that they should increase its use, but it turned out to be unexpectedly easy to introduce milk through the back door. In another instance, a father with four advanced tubercular cases in his family agreed to hospitalize the patients after an extensive explanation as to the nature of the disease, but on fuller explanation angrily withdrew permission. Other agencies working in this and similar areas experienced like difficulties. Efforts by agricultural experts to combat extensive soil erosion by getting people to reduce the size of their cattle herds resulted in an impasse, yet the available grazing for cattle was so inadequate that the milk yield was negligible and many cattle died every winter from starvation.

In each of these instances, the intensity of effort required to motivate changes was different; in some cases effort was nominal, in others considerable, and in others great. How are these differences to be explained? What information do health workers need to have about a community to enable them to predict some of the resistances they are likely to meet, and therefore plan program priorities more realistically?

THE SITUATION

Carrying Out a Comprehensive Health Program

The Zulu People

In the mountainous, wooded, and grassy country surrounding the Polela Health Centre live some 16,000 Zulu tribesmen. Their mud-walled, thatched-roofed huts are occupied mainly by women, children, and old men; the adult male population spends the major part of the year working in the neighboring towns. An occasional small store, some scattered mission schools made of mud or wood and iron, the one main dirt road through the area, the German print dresses of the women and ragged shirts of the men—these form the only outward signs of contact with western civilization. Many less apparent evidences of culture contact exist, however. Of these, the disruption of family life caused by the migrant labor system and the inadequacy of the old codes and mores in a changing world have perhaps the most important health implications.

The ancestors of these people originally belonged to a small clan of Central African Zulu tribesmen. They traveled south in the great migrations from Central Africa and in the early part of the seventeenth century settled in what is now Zululand, in northern Natal. At the beginning of the nineteenth century, the clan's chieftain, Chaka—a man of extraordinary military genius and insatiable political ambition—embarked on a campaign of imperial conquest. He conquered most of southeastern Africa and united all the various clans into one great empire, the Zulu nation. Even today the Zulus pride themselves on their warrior tradition and tend to look down upon the other Bantu peoples of South Africa.

The disintegration of the Zulu empire, started by internal dissension, ended in conflict with the whites. The last major clash occurred as recently as 1906. During the reign of Chaka, war and starvation had set in motion great waves of refugees, and clashes with the whites caused further dislocation. The people of Polela today are remnants of many clans scattered by Chaka and the European wars.

Today Zulus comprise some one and one-half to two million of the eight million Bantu inhabitants of the Union of South Africa, whose total population is about 12 million. In common with the majority of Bantu tribes of Africa, the basic unit of Zulu society has not been the individual or the married couple and their children, but the "extended" family centered around the male family head. Until recently polygamy was prevalent, and the family was an extended polygamous unit. Grown sons continued to live with their parents, along with their own wives and children. Obtaining a wife necessitated the exchange of cattle between the families of the groom and bride. This was no mere matter of buying and selling, but a kind of social contract between the two families designed to guarantee good faith and good behavior on both sides.

Today, owing partly to poverty and the relative scarcity of cattle and partly to the influence of Christianity, polygamous families are becoming increasingly rare. Furthermore, one of the effects of contact with Europeans has been the increasing disruption of Zulu family life, and today small husband and wife families, as well as "broken" families, are far more common than the extended type of family of a few generations ago.

In spite of three centuries of change wrought by contact with western culture, traditional concepts and beliefs still govern many attitudes and activities of the vast majority of people. This is certainly true in regard to health. Of particular importance is the belief that all natural phenomena, including crop failures, lightning and storms, as well as sickness, are caused by the spirits of one's ancestors.

The advent of Christianity and the increasing number of Christian converts have changed many of the outward manifestations and rituals concerning these beliefs. Today some 60 per cent of the people in this area are Christians. Christianity has done little, however, to change underlying beliefs; the vast majority of those served by the Polela Health Centre would feel defenseless in a hostile world unless they could undertake appropriate ceremonies of propitiation, however disguised for the benefit of the missionaries.

For example, it is considered essential to have a feast one year after the death of the head of a family to propitiate his spirit. This feast involves the ritual slaying of an ox and several goats. To protect the home, incantations are made over the contents of the gut of the ox, since it is believed that these contents can be used to bewitch the home if they fall into the hands of an ill-wisher. The entire kin group and neighbors assemble to dine on meat and beer. Each person eats a prescribed part of the ox, depending on his age, sex, and relationship to the family. Certain choice pieces of meat and blood are placed in a designated section of the hut for the use of the spirits.

Since this ceremony has been banned by missionaries, today converts to Christianity hold a "feast of remembrance" one year after the death of the family head. At this feast the ox and goats are slaughtered with the same rituals, the contents of the gut are protected in the same manner, the meat and blood are placed in the appropriate place for the use of the spirits, but the people eat from tables instead of sitting on the ground and sing Christian hymns while they eat those parts of the ox appropriate to their sex, age, and relationship to the family!

One effect of culture contact, however, has been of fundamental importance. Following the midnineteenth-century discovery of diamonds in Kimberley and gold in the Transvaal, the industrial revolution came to South Africa. This led to the growth of towns and cities and an ever-increasing demand for labor. The masses of Bantu peoples provided a ready source of labor for mines, industries, and domestic work. But the dominant white population refused to accept those Bantu who came to the cities as a permanent part of the urban population. This gave rise to a system of migrant labor, whereby adult males were encouraged to come to cities while their wives and children had to remain in specially designated rural "Native Reserves." Over the years, the increasing poverty of these reserves has accelerated the townward migration of the adult males, and today the majority of able-bodied adult males spend less than two months a year with their wives and families. The disproportionate sex ratio in the urban and rural areas during the major part of the year has led to ever-increasing promiscuity, illegitimacy, and a weakening of family ties, in the face of which traditional codes of morality are virtually powerless. This situation has had the further deleterious effect of increasing the incidence of venereal disease and juvenile delinquency and subjecting women to ever greater emotional strain.

These, then, are some of the main features of the community which the Polela Health Centre began to serve in 1940.

The Polela Health Centre

The staff of the Polela Health Centre was organized into a number of multi-disciplined teams, each team consisting of a family physician, a family nurse, and a community health educator (health assistant). A team functioned in a defined geo-graphical area consisting initially of approximately 100 families. Periodically this area was extended, until today each team serves between 300 and 500 families. In this area over the years, the major health problems were defined through analysis of the clin-ical records maintained by the Centre teams, augmented by especially designed surveys.

These problems were broadly classified into those needs that were "felt" and those that were "unfelt." In general, "felt" health needs were those expressed by the people themselves in the course of group discussions; for example, a desire to do something about the high incidence of infantile mortality and morbidity and a desire for healthy children. "Unfelt" needs included, among others, the totally inadequate diet, the poor state of environ-mental hygiene, the lack of immunization, and the desirability of changing some of the child-rearing practices.

Health programs were then initiated on two planes, in which the promotive-preventive and the curative aspects of health and medical care services were integrated. The one approach, community health education, was the responsibility of the health educators. Through periodic routine home visits and small group discussions, they attempted to make the "unfelt" needs of the community "felt," and to motivate people to make those changes in their way of life that were necessary to meet these needs. Simultaneously, the other approach, curative and preventive services to individuals within their family unit, was the responsibility of the doctor and nurse on the team. Each individual was offered complete periodic health examinations, followed by family conferences to discuss the health problems peculiar to that family. An illness in any of the families would be treated by the same doctor and nurse who had been endeavoring to keep them healthy.

Details of these periodic health examinations and the illnesses that had been treated were recorded in the clinical records. These records supplied one of the sets of health indices used in analyzing and assessing health problems and evaluating progress. Team meetings were held daily, and all aspects of the total program were reviewed and assessed. Future programs were evolved at these meetings in accordance with progress made or obstacles encountered. The meetings also assured the fullest possible integration between the promotive-preventive and curative aspects of the program. Thus, for example, if syphilis were found to be a major problem, the staff would arrange group discussions in the community designed to discover local concepts about the nature of the disease. The discussions would highlight differences between these concepts and those held by the Centre staff, particularly as to the relationship between syphilis and abortions and stillbirths. At the same time, facilities for treatment would be improved. While under treatment, the patient would receive further instruction from his doctor and nurse concerning the nature of his disease and the aims of treatment. A fundamental working principle was that new concepts and practices should never be imposed upon the community; rather, they should be integrated into the culture through active popular participation. The majority of the guiding principles and concepts were developed by Dr. Sidney L. Kark, founder and original medical officer in charge of the Polela Health Centre. At the time of writing he is medical officer in charge of the Institute of Family and Community Health, Durban, with which the Centre is associated.

The details of four specific areas of health action in the Zulu community served by the Centre will illustrate the general concepts that have been outlined. These will be described in the order of difficulty presented, each successive effort encountering increased popular resistance to change. Two of the illustrations involve attempts to improve the diet, one by the introduction of home-grown vegetables, the other by greater use of eggs and milk. It will be seen that the second was harder to accomplish than the first. The third effort, an attempt to control tuberculosis, proved still more difficult. Most difficult of all was an effort to control soil erosion, a condition basic to many of the health problems.

Reeducation for Better Nutrition

As already indicated, severe malnutrition was a major community health problem. Many factors served as predisposing, precipitating, and contributory causes. Food surveys indicated that the prevailing monotonous, often grossly deficient, diet was one of the major causes. The high incidence of chronic disease, particularly tuberculosis, syphilis, and recurrent bouts of dysentery and diarrhea, was another cause. Still another was the great physical effort required, particularly from women, in their day-to-day life. The program to change the food habits of the community involved a detailed knowledge of the existing diet, an analysis of the factors responsible for it, and an investigation of current attitudes and beliefs about food.

The diet consisted principally of maize (corn) prepared in numerous ways, supplemented by dried beans, negligible amounts of milk, and occasionally meat and wild greens. Potatoes and pumpkins were eaten seasonally, and millet (sorghum) was fermented to brew beer, which was consumed in large quantities. Whenever funds allowed, sugar and white bread were also bought. Even though this was a rural agricultural community, poor farming methods and poverty of the soil made it impossible for the vast majority of the people to raise adequate food supplies. About half of the families produced less than one-quarter of the maize necessary to feed themselves, and consequently a large percentage of their food consisted of refined maize meal purchased with money sent home by the migrant laborers. Furthermore, during the best month of the year, even if all the milk had been equally distributed, only one-twentieth pint per head per day would be available. In addition to extreme poverty and extensive soil erosion, factors responsible for the poor diet included certain traditions as to which foods were customary, ignorance of the nutritional values of food, inefficient use of available resources, and cooking methods that frequently destroyed a large fraction of the nutrients.

As anticipated, early attempts to demonstrate the causal relationship between poor diet and low standard of health encountered considerable skepticism. People maintained that their diet was the diet of their ancestors and had always been the diet of their people. On this same diet, had not their ancestors been strong and healthy, mighty men of valor and military deeds? It was difficult to refute this point without having any reliable information about the health of their ancestors.

A search of the available literature, however, revealed that the present diet had not always been the traditional diet of the Zulus and other Bantu-speaking tribes. Prior to the arrival of the whites, the indigenous cereal had been millet, maize having been brought into the country by the early settlers. Because of its greater yield, maize had gradually supplanted millet as the staple cereal, millet being reserved solely for brewing. Furthermore, historically the Zulus were a roving pastoral people owning large herds of cattle; milk and meat had played a prominent part in their diet. So important was milk as an article of food that no meal was considered complete unless milk was included. Milk is consumed in the form of thick soured curds, and consequently the process is described as "eating" rather than "drinking" milk. The relatively fertile nature of the land at that time and the extensive wild game resulted in further additions of meat to the diet and a plentiful supply of wild greens. Roots and berries gathered from the forests were also extensively used.

The health educators attempted to make people aware of these facts through group discussions at informal gatherings held at various places in the area. As the "key" homes came to be recognized—homes visited frequently by many people—the group discussions were increasingly held there. Most of the people did not speak English, but this was no handicap; all the health educators were Africans, and all discussions were held in Zulu. These discussions were supplemented by routine periodic home visits, during which the occupants of each house were engaged in a conversation about the diet of their ancestors as compared with their present diet.

Surprisingly enough, once the facts about the diet of "the olden times" were presented, they were readily accepted by many of the older people. Fairly frequently they would make comments such as these: "Now that you come to mention it, I remember my grandmother telling me those same things." "Yes, those were the good old days when we all had good things to eat." Almost in the same breath, however, they maintained that their present diet was traditional. Once they saw the anomaly, however, a certain measure of interest was aroused and cooperation achieved, particularly among the older people, who were more likely to remember former conditions. This was of great importance in gaining acceptance for the program. The assistance of the older group was particularly gratifying in view of the fact that this group usually forms the most conservative element in any community. At Polela the older people were those most consistently opposed to the introduction of new ways.

Interest in the subject of food was further aroused by discussion on the commonly held concepts of digestion and the functions of the different articles of diet. It was widely, though not universally, held that in some manner food entered the blood stream. What happened to it thereafter was unspecified. Greatest interest was aroused by considering how a fetus was nourished *in utero;* discussion on this point would sometimes continue for hours. Many women were of the opinion that there must be a breast in the uterus from which the fetus suckled, for as they said, "We all know the baby in the mother's womb grows, and all growing things need food, and the only way a baby can get food is through suckling." Others indicated that calves *in utero* also grow and, therefore, must be receiving food, and who had ever seen a breast in a cow's uterus? Some women maintained that the fetus was nourished by the placenta; the Zulu term for placenta literally means "the nurse." But when challenged, they were unable to explain how the placenta could feed the baby.

The result of these and similar discussions was to arouse a desire for further knowledge. When the functions of the placenta and umbilical cord were explained by use of posters and models, the interpretation was readily accepted. Some of the posters were remarkably effective in stimulating curiosity and discussion at this stage. One picture showed a longitudinal section of a uterus with a fetus *in situ*. At one discussion group, an old woman remarked indignantly, "I never believed I would live to see the day when such pictures would be shown us in public—and by a man at that!" Nevertheless, she was one of the most eager to get a good view of the poster and took a lively part in the conversation.

As concepts about the digestion and absorption of food began to change, it was possible to direct discussion to the function of different types of food. The view generally held was that all food had only one function, to fill the stomach and relieve hunger. This view was immediately challenged by a number of people, however, who maintained that certain foods gave strength and others were fattening—a bodily attribute much valued in this community. Over a period of time it became more generally accepted that different foods had different functions; the value of milk, eggs, and green vegetables especially for growing children came to be understood.

Increased interest and changing attitudes toward food created a favorable climate for the next step, a program to induce changes in diet. The results of this action program may be indicated by focusing attention on efforts to increase use of vegetables and of eggs and milk.

Increasing Production of Green Vegetables

From its inception, one of the cardinal principles of the health education program was to demonstrate how better use could be made of available resources and, by so doing, how these new needs could be met in part. Since all the homes had adequate space around them, a home vegetable garden program was initiated. A demonstration vegetable garden was grown at the Health Centre, where members of the staff could gain gardening experience and where local families could have the methods demonstrated. The more cooperative families were assisted in starting their own vegetable gardens; as the number of gardens increased, a seed-buying cooperative was initiated. The establishment of a small market where families could sell their surplus produce and annual garden competitions were some of the more successful techniques used.

In addition, cooking demonstrations were held to show how these home-grown vegetables could be cooked to suit the tastes of the community and still preserve their nutrient value. Garden surveys conducted four times a year gave an indication of the progress made at different seasons. In 1941, the year of the first survey, 100 homes were surveyed; three vegetable gardens, growing a total of five different varieties of vegetables, were found to exist. In 1951, during the same season, 1,000 homes were surveyed and nearly 800 vegetable gardens, growing a total of more than 25 different varieties of vegetables, were in existence.

Not only had this program resulted in a marked increase in vegetable consumption, but it was possible to associate it with another program aimed at improving environmental hygiene. In order to improve the fertility of the soil for vegetable growing, families were shown how to make compost in pits instead of scattering it indiscriminately. All household refuse could immediately be placed in these pits and would eventually aid in producing better vegetables.

Eggs, Milk, and Taboo

While the home vegetable garden program was thus relatively satisfactory, greater difficulty was initially encountered in attempts to increase the consumption of eggs and milk. Of those families surveyed, more than 95 per cent had fowl, and eggs were fairly plentiful at certain seasons of the year. However, eggs were infrequently eaten. There were a number of reasons for this. It was considered uneconomical to eat an egg that would later hatch and become a chicken; egg eating was regarded as a sign of greed; and, finally, eggs were thought to make girls licentious. None of these notions, however, was associated with powerful emotions, and with patience it was possible, over a period of years, to overcome to a great extent the aversion to eggs.

To accomplish this, the function of eggs in promoting growth and "strengthening" the blood was discussed during group meetings and home visits. Cooking demonstrations showing how eggs could be incorporated in the diet, particularly of infants, were held periodically in the homes and at the Centre. Well-child sessions were called "mother and baby" sessions, since both mother and child were cared for. At these sessions mothers were advised how and when to introduce eggs into their children's diet, and the reasons were again discussed. People were encouraged to buy better breeds of cocks to improve the strain of their fowl and shown how to build nests to protect eggs from dogs and small wild animals.

As a result of these efforts, eggs today form a relatively common article in the diet of infants. While the aim of the Health Centre— an egg daily for children over six months—has not yet been achieved, many of the children do get from three to four eggs a week in the productive seasons of the year. Because of the shortage in supply, adults cannot have eggs so often as their children, but eggs are bought by many families for the use of adults whenever they are available—something almost unheard of twelve years ago.

The question of milk proved a more difficult and complex problem. In addition to the extremely limited supplies available, the "eating" of milk was associated with very deep-seated and powerful customs and beliefs. Only members of the kin group of the head of a household can use milk produced by that man's cattle. In fact, one of the methods of establishing relationship to a family is to request milk on entering the hut. While this restriction applies equally to men, women, and children, so that no family could supplement its milk supply from another family outside the kin group, the situation is more complex in the case of women.

During her menses or when pregnant, a woman is thought to exert an evil influence on cattle and may not pass near the cattle enclosure or partake of any milk. This applies even in her own home. Since it is usually impossible for men to know when a woman is menstruating, it is customary to exclude milk from the diet of the majority of girls once they have passed puberty. When a woman marries and goes to live with her husband's family group, she falls under a double restriction. Not only is she a woman, but she is now in the home of a different kin group. Consequently, of all people in the community, married women are most rigidly excluded from partaking of milk. The only conditions under which a married woman might have it are these: if her father presented her with a cow at the time of her marriage, she could use the milk; or if her husband performed a special ceremony involving the slaying of a goat, she would be free to use milk in his home. Because of the poverty that prevails, neither of these two procedures is common in this area today.

The reasons for these customs are lost in the mists of antiquity, not even the oldest people in this community being able to explain them. "This is our custom, and this is how it has always been" is the only explanation offered. In all probability it is likely that the customs are closely related to native religious beliefs centered around ancestors. Even today when some 60 per cent of this community are Christians, ancestors play a very important part. A person feels himself to be dependent upon the good will of his ancestors to protect him from all manner of ill luck, ill health, and misfortune. The link between a man and his ancestors is his cattle, and ceremonies of propitiation involve the slaying of cattle. Accordingly, anything that might have an evil influence on the cattle would anger the ancestors; in addition, a married woman continues to have her own set of ancestors and must not interfere with her husband's.

Whatever the underlying reasons, it soon became evident that the taking of milk by girls and especially by married women had powerful emotional connotations. In the face of those deep-seated beliefs, no mere conviction of the nutritional value of milk could be expected to change the practice. This became an important problem, since the nutritional state of expectant and lactating mothers was a subject of major concern to the Health Centre, and these were the individuals most rigidly excluded from using milk. Fortunately, it was possible to overcome this difficulty to a considerable extent by introducing powdered milk into the area. Even though people knew that this powder was in fact milk, it was not called milk in Zulu but was referred to as "powder" or "meal" and accepted by all families without protest. Even the most orthodox of husbands and mothers-in-law had no objection to their wives or daughters-in-law using this powder, and each year a greater number of people have bought milk powder to supplement the limited amounts which could be prescribed by the Health Centre. Cooking demonstrations designed to show various methods of incorporating this powdered milk into the diet increased its popularity. For some years now the Health Centre has been prescribing 800 pounds of milk powder every month, and this supply falls far short of the mounting demand.

While the introduction of milk powder has provided a partial solution to the problem of increasing milk consumption, it is by no means a complete answer. Many people, particularly the women, still do not make the best use of available milk supplies.

The Problem of Pulmonary Tuberculosis

While the problem of inadequate egg and milk consumption was more difficult to overcome than that of vegetables—and is still not entirely solved—the resistance encountered in the attempt to combat pulmonary tuberculosis was even greater. The difficulty in controlling tuberculosis stemmed mainly from reactions of the people toward the disease, although technical difficulties associated with case-finding procedures and therapeutic techniques were also involved. The recent advent of drugs that produce more dramatic results has been of immeasurable value, not only in treating cases but in changing local concepts of disease.

As already stated, pulmonary tuberculosis was a potent factor contributing to the poor nutritional state of many people in the community. At the same time, tuberculosis was itself a reflection of this poor nutrition. While it is difficult to give an accurate figure of the prevalence of this disease due to inadequate case-finding facilities, it is estimated that there are 15 cases of active tuberculosis per 1,000 population in this rural area. In a recent survey of roughly 100 families, one home in every four was found to harbor an active case, including primary tuberculosis in children. In addition, tuberculosis is now one of the leading causes of death in this community. Of even graver importance, there is every indication that during the past twelve years the incidence of the disease has increased rapidly, and it would appear that this area is suffering from an epidemic of tuberculosis.

Many factors have been responsible for this rapid spread and the failure of the Health Centre to control the disease. These include continuous introduction of new cases into the area by returning migrant laborers, the lack of isolation facilities, the difficulty of adequate case-finding in a mountainous rural area, and the poor nutritional state of the people. None of these aspects, however, has proved so great a handicap as the intense resistance and noncooperation of the people in regard to tuberculosis control. Reluctance is manifested mainly in the case of adult patients, there being far more cooperation where a child is the sufferer. It has been the general experience at the Centre that even though an individual may have been attending the clinical sessions at the Health Centre for several years, an announced diagnosis of tuberculosis would terminate attendance. Some of the reasons for this lack of cooperation are to be found in local concepts and attitudes concerning tuberculosis.

According to the Zulus, any disease associated with labored breathing, pains in the chest, loss of weight, and coughing up bloodstained sputum is attributed to the machinations of an ill-wisher. This person causes poison to be put in the victim's beer or food; he may do this personally or through the services of a "familiar" over which he has control. This poison is not excreted through the bowel but remains indefinitely in the stomach causing a person to vomit blood and lose weight. Eventually the influence of the poison affects the lungs and causes pains in the chest. The treatment consists in taking an emetic specially prepared by a "witch doctor" skilled in treating this disease. Once the emetic causes the poison to be vomited, the patient will be cured. If he is not cured, not enough of the poison has been brought up.

It is maintained by the Zulus that this syndrome is one of the oldest known to them and that cases occurred frequently, long before contact was made with the whites. Objective evidence, however, indicates that tuberculosis was extremely rare, if not absent, among the Zulu and other Bantu tribes until comparatively recent times. In discussing the history of tuberculosis in South Africa, one authority has this to say: "Up to the time of Livingstone who in his 'Travels and Researches in South Africa' states categorically that tuberculosis did not exist among the tribes, there is no evidence that clinically recognizable tuberculosis among the Bantu was other than a rarity."[1] It is likely that this syndrome originally was produced mainly by cases of pneumonia and congestive cardiac failure.

People in this community were thus firmly convinced that patients presenting symptoms of pulmonary tuberculosis were suffering from a disease that had always been treated by their own medical men, and about which a white doctor could be expected to know little. In addition, it was known that if a diagnosis of tuberculosis was made, hospitalization would be advised. The nearest tuberculosis hospital is 100 miles away, and since the majority of patients who had agreed to be hospitalized had been practically moribund before giving their consent, it was generally accepted that hospitalization was synonymous with death. The worst feature of such a death was that it would occur in a strange place, many miles from home, relatives, and the protection of the ancestors. Even if a patient refused hospitalization, it was known that strenuous efforts would be made by the health workers to isolate him, and what could be more unreasonable than to separate an individual from his friends and relatives at the very time he most needed their presence to comfort and cheer him and assist in his recovery?

A firm belief in the efficacy of the indigenous medical methods in treating such diseases was thus coupled with an intense fear of accepting a diagnosis of tuberculosis. It must be admitted that the prevailing concepts constituted a logical chain of thought. Granting the original premise, that an ill-wisher had poisoned the patient, it could logically follow that such poison would cause vomiting, eventually bloodstained, and a loss of weight. Further,

[1] Gale, G. W., "The History and Incidence of Tuberculosis in South Africa," *The Leech*, vol. 16, August, 1945, p. 7.

the obvious treatment would be to give an emetic; since this was no ordinary poison, a special emetic prepared by a skilled person would be required.

Only a limited number of approaches appeared feasible in any attempt to alter these concepts. It would be extremely difficult, if not impossible, to convince people that the original premise was false. No one ever saw the ill-wisher put poison in the food; it was just automatically assumed that this was the case. Assuming this premise, the rest of the argument was difficult to refute. One vulnerable point was the belief that the influence of the poison spread from the stomach to the lungs and caused pains in the chest and coughing (recognized as an essential feature of the syndrome). The health education program decided to exploit this weak point, demonstrating that the lungs were separate from the stomach, and presenting an alternative and equally logical set of deductions for consideration. That no connection existed between the lungs and stomach was demonstrated by means of models, posters, and reference to the anatomy of cattle and goats. It was then suggested that the "poison" responsible for the disease could be inhaled rather than swallowed, and that its dissemination might be a matter of accident rather than design. Once inhaled, this "poison" would attack the patient's lungs and could be spread unknowingly by that sufferer in turn.

As can be imagined, this type of education was tedious and demanded great patience and prolonged discussion. Fortunately, the community programs were directed mainly toward healthy people. The majority of people involved were not tubercular and thus the element of intense fear was not present. It was the responsibility of the doctors and nurses to demonstrate their ability to treat the disease should any person contract it. Prior to the advent of the new antibiotics, this was a very difficult task, since no short-term dramatic results could be anticipated. The use of these newer drugs has materially assisted the entire program by giving people more confidence in the ability of their doctor and nurse.

In the course of time, a slight decrease in the resistance of the community could be detected. Progress was painfully slow, however, and only by accident was it realized that there was yet another powerful reason preventing the acceptance of a diagnosis of tuberculosis. During a family consultation this additional factor was brought to light in a dramatic fashion.

Four years ago, a daughter of this family had married and contracted tuberculosis in her married home. Her disease had been diagnosed by the Health Centre, but all recommended treatment had been refused. Subsequently, the daughter returned to her maiden home; it was presumably thought that the influence of her ill-wisher was too powerful at her married home. Over the years, eight individuals became infected in her maiden home, four of them dying. With four more of his household seriously ill, the head of the family eventually agreed to discuss his plight with the Centre doctor.

It was known that this man was a part-time "witch doctor," one who was skilled in the arts of Bantu medicine but practiced his profession only occasionally. The consultation opened with a long discussion of Bantu concepts of disease, the father wishing to be convinced that the doctor knew both aspects of the problem—not only the medicine of the whites. Fortunately, the doctor came out of this "quiz" relatively well. After another hour and a half of conversation, the father pronounced himself satisfied. He said he would accept the doctor's recommendations and hospitalize the patients. The doctor then decided to give a résumé of the course of the disease through the family, beginning with the return home of the married daughter suffering from tuberculosis.

This review brought surprising results. Instead of reinforcing the father's decision, as was intended, it suddenly made the old man completely uncooperative; he withdrew his consent for hospitalization. Eventually, after long and patient discussion, the reason for this anger was discovered.

By suggesting that the daughter had started the disease process in this family, the doctor in effect had accused the daughter of possessing the power to spread disease. In this community only sorcerers and witches are recognized as having that power. When the full implications of the doctor's concepts became clear to him, the father realized that by accepting them he would be party to agreeing that his daughter was a witch. Eventually it was possible to obtain consent for hospitalization once more, but only after withdrawing the suggestion that the daughter was in any way responsible for the spread of this disease.

Effects of the Combined Approach

One of the more successful features of both the nutritional and tuberculosis programs was the combined use of clinical sessions and neighborhood health education, the one reinforcing the other. A major goal of the health education program was to convince parents of the importance of regular prenatal and well-child care. The techniques employed here were based on the same principles that governed the programs already described. As a result, the percentage of expectant mothers attending the prenatal sessions increased from fewer than 20 per cent in 1943 to more than 80 per cent in 1952. Similarly, the percentage of mothers who made use of the regular mother and baby sessions increased from a negligible percentage to more than 85 per cent in 1952. At the mother and baby sessions, detailed dietary advice was given to mothers by the family nurse and doctor. Women who had already been exposed to neighborhood health education programs now found this general knowledge applied specifically to themselves and their children.

In the sphere of nutrition, the combined programs yielded dramatic results. An infant mortality rate of 276 per 1,000 live births has been reduced in ten years to just under 100. The major factor influencing this reduction appears to be the improved nutritional state of the babies. Vital statistics available from other parts of Bantu South Africa show that this trend is not general.

Further results are equally evident. The incidence of gross cases of nutritional failure such as pellagra and kwashiorkor has dropped markedly; the incidence of kwashiorkor fell from 12 or more cases a week to fewer than 12 cases a year. The average year-old baby at Polela today weighs two pounds more than the average baby did some six years ago. In addition, the diet of infants has changed quite radically. In 1941 a one-year-old Zulu baby was fed breast milk and maize products. This diet was supplemented seasonally with wild greens, pumpkins, potatoes, and negligible amounts of milk. Today, besides breast milk and maize products, a baby receives powdered milk, eggs, tomatoes, spinach, cabbage, pumpkins, potatoes, peas, fruit in season, and millet.

One index of the greater difficulty experienced in controlling tuberculosis is that no significant decrease in the prevalence of the disease or in mortality rates has yet appeared in spite of the fact that efforts to curb tuberculosis were equal to or greater than those in the nutritional field. What has occurred, however, is a marked change in the attitudes of the people and greater cooperation. This has been evidenced by the increasing willingness of tubercular patients to seek treatment at the Centre. Further, while people at first refused to submit to x-ray examination, the present demand for x-ray services is greater than the Centre can meet. These changing attitudes, along with recent therapeutic advances, in all likelihood will produce improvements in the tuberculosis situation within the next few years.

Health, Soil Erosion, and Ecological Balance

The varying degrees of success achieved by the Polela Centre's programs show that change has been possible in spite of difficulties. A greater effort was required to produce less change in controlling tuberculosis than in improving diet; similarly it was more difficult to effect change in relation to milk and eggs than in regard to vegetables.

However, the relative success of these programs cannot disguise the fact that the critical circumstance associated with the low standard of health in the Polela area is soil erosion, which continues unchecked. Indeed, the very successes attained by the Health Centre will eventually aggravate the problem by increasing the pressure of population on the limited land. Soil erosion is not only the most critical factor in the overall program of improving standards of health; it is also a problem which cannot possibly be solved by a health agency acting alone. Many different approaches have been made to the question of soil conservation in native reserves in South Africa. In this community the two main features of the conservation program have been attempts to improve agricultural practices and to prevent overstocking and overgrazing by cattle.

In an effort to improve farming practices, Africans have been trained in agricultural colleges as "agricultural demonstrators" and stationed in native reserves among their own people. To prevent overstocking and overgrazing, the right of entry of cattle into an area has been strictly controlled and strenuous efforts have been made to persuade cattle owners to reduce the size of their herds. In spite of these and all the other procedures that have been tried, soil erosion is increasing at an alarming rate. Some of the efforts, particularly in regard to reducing the number of cattle, have had the unfortunate effect of increasing hostility and resistance. Explanations for this unhappy state of affairs must be sought in the natural and cultural history of soil erosion in South Africa.

Originally the Bantus were a roving pastoral people owning large flocks and herds. They would farm a plot of land until it was exhausted and then migrate to a more fertile area. From the latter part of the nineteenth century, their right of movement has been restricted and rural Africans have been confined in reserves. In these reserves, families had relatively small plots of land which they cultivated season after season without changing their original agricultural practices. Returning little of the waste products to the soil and oblivious to crop rotation, they have steadily deteriorated the fertility of the land.

Furthermore, the use of migrant labor in all industries and domestic work has drained the men from the fields, and in consequence the care of the land has become the job of women and children. Increasing poverty of the reserves in turn has accelerated the migration of men to the towns, further aggravating the situation. Since women in Zulu society have the legal status of minors and lack authority to change existing practices, it is not surprising that the efforts of the agricultural demonstrators have been of so little avail, women and children being their only audience for the greater part of the year. Thus, poor farming methods continue unabated, perpetuating the vicious cycle of deepened poverty, longer absences of the men to work for wages, and decreased possibilities of altering prevailing agricultural practices.

Additional forces abet this downward spiral. One is the mountainous nature of the land which makes large tracts unsuitable for agriculture even if modern technology were available. Another is the overcrowding of the reserves by man and beast. Still others are the destruction of the soil cover by deforestation to obtain fuel and burning pastures in spring to hasten the appearance of green grass in order to relieve starvation of the animals.

The efforts of administrators to ease this pressure on the land have centered mainly on attempts to control the cattle and reduce their number. Much hostility has been aroused by these methods, largely because insufficient account was taken of the function of cattle in Zulu culture. People with European background have found it easy to assume that the major uses of cattle are to produce milk, to serve as draught animals, as an index of wealth, and— among native Africans—as payment for the "bride price" necessary to obtain a wife. Accordingly, it has also been assumed that fewer cattle of better stock would be acceptable, since they would produce more milk. Compensation for reducing the herd could be made in cash, which should also become an index of wealth, and a wife could then be obtained by a cash transaction or payment in kind.

All these assumptions overlook the deep symbolic value of cattle. The transference of cattle involved in a marriage is more than a matter of buying or selling a wife. To the Zulus, it guarantees the good behavior of both marriage partners, for which the families of the bride and groom hold themselves responsible. Moreover, since cattle form an essential link between a man and his ancestors, loss of cattle means a weakening of this bond, leaving one defenseless in a hostile world. Finally, the deep attachment of men for their cattle must not be underestimated. Any man in this area could, without hesitation, describe each of his cattle in minute detail, depicting not only appearance and color but character and habits as well. Many Zulu men probably know far more about their cattle than they do about their children.

Thus, it is evident why attempts at cattle reduction should encounter resistance. But even if this reduction were accomplished, the problem would scarcely be solved in view of the many additional and interrelated factors responsible for the accelerating soil erosion. Furthermore, while the reduction of the number of cattle might ease the pressure on the land to some extent, stock limitation alone would have unfavorable effects on the health of the people unless this move was part of a much more comprehensive program. Initially, stock reduction would mean a still further limitation of the already inadequate milk supply, since pedigreed cows could not survive without good pastures. The numbers of oxen available for draught purposes is already limited, inasmuch as most of the cattle are owned by only a few families. Many families, therefore, have to borrow oxen from their neighbors for plowing. The delay in plowing some of the fields results in frequent crop failures caused by early frosts; a further reduction in cattle would only aggravate this situation.

It thus becomes apparent that soil conservation, on the scale necessary in this area, is beyond the scope of a health agency. It would require a broadly based community program integrating the activities of various agencies and a thorough knowledge of relevant social and cultural forces.

IMPLICATIONS

While no attempt has been made to present an exhaustive discussion of all the factors involved in maintaining health, enough has been said to show that the improvement of health conditions cannot be conceived as an isolated effort; rather, it must be seen in its total context. In the Polela area this context includes economic, political, and ecological considerations, as well as many features of the local culture.

Recognizing that most health problems among these people are fundamentally related to soil erosion, poverty, and the system of migrant labor, one can envision a solution that makes maximum use of local resources. Specifically, such a plan would begin by building a dam across the river that flows through the valley, using the impounded water to irrigate the lower flat slopes. In this way, crops could be grown the year round, and not merely during the wet summer months as at present. The rest of the area, which is too mountainous for extensive cultivation, could be put into timber. The climate is eminently suitable for pine trees, and within ten to twelve years these would begin yielding returns. Once the timber was mature, after eighteen years, hydroelectric power could be developed from the dam to start timber industries.

Such a scheme would check soil erosion and gradually restore fertility. It would also provide sufficient occupational opportunities to slow down the migration of men to the towns. The increased productivity of the area would offset the population increase that would come with improved health. Under these circumstances, a comprehensive health program could be expected to yield enduring results. While this kind of program would appear to solve many community problems, the power to implement it obviously far exceeds the scope of a health agency. This being so, it becomes the obligation of the health agency to attempt motivating other agencies to cooperate in carrying out some such scheme, and at the same time to recognize realistically the magnitude of changes that are possible through its own efforts.

Once a health agency has delineated those areas in which change is feasible, it is important to distinguish tasks in terms of the amount of effort that will be required to overcome local resistance. It has been shown that the control of tuberculosis among the Zulus was more difficult than the improvement of diet. Within the dietary program, it was more difficult to increase the consumption of milk and eggs than vegetables. In all the programs it was necessary to bear in mind the limiting factors of low productivity and the system of migrant labor, which would permit changes only up to a certain point.

It will be readily appreciated, however, that improving the productivity of an area by itself would not automatically solve all health problems. A comprehensive health program closely integrating neighborhood health education with medical care has proved effective in the Polela area even though certain conditions beyond the control of the health agency have set limits to the changes that could be effected. The techniques developed by the Centre have been found useful, not only in this particular community but in other communities of South Africa as well.

In addition to combining the promotive-preventive approach with the curative approach, new ideas have been communicated to the people with lasting results. This happened because the new ideas were brought into correspondence with existing ideas, rather than being imposed from above. As a result, there have been increased cooperation and confidence in the Health Centre on the part of the community. To achieve these ends, the small-group discussion method was found to be much superior to a mass approach. It in turn has necessitated operating in a limited sphere and gradually increasing the area of influence centrifugally. Attempts were made to build into the programs themselves techniques for appraisal and evaluation. This has been a constant feature of the work of the Centre, rather than a spasmodic occurrence.

SUMMARY

Examples from the work of the Polela Health Centre serving a Zulu community in the Union of South Africa illustrate the different degrees of resistance encountered in trying to make a variety of changes in the health status of the people. Changes were progressively more difficult to effect in these four aims: improvement of diet by the cultivation of vegetable gardens, increasing the consumption of milk and eggs, the control of tuberculosis, and, finally, soil conservation, which is basic to problems of health.

Thorough understanding of local ways and values and the importance of fitting new ideas into the existing cultural framework of the people were shown to be essential if lasting results were to be achieved. The experiences of the Centre demonstrated the advantages of an integrated service wherein the promotive-preventive and curative aspects of health practice are combined and made the responsibility of the same team.

SELECTED REFERENCES

Cohn, Helen D., "The Educational Nurse in Health Centre Practice," *Health Education Journal* (Central Council for Health Education, Tavistock Square, London), vol. 8, October, 1950, pp. 178–184. A nurse cites in detail the case of a Bantu family served by one of the health centers to illustrate the necessity of integrating promotive, preventive, and curative work.

Gluckman, Max, "The Kingdom of the Zulu of South Africa" in *African Political Systems*, edited by A. Meyer Fortes and E. E. Evans-Pritchard. Oxford University Press, London, 1940, pp. 25–55. A scholarly analysis of Zulu power structure and the effect upon it of European impact written by a primary anthropological authority on the Zulu.

Kark, Sidney L., "Health Centre Service: A South African Experiment in Family Health and Medical Care" in *Social Medicine*, edited by E. H. Cluver. Central News Agency, Johannesburg, 1951, pp. 661–700. A comprehensive background article on the Polela program, its scope, its development, and the respective functions of team members—doctor, nurse, and health educator.

Kark, Sidney L., and John Cassel, "The Pholela Health Centre: A Progress Report," *South African Medical Journal* (Johannesburg), vol. 26, no. 9, 1952, pp. 101–104 and 132–136. A report of specific programs, techniques, and results.

Krige, Eileen J., *The Social System of the Zulus*. Longmans Green and Co., New York, 1936. Zulu past and present, based mainly on a survey of published sources.

Richards, Audrey I., *Hunger and Work in a Savage Community*. The Free Press, Glencoe, Ill., 1948. A British anthropologist with extended field work in Africa provides a compact and readable outline of Zulu life in the course of following out the implications of the Zulus' "nutritional system."

Simons, H. J., "Race Relations and Policies in Southern and Eastern Africa" in *Most of the World*, edited by Ralph Linton. Columbia University Press, New York, 1949, pp. 271–330. A competent regional survey emphasizing contemporary economic and racial conditions.

Case 2

MENTAL HEALTH EDUCATION IN A CANADIAN COMMUNITY

by John Cumming and Elaine Cumming

In areas where technological advances are pushing problems of malnutrition and infectious disease into the background, the perplexing problem of mental illness looms ever larger. New departures in service and research are being undertaken in the hope of finding effective controls. Among these are trial programs of psychiatric consultation to personnel in key services and agencies of the community, such as the Wellesley program of social psychiatry described in the case study by Dr. Naegele, Case 11. Public education, the subject of the Cumming case, represents another approach to the problem.

In recent years a number of systematic surveys have been made to ascertain popular conceptions of mental health. More numerous have been efforts to enlighten the public by means of mass media and group discussion. Seldom, however, have careful attitude surveys been coupled with educational campaigns in order to study the relationship between propositions advocated by the educators and assumptions entertained by the public, and to measure the effectiveness of educational programs. This is just what the Cumming team did in a Canadian community. The clear evidence they produced of their failure to alter attitudes toward the mentally ill is a mark of their success in designing an instructive experiment. Their retrospective self-criticism, combined with analysis of the reasons for resistance and resentment, sheds needed light on the wisdom and method of educating the public in matters of mental health. Their findings in a Canadian town apply with equal force to communities in the United States.

The citizens of Prairie Town do not believe in sorcerers as do the Zulus described by Dr. Cassel in the preceding case study, but their convictions about the mentally ill are no more rational and are just as deeply seated. Both cases point to the same conclusion: as a guide to health education, it is insufficient to assess popular beliefs in terms of their scientific accuracy; it is also necessary to know the functions they perform for those who hold them.—EDITOR

THE PROBLEM

Unexpected Outcome of an Educational Experiment

In 1951 an experiment in altering popular attitudes toward the mentally ill was launched in Prairie Town, a community in a western Canadian province. The project grew out of a desire on the part of the province's Department of Public Health to extend its usefulness by entering the field of preventive psychiatry. We who were working in the psychiatric division of the Department pondered how to make a beginning in this direction. One possibility considered was that of early case-finding. But our mental hospitals were already overcrowded and our recently established outpatient clinics had long waiting lists of people eager to be helped.

A more appealing plan, we reasoned, was to develop a program of education that would give people in the community a better understanding of mental illness and of current knowledge about child development, delinquency, and allied subjects. In the long run such an educational program might possibly decrease the incidence of mental illness. But whether or not this would prove true, it did seem that bringing about a more tolerant popular attitude toward those who had been in mental institutions might well speed the process of psychiatric rehabilitation and lower the high relapse and readmission rate. Discharged mental patients usually encountered a generalized attitude of fear, suspicion, and rejection on returning to their community. Our public health nurses knew this from their efforts to help former patients readjust to their home surroundings, and we knew it from stories told us by former patients.

Aided by a generous grant from the Commonwealth Fund, we carried out the Prairie Town experiment. We prepared the ground slowly and carefully. Then for six months we utilized all local facilities in a concerted effort to bring about a measurable change in attitudes toward the mentally ill. By means of questionnaires and interviews we tested a sample of townspeople twice, once at the beginning of the intensive campaign and again at the end. After our educational experiment was over, we had time to analyze and compare the two sets of test material. The tests showed that no significant change in attitude had occurred.

We had been unable to effect any evident change in attitudes toward the mentally ill. Attitudes toward us, on the other hand, had undergone a very evident change. The people of Prairie Town, initially friendly and cooperative, had become increasingly aloof as the months went by, despite every effort on our part to be tactful and friendly. From apathy they resorted to withdrawal; and when our interviewers returned to Prairie Town at the end of six months to administer the retest, they were dismayed at the outright antagonism they encountered. Our well-intentioned efforts to alter attitudes had apparently produced side-effects that we had not bargained for. What was the connection between the negative outcome of our educational program and the positive hostility that was aroused? What does this connection reveal about the needs served by popular concepts of illness?

THE SITUATION

An Effort to Alter Mental Illness Concepts

The Community of Prairie Town

Prairie Town is located about 50 miles from Prairie City and was chosen mainly for reasons of convenience. It can be reached both by transcontinental railroad and by a good highway which is kept open and free from snow all winter, an important consideration in this part of the world. This area of the province is mainly Anglo-Saxon in origin, and Prairie Town is an old and stable community. Thus, project workers did not have to deal with language difficulties or a shifting population.

Prairie Town is mainly a distributing center. Many residents are farmers who own homes in the town as well as farmsteads in the surrounding area. Most residents have lived in the town for many years; many were born there. It is a wealthy town for this part of the country, proud of its modern facilities, including sewer and water systems, which are unusual for a prairie town of 1,350 persons. People of Prairie Town are essentially conservative and individualistic. When the library board canvassed the town for donations for a small building to house the library, they could not raise the necessary $400, despite the fact that three people in town are reputedly near millionaires. One of these said to the canvasser, "If people want to read books, let them buy them themselves." The town has one movie house and a weekly newspaper. Community recreational facilities are poor. Both the grade school and the high school are old and inadequate, in marked contrast to Prairie Town's many fine homes with well-kept grounds. Many streets are lined with stately trees, carefully planted and cared for, something seldom found in other prairie towns. Most of the better homes have large flower gardens, and local pride in the appearance of the town is reflected in the commonly used slogan, "Prairie Town, the beautiful."

However, when Prairie Town citizens use this slogan, they do not mean to include that part of town known as Germantown. Germantown contains no Germans but was so named, according to a local story, during World War I, when the term "German" was applied to any unpopular group. Germantown is a collection of tiny wooden and tar-paper-covered houses on the east side of Prairie Town. It is inhabited mainly by Metis, a French-Indian cross comprising about 5 per cent of the population, and by a few other depressed minority groups. Germantown families are not served by the sewer and water facilities of which Prairie Town is so proud. Prairie Town is a wealthy town, but it is also a town of contrasts.

In Prairie Town there are a large number of organizations, social clubs, church groups, choirs, sports clubs, service clubs, and fraternal organizations. A local agricultural agent who proposed building a community center surveyed these groups and counted more than 70 organizations. The groups show a high degree of overlap in membership and direction, but there are also many people in town who belong to only a few organizations or to none. The town is set off from others around it by two government agricultural and experimental stations. Personnel of these installations contribute a small group of high technical education to Prairie Town's population. These people have a social life largely confined to their own numbers, and while respected by the townsfolk, they are not included in the informal groupings of the town.

Our survey revealed two main types of people in Prairie Town. One segment of the town places a high value on the puritan virtues: honesty, hard work, thrift, good housekeeping, and a God-fearing religious life. The values of the other segment, more educated and better housed, center on "community service"; men of this group want to be known as good mixers and proficient businessmen and prefer that their wives be active in community affairs as well as proficient in housekeeping.

A Mental Health Educational Campaign

In planning the educational campaign before coming to Prairie Town, we had postulated that people tend to reject the mentally ill because of fear, ignorance, and guilt. Experience has shown that the average layman thinks that most persons who become mentally ill are violent; this is believed not only by those who have had no direct contact with the mentally ill but also by many who have. The latter seem to accept the general belief rather than trust their personal experience.

In addition to this explicit fear, we thought, people may have a less conscious fear of becoming mentally ill themselves, since causative factors are so general and so imperfectly understood. This fear may be created by a little knowledge. We found, for example, when teaching student nurses in the psychiatric department of a general hospital that they had a great deal of anxiety because in some respects they could see little difference between the mentally ill and themselves, and because they could find in themselves many of the psychological mechanisms used to explain mental illness.

Many people who have placed friends or relatives in an institution feel relieved at being absolved of their responsibility. To acknowledge that such institutions are socially undesirable or physically inadequate would provoke a sense of guilt; the easier course is to remain blind to the facts. Relatives of mentally ill persons often keep reassuring themselves that institutional care is "the best thing" for their relatives, and that the institution in question is at least "better than most others." Another way to redirect guilt is to attribute to minority groups traits about which the "projecting" individual feels ambivalent. This mechanism is well known in racial prejudice, and we assumed it to be partly responsible for some of the distorted concepts about the mentally ill. We reasoned that some of the violent impulses attributed to the mentally ill might in fact be projections of a normal person's unconscious urges.

On the assumption that misconceptions about the mentally ill were tied in with deeper emotions such as fear and guilt, we regarded the task of community education as a delicate undertaking. We would have to avoid assuaging some fears at the cost of arousing others. For example, if we were to stress the point that mental hospitals, contrary to widespread sentiment, are not an ideal setting for inducing recovery, we might thereby increase the amount of guilt felt by those with hospitalized relatives.

We knew that we would often be questioned on the nature of mental illness, the characteristics of the mentally ill, conditions in mental hospitals, and treatments for these disorders. To evade these questions would in itself produce suspicion and anxiety; therefore, we decided that when they did arise they should be answered honestly, sympathetically, and with a minimum of sensationalism.

We undertook to teach three basic concepts: first, that there is a very wide range of human conduct that can be considered "normal"; second, that behavior does not "just happen" but has determinate causes and can therefore be understood if one knows the factors involved; and third, that the borderline between "abnormal" and "normal" is vague and arbitrary.

Although our primary backing came from the provincial government, it was decided to align the program with the Canadian Mental Health Association, a voluntary nonprofit organization, so that we would not be considered an agency of government. We expected Prairie Town to be a conservative town where there would be a great deal of opposition to the liberal ideas of the current government. We used as a rationale for entering the community the idea that we were trying to establish what the term "mental illness" meant to a group of typical citizens. The project team included a psychiatrist and a sociologist as senior workers, and six trained interviewers. Some of these personnel stayed in Prairie Town for extended periods of time, and others came to the community from their base in Prairie City when their special services were required.

Initial contacts in the community were established without too much difficulty. On a bright day in late August we drove the 50 miles from our Prairie City base to Prairie Town. Our first stop was at a local store, whose owner we already knew. We explained to him that we were interested in learning what the townspeople thought about the mentally ill. During our discussion, he posed a question which we were to hear many times: "Why do you want to know what we think; why not go to the experts?" To this question we developed a standard reply; we countered with the question, "Who sends people to mental hospitals?" In answering this, people usually placed the responsibility on the local doctor, but when we next asked why the mentally ill person had been taken to the doctor in the first place, they usually recognized that ultimate responsibility rested with the family and neighbors of the ill person. We told the storekeeper that many experts felt that some of the patients in mental hospitals might not be so ill as people who remained harmlessly in the community, and pointed out the role of community beliefs and attitudes in bringing about this situation.

From the storekeeper we got a list of people who were influential in the community. The list included not only town officials but many executive officers of local clubs and organizations. Over a period of about a week we called on each of these. We talked about our survey, asked for permission to attend their club meetings from time to time, and volunteered to help plan their programs for the coming winter. Their response, in general, was polite and friendly, but they seemed a little puzzled. They accepted our purposes intellectually but had difficulty understanding why we wanted to collect information without any immediate practical use in mind. We did not yet realize that this type of research is considered a normal occupation by very few people.

When our initial rounds were completed, we had a chat with the proprietor of the local weekly newspaper and gave him a release concerning our program. He promised to cooperate and in the months that followed gave us wholehearted assistance. News stories and articles we furnished appeared in his paper almost every week, in addition to paid notices advertising various facets of our educational program. The proprietor also gave us editorial support on several occasions.

We tried to reach as many people as possible. We used all means and resources usually called into play in such campaigns: motion pictures, pamphlets, special books placed in the local library, notices in the local newspaper, radio broadcasts, speakers, and small group discussions with competent discussion leaders. Not wishing to make this an impractical experiment, we included no items in our program that could not be obtained by an interested and informed citizenry at a cost within their local means. While we promoted a great deal more "mental health" activity than has ever before been induced in a community of comparable size to our knowledge, a similar educational campaign could be produced again without calling for special outside funds.

The first group to become interested in our program was the local Parent-Teacher Association. The president of the group invited us to its first executive meeting, during which the forthcoming winter's program was to be planned. We attended two executive sessions and were disappointed to find that the quorum necessary for decisions was not present at either meeting. We felt that this was partly due to the fact that the P.T.A. was a new and relatively weak organization, but we were soon to find this pattern of reaction recurring as we met with other groups and executives. We began to believe that the whole town was suffering from some sort of apathy. Only later when we saw the energy and enthusiasm devoted to other town projects did we realize that this "apathy" was in some way connected with what we were trying to do.

Later on, however, the P.T.A. became a source of strength to us. It accepted our help in planning the winter program and joined us to co-sponsor a three-day festival of educational films on child care. It also did a good deal of work in helping us produce a series of 12 half-hour radio programs in which local children and adults held panel discussions on children's problems. These programs were popular and had a good listening audience.

Community "apathy" was evidenced in other situations. Some local citizens felt it might be useful to form a group to discuss the development and mechanisms of human personality. We were quite eager to help with this. First, we talked over the idea informally with a few people and then called a meeting to discuss the formation of such a group. It was decided that the theme of the discussions would be "Why I am as I am" and that the group should meet every second week throughout the winter. Several came to the organizational meeting without specific invitation; 14 persons were present. Enthusiasm seemed to be high and almost everyone claimed to know of others who would be interested. Expecting a large turnout, we arranged for two other specialists from Prairie City to attend the first meeting so that the participants could divide into small discussion groups with one informed person in each group. When we arrived at the rather large meeting room, we found a total attendance of five persons. Although this group eventually grew larger, the small initial turnout typified community response to our educational efforts.

Another form of "apathy" was evidenced during the history of this discussion group. Peak attendance at meetings grew to about 35, but with the exception of a few faithful participants the composition of this group was constantly changing. Thus, five or six newcomers would be present at each meeting, and five or six who had attended previously would be absent. This same pattern occurred at meetings of other groups, although it was more pronounced in this group that continued to meet throughout the whole winter.

It became apparent that our use of written material was not very successful. The local newspaper, as noted, was especially cooperative and printed whatever material we furnished. However, there was little evidence that these stories were widely read. Similarly, the demand for the pamphlets we offered at meetings and advertised in the newspaper or on the radio proved to be very slight. It seemed that the citizens of Prairie Town were not a pamphlet-reading people. On the other hand, about a dozen popular books on mental health topics we placed in the local library had a very good circulation as compared with the usual rate for new books. The library board, incidentally, felt that any more books on mental health would have caused an imbalance in this direction. Perhaps with some justice, the board had classed these books with those donated by various religious organizations setting forth their doctrines.

Apathy, Anxiety and Hostility

The sparse attendance at meetings, the rapid turnover of discussion groups, and the apparent neglect of our printed educational materials—all these we at first attributed to apathy. As the program progressed, however, we began to realize that what we had interpreted as a general lack of interest in our message and as indifference to our program was actually something very different and far more active. The educational program itself was creating unrest and anxiety. When we first came to Prairie Town, the people were polite and friendly. These attitudes changed slowly and subtly; only in retrospect were we able to put together certain incidents and events as evidence of mounting anxiety.

As already indicated, on entering the town we had told people that our object was to learn what an average community thought about mental disease. In retrospect, we believe that few of them were completely satisfied with this explanation. One way of expressing their puzzlement was to joke about our stated purpose. One man said, "Well, I guess you're here because you found out we're all crazy."

The next evidence of the community's discomfort at our presence was a series of rumors that swept the town. One was that "the government" had sent out the research team to investigate attitudes toward mental illness because "they" were thinking of building a new mental hospital in Prairie Town. This rumor, while quite unfounded, was not unreasonable in light of the avowed purpose of our program and the content of the questionnaires. The next rumor was less logical: the survey was said to be a "plot" of the Roman Catholic Church. The grounds for this rumor were difficult to find; the local Catholic clergy was definitely, if not actively, opposed to our program. The only possible basis we could see was the fact that a member of the Parent-Teacher Association, which was working with us, was a Roman Catholic. About 15 per cent of Prairie Town is Roman Catholic.

The faltering attendance at the citizens' study group and the lack of enthusiasm for other aspects of our work have already been cited. As the months went by, people increasingly claimed that "other interests" took precedence over those of our program. One man, asked why he ceased attending an activity sponsored by the project, said, "People say there's nothing to do in Prairie Town, but you could keep going morning, noon, and night if you belonged to everything." During the latter part of the program, we helped a local organization sponsor two very good commercial films, one of which dealt with a mental health topic. Ordinarily Prairie Town attends its local theater faithfully. Since the proceeds of the showing were to go to the local sponsoring organization, representatives sold tickets from house to house. There was no competing event in the town, but despite this the theater was less than half full, an attendance smaller than would be expected from an ordinary poor film on a bad night.

During the early part of the program, the Civil Servant's Association requested us to provide a speaker for one of its meetings. We decided to show the group an educational film on mental health called "Breakdown," made by the National Film Board of Canada. The main incident of the film was the sudden schizophrenic breakdown of a young woman of twenty-three. Knowing from previous experience that the film disturbs some viewers because the heroine's breakdown seems to be "uncaused," we decided to counteract the anxiety thus aroused by conducting a discussion immediately afterward to explain the cause of the breakdown. Although these discussions were held, the Association voted at its next meeting not to have any more mental health films or speakers, despite a previous commitment to present a series of mental health programs.

The most dramatic evidence that our educational program was generating anxiety came from a local citizen who had been closely associated with the project. June was an intelligent, alert woman of about thirty-five. She was very active in civic affairs and had been instrumental in forming the P.T.A. in Prairie Town. From the start of our project she welcomed our aid in planning P.T.A. programs, and as time went on became more involved with the activities and materials of our campaign. She had done a great deal of voluntary work, and when the pace of our program was accelerated in midwinter, we decided to employ her as a paid part-time worker. In late winter she became upset. She began to warn us that it would be better if we stopped certain of our educational activities, saying that they had "run their course" and that "everyone is so busy at other things." Shortly afterward, our staff headquarters in Prairie City received several urgent long distance calls from June. She became so highly agitated that it was necessary to admit her to a psychiatric unit where she was given intensive treatment for a state of acute anxiety. Again, in retrospect, we feel that her association with our anxiety-producing program had caused tension between her and her friends, which had led to her temporary instability.

Not until the program reached its end did the increasing anxiousness of the people of Prairie Town manifest itself in overt hostility to our project. When the interviewers returned to Prairie Town at the end of six months to conduct the second interview of our before-and-after series, they were disconcerted by the coldness of their reception. Those interviewed were guarded and cautious. They asked questions such as this: "What happens if I give the wrong answer?" Some kept threatening to break off the interview. One man of considerable influence in Prairie Town, who was scarcely involved with any phase of our program but who had noted its general effects, said to us, "You've sure got this town by its ear." He added that he was amazed at the intensity of the excitement and anger in the community. There is little doubt that the people felt our project was directly responsible for June's temporary breakdown.

Not only did the interviewers meet with reluctance to cooperate, but with active and angry refusal as well. They had been in Prairie Town only a few hours when the wife of one of the original members of the study group telephoned and declared curtly that she did not wish to be interviewed, refusing to give any reason. Shortly afterward her husband, an agricultural scientist who had been an early and active member of the study group, telephoned us and similarly refused to be interviewed. We told him that he had no reason to assume he would be interviewed again since our reinterview sample was different from the original sample. This assurance had little effect. In ten minutes he burst into the hotel room occupied by the project staff and said angrily,

"Withdraw my name from anything you have it on." We again declared we would not involve him in any way and asked why he felt as he did. "There's no reason," he said, "I'm just not interested, let's put it that way, I'm just not interested," and left abruptly.

Finally, as if representing the feelings and wishes of the community as a whole, the mayor of Prairie Town approached one of our interviewers and inquired what he was doing there. He proceeded to question him at length as to his credentials and his right to conduct the interviews. Then he said, "We have had too much of this sort of thing. We are not interested in it in this town any more. The sooner you leave the better." Although the mayor was finally mollified, it was evident that we had worn out our welcome in Prairie Town! It is significant that it was not the education team who felt this hostility, but the interviewers who were virtually unknown in the town. Thus, it appears to have been hostility to the material rather than to the people who carried it.

At the end of our educational program, when both the attitude questionnaire and the intensive interview were administered a second time, there was some falling off in the number of people returning the questionnaire, but it was not enough to bias the results to any appreciable extent. Similarly, fewer people were willing to submit to the interview on this second occasion, but our sample was not significantly affected by this difference. Results were surprisingly clearcut. After an intensive educational campaign of six months, virtually no change had occurred in attitudes toward or beliefs about the mentally ill.

It could not possibly be argued that we had not touched our community, that our message had simply failed to reach the 900 adults in Prairie Town. The intensity of response to our program was amply evidenced by the man who commented, "You've sure got this town by its ear." The widespread and openly manifested hostility that greeted our returning interviewers could scarcely betoken indifference or ignorance. The people of Prairie Town knew we were there, knew that we were trying to change their ideas, and refused stubbornly and actively to accept that change. It was evident that we had been trying to change ideas that were very deeply and firmly held and that the more energetically we tried to dislodge them, the more tightly people held onto them and the angrier they became at us for trying to take them away.

The results of the attitude questionnaires and interviews, systematically analyzed after we had left Prairie Town, revealed that some of our efforts had been misdirected. The primary purpose of giving tests before and after the educational campaign was to ascertain whether and in what respects our experiment had succeeded in changing popular attitudes concerning mental illness. As it turned out, the interview material also served another purpose; it supplied clues that enabled us to understand why our attempts had incurred hostility. What did the test show?

Attitudes Toward Mental Illness

After we had become well accepted within Prairie Town and before beginning our educational program, we persuaded several local groups to help us distribute a two-page mimeographed paper-and-pencil questionnaire. One Monday afternoon a copy of this questionnaire for each adult was distributed to every house in town. The volunteers also distributed a reprint of an editorial from the local paper urging cooperation with our project. Later that evening the same group picked up the filled-in questionnaires.

At about the same time a group of six psychologists and social workers trained as interviewers administered a long interview schedule to a carefully randomized sample of 100 adults. The interview schedule was much more intensive than the questionnaire and sought information on a wide variety of topics relating to mental illness. The interview schedule was developed by the National Opinion Research Center of the University of Chicago under the direction of Dr. Shirley Star and has been administered in the United States. The interview reached fewer people but at a deeper level than the questionnaire. The two research instruments, when the data were later analyzed, produced a fairly detailed picture of how the people of Prairie Town felt about the mentally ill.

The questionnaire was answered and returned by 540 people, or about 60 per cent of the adult population. It consisted of a number of yes-or-no questions on two topics: whether people were willing to associate with those who had been mentally ill and under what circumstances; and whether they felt in any way responsible for causing mental illness or caring for the mentally ill.

Answers to the questionnaire items on willingness to associate with former patients revealed wide variation in attitudes, roughly corresponding to the different social and economic positions of community members. In general, the community-minded people —who tended also to be younger and better educated—appeared more willing to associate with those who had been mentally ill than did the "puritan" group, who tended to be in lower economic brackets and less well educated. Willingness to associate with former patients depended on the intimacy of the association. For example, 78 per cent replied they would not object to having a discharged mental patient in their club but only 32 per cent said they felt it would be possible to fall in love with someone who had been mentally ill. Thus, data from Prairie Town supported our assumption that people tend to fear and avoid the mentally ill. The questionnaire further indicated that degrees of proximity varied with type of respondent and type of situation in which association occurred. Of course, it is likely that in an effort to appear enlightened and tolerant, some respondents expressed greater willingness to associate with the mentally ill than they really felt.

Answers to the questions on responsibility also showed wide variation, but this was not related to social and economic differences. Rather, it depended on one's notions as to the cause of mental illness. Those who believed that the causes of mental illness were primarily biological did not feel so responsible for the mentally ill as those, for example, who believed mental illness was mainly due to social and economic factors.

The interview schedule was administered to a sample of 100 adults, as already mentioned. Most of the questions were "open-ended," permitting people to express their opinions quite freely. The interview material was typed in detail and stored in Prairie City until it could be analyzed at leisure after the educational campaign ended in Prairie Town. When the results of the interviews were finally processed, this paramount impression emerged: popular thinking about mental illness appeared confused and inconsistent. Conceptions of the nature, cause, and treatment of mental illness seemed hazy and frequently contradictory. In general, the people tended to regard as "normal" a much wider range of behavior than psychiatrists would. Behavior that would seem clearly pathological to a psychiatrist would be dismissed by many respondents as "just a quirk" or by saying "he'll get over it" or "it takes all kinds to make a world."

As part of the interview, six "cases" were briefly described, each typifying a different form of mental illness according to psychiatry. These were presented as specific individuals. Only their behavior was given; no psychiatric labels were attached. Most of those interviewed agreed that the description intended to exemplify a paranoid schizophrenic was indeed that of a person who was "mentally ill." But for each of the other five cases, a majority of the people denied that the person described was mentally ill. Between 65 and 75 per cent rendered the judgment "not mentally ill" in the cases representing respectively a chronic alcoholic, a woman with simple schizophrenia, and a man diagnosed clinically as "a depressive with underlying suicidal tendencies," although more than half the respondents agreed there was "something wrong" in each of these three instances. Only 4 per cent thought the case of a delinquent boy reflected "mental illness," and many found the behavior of a compulsive girl with phobic features praiseworthy because of her excessive care concerning details.

The question "What is mental illness?" drew a wide variety of answers. Most respondents tended to make a sharp distinction between insanity or mental illness—considered serious and virtually incurable—on the one hand, and "nervous" disorders—less serious and amenable to treatment—on the other. However, in citing symptoms, they tended to attribute the same symptoms to both types. Asked to characterize mental illness, they cited a wide range of attributes: unpredictability, violence, irrational behavior, anxiety states, withdrawal, depression, and others. Of these, "unpredictability" was most frequently cited.

However, it appeared that the single most important criterion for adjudging a person sane or insane was whether or not he had been institutionalized. A mentally ill person was someone whom doctors had acclaimed mentally ill by placing him in a mental hospital. Thus, it can be inferred that the same behavior that was judged "normal" in a nonhospitalized person was judged "abnormal" in one who had been hospitalized.

Notions of the cause of mental illness appeared to be unsystematic and often mutually contradictory. Many factors were cited as capable of causing mental illness, ranging from purely biological factors to bad social conditions. In general, the human organism was visualized as a machine in very delicate balance, easily upset or put out of order. A small number of people attributed mental illness to moral dereliction, a punishment for failure to live a clean and moral life.

Conceptions of cure of mental illness were related to ideas of its cause. Those who saw biological factors as causing mental illness tended to believe that it could be readily cured by a doctor or a nerve specialist, who would fix up the "nerves" that had gone wrong. Those espousing moral causality felt that mental illness could be cured by returning to correct moral behavior and seeking salvation.

Almost everyone expressed great confidence in the effectiveness of mental hospitals as agencies of cure. If the machinery of the body was easily thrown out of kilter, it could as easily be righted. This picture of mental illness as something readily cured by doctors and hospitals appeared to contradict the conception of mental illness as essentially incurable. Similarly, the picture of mental hospitals as highly effective agencies of cure appeared inconsistent with the tendency to class as "mentally ill" only those who had been hospitalized.

Attitudes to the mentally ill expressed during the interview were similar to those revealed by the paper-and-pencil questionnaire. Half of those interviewed felt that insane people were dangerous to be near. More than two-thirds claimed that while they personally would not feel differently toward someone who had been mentally ill, others would; it is likely that the attitude attributed to others was really their own.

Why the Hostility?

It will be recalled that an important motive for trying to change popular attitudes toward mental disease was our conviction that misconceptions about the cause and nature of mental illness were harmful to discharged patients, tending to drive them back to the hospital. It will be recalled that our educational program aimed to replace erroneous conceptions with three basic ideas: the range of "normal" behavior is wider than is generally realized; abnormal behavior does not just happen but is caused and therefore subject to change; abnormality and normality are not two separate and unrelated states, but rather differing manifestations of the same kinds of behavior.

The results of our attitude questionnaires and interviews showed us that some of our educational efforts were misdirected. The "fit" between their set of ideas and ours appeared haphazard and unsystematic. Apparently the people of Prairie Town not only already believed that a wide range of behavior was "normal," but were willing to accept as normal an even wider range of behavior than were most psychiatrists. As to our next point, that disturbed behavior is "caused," the people of Prairie Town already knew this. They differed from medical personnel in that they imputed a different set of causes—a set more ramified and inclusive and yet less logically consistent than medical notions of etiology. It was our third idea—that there is a gradation rather than a sharp division between normality and abnormality —that diverged most strikingly from popular conceptions.

It was our hope that the net result of our program would be to make people more accepting of the mentally ill and more willing to act toward them as they did toward "normal" people. It was precisely this result that the people of Prairie Town seemed determined to prevent. Their ideas about mental illness and the mentally ill appeared inconsistent and often illogical when judged in terms of our ideas; but looked at in their own terms they were consistent, even reasonable and necessary. The whole set of ideas, beliefs, and attitudes about mental illness held by the people of Prairie Town was a response not to considerations of empirical truth, but rather to the needs of the community. For the community of Prairie Town, it was far less important to know the detached "truth" about mental illness than to have some workable way to handle the difficult problem of mental illness. A crucial element in their method of handling this problem was belief in a black-and-white difference between the sane and the insane, and the concomitant conviction that the mentally ill must be removed from the community. These popular ideas were diametrically opposed to those our educational program sought to teach. As we worked to undermine them and replace them with "correct" ideas, people became increasingly upset and angry. Why should this be so?

From the point of view of the people of Prairie Town rather than from a scientific or clinical standpoint, their ideas concerning the nature, cause, and treatment of mental illness formed a consistent pattern, one we can call the "pattern of denial and isolation." Many aspects of the behavior of the community became meaningful once we began to view them in the context of this pattern. Briefly, the pattern is this. People tend to deny the existence of abnormal behavior for as long a time as they possibly can. When behavior becomes so deviant that it can no longer be tolerated or construed as normal, people act to isolate the mentally ill person, both physically and conceptually.

The attitudes expressed in the questionnaires and interviews, as well as the observed behavior of the people of Prairie Town, testify to this pattern. Responses to the psychiatric cases in the interviews showed that the people tended to deny the existence of disturbed behavior, to "normalize" what was clinically mental illness. A very wide range of behavior was accepted as "normal." Having a wide and heterogeneous conception of the cause and nature of mental illness helps to maintain this acceptance. However, once a person is definitely categorized as "mentally ill," usually because he has been hospitalized, people's attitudes sharply reverse themselves. Instead of saying in effect, "He's just about like everyone else," people say, "He's very different from everyone else and must be separated from normal people." The attitude questionnaire showed that people wished to avoid close contact with the mentally ill. It also showed a considerable fear of disturbed persons, as we had anticipated, along with a tendency to be ashamed of that fear.

The feeling that mental hospitals are good places and will cure the mentally ill is connected with the desire to put out of one's mind all thoughts of a mentally disturbed friend or relative. Once a person is placed in a mental hospital, he is "put away" both physically and from one's thoughts, and the picture of the mental hospital as a desirable place helps to assuage the guilt a person might feel at so isolating a friend or relative. Once a person is admitted to a hospital, he is virtually deserted by friends and relatives, as if contact were somehow contaminating and dangerous.

It is evident that this whole complex of beliefs and attitudes is a product of the community's attempt to solve a perplexing problem. At the core of this solution is the need of the community to separate itself from deviant people. The people themselves indicate that "unpredictability" of behavior is the basic reason they fear the mentally ill, but since most of the mentally ill are scarcely less predictable than anyone else, it is likely that people equate deviation from behavioral norms with unpredictability. The pattern of denial and isolation arises from the attempt on the part of the community to maintain its code of conduct and hence its own integrity by protecting itself from deviant behavior.

The reasoning runs like this. There are two main kinds of people—people like you and me, and the mentally ill—and there is a sharp line between them. When a person's quirks, odd habits, "different" behavior, funny actions are still reasonably close to those of most people, he belongs in the ranks of the sane. The community tries to keep him there by "denying" as long as possible that such behavior constitutes mental illness. But if the behavior of the disturbed person produces some conspicuous result—a breakdown, commitment to a psychiatric ward, an undeniable breach of the laws of society—the community then mobilizes to protect itself and its rules of conduct. It does so by suddenly branding the disturbing person "insane," a verdict carrying the sentence of banishment. He is now in a completely different category from "normal" people and must be treated differently. The community, in order to maintain the sanity and balance of its members, must dissociate itself from the now dangerous deviant.

It may now be understood why our educational efforts caused so much disturbance in Prairie Town. In our attempt to produce a more permissive climate for former mental patients, we conveyed the idea that they were pretty much like everyone else, and that there was no sharp line dividing the sane from the insane, but rather a continuous range of behavior. In stressing this idea we were hammering directly at the core of the community's own solution to the problem of the mentally ill. Our problem was not theirs. We were concerned with the cure of the mentally ill, the people of Prairie Town with the stability and solidarity of their own community. In striving to achieve our purpose we violated theirs.

From our therapy-centered viewpoint it was evident that mental hospitals are not the best means for curing the mentally ill; the hospitalized patient is maintained in an artificial situation isolated from the beneficial influence of normal social intercourse. In trying to educate the community to this point of view we challenged a basic part of their solution to the problem of mental illness. The community "solves" this problem by putting the mentally ill in a class apart and keeping them in isolation, but underneath it is uncomfortable about this solution. Doubts as to whether this is really the right way come to the surface from time to time. People cope with these doubts by reassuring themselves and one another that the mental hospital really is the best place for anyone mentally ill; that people are cured there; and that their hospitalized friend or relative is really being helped much more than if he remained in the community. We have noted the almost pathetic eagerness of the relatives of hospitalized mental patients to assure themselves that this was a good hospital, or at least better than most others.

By informing the people that many mental hospitals were in fact overcrowded, inadequately staffed, and maltherapeutic, we were destroying the device people used to assuage their guilt over having exiled their relatives. If people accepted our assertion that mental hospitals were undesirable or even harmful, they would have to face their own inner feelings of guilt and shame, feelings that had been kept in check by their motivated evaluation of the mental hospital as a "good" place.

In short, Prairie Town's pattern of beliefs and attitudes toward mental illness was not merely a patchwork of half-truths, fallacies, and inconsistencies, as appeared from a first inspection of the interview data; it played an important part in preserving the well-being of the community and the peace of mind and self-esteem of the average individual. When they sensed that our educational program was a concerted attempt to weaken and dislodge these protective beliefs, the people of Prairie Town became disturbed and anxious and warned us indirectly to soften our message and relax our efforts. When we persisted, their anxiety went over into active hostility. To protect itself, the community mobilized to eject the disturbing forces.

IMPLICATIONS

We all live our lives upon certain cultural assumptions about the nature of disease, the proper way to raise crops, what are wholesome and unwholesome foods, and a myriad of other attitudes and beliefs. It is reasonable to suppose that these are organized into a workable interrelated pattern. Thus, any sudden onslaught on a particular set of beliefs, whether they concern diet or mental illness, may cause considerable dislocation in this whole system. However, attempts to change beliefs and attitudes will probably go on and we can only hope that this will be done more and more skillfully so that the process will become less uncomfortable both for the educator and for the public. What can our experiences in Prairie Town teach us about planning and carrying out similar programs in the future?

The Program in Retrospect

Reviewing the total program, there are a few things we are glad that we did as we did. Among these was our gradual and unobtrusive entry into the community. We feel sure that this town could not be taken by a frontal assault. The fact that we offered to aid the various organizations in planning their programs facilitated cooperation. Establishing contact with and explaining our program to key figures in these organizations before our publicity campaign began helped in gaining their cooperation. We were wise to have dissociated ourselves from government and any specific organization already in the town and to have avoided identification with any particular group or person until we could gauge how well they were accepted by their fellow citizens.

There are several factors which we might have anticipated, but did not. For one thing, we had no moral purpose in our stated aims. If we had had such a purpose, greater cooperation would probably have been forthcoming from the various religious groups. In addition, we had no real program of action. That is, we did not, for instance, realize until too late that there was a considerable force in the community that favored building a common recreation center. To have allied ourselves with such a cause early would perhaps have given more meaning to our campaign. Furthermore, although we had anticipated some anxiety, we were perhaps not sufficiently zealous in seeking signs of it as the program progressed or quick enough in reading those presented to us. Further, we had no suitable program, if such is possible, for dealing with this anxiety as it arose.

Other conditions could have been made evident only by more thorough advance investigation of the community. Had such a study been made we would have been aware, for instance, that the town was divided rather sharply into a low education group, which included the Metis minority, and a middle and upper educational group. We would have learned in advance that there were two segments within the educated group—"joiners," who made up the membership of most of the town's 70 organizations, and those who admired the puritan virtues and stood apart from most organizations other than the Protestant churches. This knowledge would have alerted us to the difficulty of trying to reach the whole population through these 70 organizations.

Moreover, we would have become aware of the sharp Protestant-Catholic schism in the town, which had been made more intense by the militant activity of a recently appointed priest. We would have found that the dominant Protestant minister had accepted a call to a city church and would probably not be much interested in innovations, and we would have been dubious of the possibility of working simultaneously with Catholics and Protestants. We might have concentrated on working through the Catholic Church to reach the low education group while attempting to reach the other educational groups through secular organizations.

An advance community survey would have revealed that the technically educated workers in the government agricultural stations were a group separated from the rest of the community. The town regarded them with mixed feelings, and while they could have damaged the program if they felt slighted, close identification with them could alienate other sectors of the community.

Other factors could not have been anticipated, although better knowledge of the community might have made them easier to cope with. Such an unforeseen event involved the local priest. A very cordial relationship was initially established, and there was every likelihood of getting his cooperation in working with the Catholic portion of the community. However, just about the time our program began, a psychiatrist in Montreal made a radio speech in which he implied that religion was detrimental to mental health, and about the same time a West Coast mental health group brought out a pamphlet on masturbation, describing it as a normal and natural part of childhood. These two claims drew a sharp official rebuke to mental health organizations by a high church official, and the cooperation of the local priest disappeared almost overnight.

Similarly, one cannot anticipate the weather. An unusually wet autumn delayed harvesting operations and kept many resident farmers out of town almost a month later than was usual, while a warm dry spring had a similar detrimental effect on the terminal part of our program.

Limits for Health Education

Our experience in Prairie Town may be summarized under four general points. Each of these poses questions for the health educator. First, we found, as others have, that mass media were less effective than group contacts. But in working with groups, we faced the problem that organized groups in Prairie Town were composed of and controlled by a relatively small portion of the total community. What are the techniques by which we can reach the less-educated groups in these communities? How does one present complicated ideas to people who are relatively unable to integrate them into their own experience?

Second, it became evident that people were motivated toward learning only when they felt that the material applied to them personally. How are people to be motivated toward learning without "scare" techniques ("one person in 20 will spend time in a mental hospital"), since scare techniques inevitably produce undesirable side-effects? This point would seem obvious from the upsurge of phobias and anxiety states centering around cancer and syphilis after educational programs of this type have been attempted.

Third, we can speculate as to whether a tangible action program or a treatment clinic introduced in the program might have produced more motivation to learn new attitudes and helped to reduce anxiety. If such extension of a project is sometimes advantageous and sometimes detrimental, are there criteria for judging when such extension is advisable and when it is not? When does extension of a program make it more vulnerable by providing more areas in which to make mistakes?

Finally, our experiences in Prairie Town made it abundantly clear that any energetic attempt to change attitudes and beliefs will produce anxiety. To some extent this is true even for areas of apparently minor importance, such as attitudes toward the use of powdered eggs or a new kind of seed corn. But this phenomenon becomes increasingly evident as one begins to deal with beliefs and attitudes closer to the core of a people's culture. The pattern of beliefs surrounding mental illness is certainly close to this core because it touches the very network of interpersonal relations that binds a community together. Any attempts to change existing attitudes in so vital an area must be approached with caution. There seems to be little doubt that anxiety will be aroused no matter how carefully one plans or how cautiously he proceeds. Would virtually the same results have occurred had we based our program in Prairie Town on better knowledge of the community and more sophisticated assumptions, avoiding the various practical and organizational pitfalls just cited and spreading our educational program over years rather than months?

This poses questions for the worker attempting mental health education. Can the anxiety associated with efforts to touch this area be lessened by moving more slowly, working less intensively, using different techniques, or confining such education to optimally receptive communities? Can a set of techniques be developed for handling this anxiety? Can it be controlled and made to facilitate rather than disrupt the learning process? Is it wise to attempt such a program at all? If "erroneous" beliefs about mental illness in fact fill a critical social need, should the effort be made to change them? Will the benefits accruing to the mentally ill outweigh the possible "cost" to the community in augmented insecurity about its own sanity and standards? If misconceptions about the mentally ill serve to reaffirm the solidarity of the sane, how can health workers best avert the risk of disrupting this solidarity? The case of Prairie Town has not answered these questions nor could it answer them, but it has shown clearly that they must be asked.

SUMMARY

A six-month educational program designed to alter popular attitudes toward the mentally ill was carried out in a small Canadian prairie town. Questionnaires and standard interviews were administered before and after the educational program to measure its effects. The tests showed no appreciable change in beliefs about mental illness or attitudes toward the mentally ill as a result of the program. Interviews and other data pointed to the existence of a community "pattern of denial and isolation" as a method for dealing with the threat of mental illness: the existence of abnormal behavior is denied as long as possible; when denial is no longer feasible, the degree of abnormality is exaggerated and the ill person is isolated socially and conceptually, as well as physically. Although malfunctional in reference to the rehabilitation of the mentally ill, this pattern appeared functional in reference to the maintenance of community solidarity. Efforts to change parts of this pattern by education produced anxiety and hostility. The Prairie Town experience indicates that mental health educators must carefully take into account the social function of beliefs about mental illness, anticipate the occurrence of anxiety, and prepare themselves for difficulty and slow success.

SELECTED REFERENCES

Cumming, Elaine, and John Cumming, *The Blackfoot Project:* An Experiment in Mental Health Education. (In preparation for publication by Commonwealth Fund.) A fuller description and analysis of the Prairie Town experiment. Blackfoot and Prairie Town are two pseudonyms for the same community. The details of the study are given and the implications of the results are spelled out.

Cumming, John, and Elaine Cumming, *Affective Symbolism, Social Norms, and Mental Illness.* (In preparation.) An attempt to define some of the variables that assist in determining when a person will be considered mentally ill by his friends and acquaintances and how these variables are related to the toleration of the symptoms of mental illness by lay people.

Davis, Kingsley, "Mental Hygiene and Class Structure," *Psychiatry,* vol. 1, February, 1938, pp. 55–65. This classical essay in the sociology of knowledge examines the assumptions underlying the mental health movement in the light of its goals.

Hollingshead, A. B., and F. C. Redlich, "Social Class and Psychiatric Disorders" in *Interrelations Between the Social Environment and Psychiatric Disorders,* Milbank Memorial Fund, New York, 1953. In dealing with differential rates of mental illness by social class, this article, along with other works by these authors, opens up the possibility that there exists a different toleration of deviance among socioeconomic strata.

Merton, Robert K., "Manifest and Latent Functions" in *Social Theory and Social Structure.* The Free Press, Glencoe, Ill., 1949, pp. 21–81. An analysis of how elements in a society which seem at first glance disruptive may have latent functions which make them valuable to the integration of that society.

Parsons, Talcott, and Renée Fox, "Illness, Therapy and the Modern Urban American Family," *Journal of Social Issues,* vol. 8, no. 4, 1952, pp. 31–55. An analysis of how the handling of physical illness is woven into the fabric of modern urban life. Attitudes toward illness reflect in many ways the type of society in which they are generated.

Star, Shirley A., *The Dilemmas of Mental Illness:* An Inquiry into Contemporary American Perspectives. (In preparation for publication by Commonwealth Fund.) An exhaustive analysis of public attitudes toward mental illness, based on a research project of the National Opinion Research Center.

Case 3

WATER BOILING IN A PERUVIAN TOWN
by Edward Wellin

To evaluate their success in South Africa, Dr. Cassel and his colleagues compared infant mortality rates and incidences of gross nutritional failure before and after nine years of public health work; the results were impressive. By a similar before-and-after comparison, the Cummings were able to document the fact that their six-month campaign to alter mental health attitudes had failed to produce any significant change. In evaluating the results of a rural hygiene worker's attempts over a two-year period to persuade Peruvian housewives to boil their drinking water, Dr. Wellin likewise had access to before-and-after data. Out of about 200 households the number of women who regularly boiled their drinking water rose from 15 to 26. Little significance could be attached to these numbers, however, in the absence of a standard against which to measure the worker's efficiency, especially since she was trying with varying success to introduce other health innovations over the same period of time.

A more meaningful approach was to compare the motives and circumstances of the women who boiled the water with those of women who did not. The biographical comparisons which comprise the heart of Dr. Wellin's intensive study of a restricted subject show the extent to which culture and ecology control the motivations of individuals even in apparently simple matters such as accepting competent advice to boil contaminated water. They also show the selective effects of social distinctions within the community, and the case is thus akin to those in Part IV of this volume. —EDITOR

THE PROBLEM

Evaluating the Results of a Rural Hygiene Project

Nelida is a rural hygiene worker whose full-time job is visiting households in the small town of Los Molinos in order to help the people improve their hygiene. The water in Los Molinos is contaminated. There is no sanitary water system, nor is it economically feasible to install one. The residents, however, could hope to lower the incidence of typhoid and other water-borne diseases by regularly boiling water before consuming it.

When Nelida first took up residence in Los Molinos, only a few of the 200 households were already boiling their drinking water. As one of her duties, Nelida has been trying tactfully and by indirection to persuade others to adopt this practice. She has been aided in her work by Dr. U, a health department physician who has visited the community to give public talks on topics of health and hygiene. After two years in Los Molinos, she has succeeded in getting 11 more families to boil water. Most of the families still drink unboiled water. The health department wonders what these figures mean. As health professionals see the situation, Nelida has only to prevail on housewives to add a simple habit to the sequence of preexisting water habits, that is, to get them to boil their drinking water sometime between securing and consuming it. Surely this task should not be so difficult. Why, then, have so few been persuaded and so many not?

These questions confronted the writer when he came to Los Molinos in 1953 after having spent more than two years studying the characteristics of other communities in the Ica valley. For many weeks the author interviewed Nelida and local townspeople and observed daily routines. The task of discovering systematic differences, in which Nelida was a keenly interested partner, proceeded slowly and with difficulty. It was finally accomplished to the reasonable satisfaction of the writer, but not before taking into account an unexpected number of social, cultural, and situational factors whose bearing on water boiling was not always evident on first inspection.

There were indeed differences between those who boiled their water and those who did not, but these differences were not simple. Among water boilers, as among nonboilers, there were often different and even opposing motives for the same end-product behaviors.[1]

[1] The writer is indebted to the Rockefeller Foundation and to the Pan American Sanitary Bureau (WHO) for supporting the field work which made this case study possible. Preparation of materials for publication was facilitated by a grant from the Laboratory of Social Relations, Harvard University.

THE SITUATION

Differences Between Women Who Boil Drinking Water and Those Who Do Not

The Hygiene Worker and the Health Department

Nelida is one of more than 20 hygiene visitors of both sexes employed by the Ica Departmental Health Service (IDHS), a regional agency of Peru's Ministry of Public Health and Social Welfare. The IDHS was launched in 1945 as a pioneer Peruvian effort to establish a regionally autonomous health department with a well-rounded program and an adequate complement of full-time personnel. Its inception and development were inspired and counseled by Dr. J. L. Hydrick, representative in Peru of the Rockefeller Foundation's Division of Medicine and Public Health and author of the volume *Intensive Rural Hygiene Work in the Netherlands East Indies*. Although it has received considerable aid from the Rockefeller Foundation and other international health agencies, the IDHS is managed by a Peruvian directorate and is supported mainly by Peruvian funds.

The IDHS operates out of the city of Ica, where it maintains administrative headquarters and a variety of installations and services. It enjoys a reputation, even outside Peru, both as a sound and efficient health department and as an important experimental departure from conventional lines of health administration and practice; the use of hygiene visitors is but one of a number of innovations.

Hygiene visitors are natives of the Ica valley who have taken courses of training extending over a year or more before being assigned to live and work in specific communities. IDHS policy is to recruit hygiene visitors from social levels or cultural groups similar to those with which they will work. They receive instruction in such topics as hygiene, communicable diseases, environmental sanitation, nutrition, dental care, and domestic economy. In addition to lectures and discussions, the training places heavy emphasis on role-playing techniques to teach the practical art of home visiting. Once assigned to a community, hygiene visitors report weekly to administrative headquarters for control and additional training.

Dr. U's occasional talks in Los Molinos are designed specifically to convey health information to the community. They are well attended and include such topics as modes of disease transmission, dangers of contaminated water, and the preventive value of boiling drinking water. Nelida has the job of getting families to apply good health habits in their daily routines. Other categories of IDHS personnel help to *inform* people on health matters; the hygiene visitor tries to motivate them to *apply* the new information. She makes regular and repeated home visits, during which she converses with housewives and other members of the family. She attempts both to make people aware of health problems and tactfully to suggest realizable ways of handling them. She does not lecture housewives and tries not to give unsolicited advice. Nelida works out of a hygiene center, an adobe building in Los Molinos rented by the IDHS.

Nelida is a buxom married woman of twenty-five with one child. She was brought up in an Ica valley community and comes of a family not very different from most Los Molinos families of moderate means. In 1951 the IDHS assigned her to work exclusively in Los Molinos. Other health personnel—physician, dentist, nurse, trained midwife, sanitary engineer, sanitary inspector, immunizer—come to Los Molinos, but only at intervals in the course of work in scores of Ica valley communities.

The Town of Los Molinos

Los Molinos is one of several hundred rural communities in the valley of Ica, a coastal region about 200 miles south of Peru's capital city of Lima and connected with it by the Pan American Highway. The valley is one of 40-odd oases which interrupt the rainless, sun-baked desert of the Peruvian coast. To the west is the Pacific and to the east tower the Andes. A river which flows only during the four- to five-month rainy season in the Andean highlands is the valley's prime source of water and its life's blood. Nature in the region is a study in contrast between rich agricultural oasis and encompassing desert, between aridity in July and fertility in January. Culture, too, shows sharp contrasts. Agriculture ranges from primitive subsistence farming to large-scale commercial cultivation. In communities like Los Molinos, one finds rude cane and adobe huts, traditional saint cults, native curers and lay midwives, and a complete absence of sanitary water or sewage systems. In the city of Ica, only 15 miles away, there are architect-designed dwellings, the Rotary Club, physicians and hospitals, and a relatively efficient water and sewage system.

Most people of Los Molinos are peasants. Some own individual family plots, but the majority work as field hands for local plantations. The plantations are given over mainly to cotton fields and vineyards; family plots grow beans, squash, corn, and fruits. Los Molinos has a population of approximately 1,000. The physical core of the town consists of two long rows of houses lining a dirt road. About midway is the town's main square, a large cleared rectangle bordered by the Catholic Church, the Civil Guard post, municipal quarters, the public well, and the dwellings of the more prominent families. Most houses are uniformly drab adobe and mud-plastered cane structures—dirt-floored, windowless, one-storied affairs.

Los Molinos is predominantly *cholo*, a term which has racial, cultural, and social meanings and corresponds to the term *mestizo* used in other parts of Latin America. Cholos are racially mixed, basically Indian with some Spanish admixture. They follow a way of life which is not Indian, Spanish, or modern western, but a vigorous mixture of the three. Socially, they rank low in Peru's social geography, just a cut above Negroes and highlanders. More than two-thirds of the community are cholo, and the remaining one-third is split between highlanders and Negroes. Highlanders are similar in racial makeup to cholos but are looked down on by coastal cholos; their native tongue (Quechua) and highland clothing are derided. The town's Negroes are descendants of slaves introduced several centuries ago by slave-trading Spaniards. Cholos, Negroes, and highlanders all speak Spanish, although recently arrived highlanders do so with a noticeable accent.

Economic distinctions are also recognized within the town. About ten families are prosperous. The rest are about equally divided between moderately well-off and poor. These distinctions are all relative; from an outsider's point of view they might be considered three grades of poverty. Economic and ethnic distinctions enjoy only gross correspondence with each other. Cholos are found along the whole economic range; Negroes are mainly at the economic bottom; and highlanders distribute about evenly between moderate and poor. Although Los Molinos is regarded by Ica, only 15 miles away, as an undifferentiated community of poor cholos, closer inspection reveals it to be rather highly differentiated.

Water rusts no pipes in Los Molinos. It is borne directly from stream and well to large earthenware containers in the household by means of cans, pails, gourds, and casks. Children are the most frequent water carriers. It is considered inappropriate for males and females of courtship age and married men to carry water, and they seldom do. There are three sources of water: a seasonal irrigation ditch, a spring, and a public well. All are sedimented in various degrees, subject to pollution at all times, and show contamination whenever tested. Of the three, the irrigation ditch is most favored. It is close, running parallel to the main road about 50 yards distant; children can be sent to fetch its water; it has the virtue of being running rather than stagnant; and it inspires complex devotion for its annual rejuvenation of the Los Molinos soil. People like its taste. It is only seasonal, however, running from about December to April and is part of the ramified irrigation system feeding off the River Ica.

The spring lies a mile or more from the center of town; it is a year-round source and is used by many families when the ditch is dry. Several local men who are professional water sellers fill their casks and load their burros at the spring and peddle the water to housewives. During the dry-ditch season, most families deal with the water sellers; only women and children of the poorest families make the formidable trip to the spring on foot. The public well, although a year-round source, is used regularly only by families living nearby. Most Los Molineros dislike the taste of its water.

Nelida's objectives include efforts to get people to install and properly use privies, burn garbage daily, control house flies, and report suspected cases of communicable disease promptly. She also tries to get housewives to boil drinking water. When Nelida first arrived, she discovered that 15 of the 200 households were already boiling water daily and that every household boiled water on occasion, particularly when family members were sick. During the next two years, she paid several visits to every home but devoted especially intensive effort to 21 families. She visited every one of these selected families between 15 and 25 times. Of the 21 housewives, she has induced 11 to boil water regularly. Let us look at the people behind these figures by describing six housewives, typifying different responses to water boiling. Mrs. A and Mrs. B were already boiling their drinking water when Nelida arrived. Mrs. C and Mrs. D began doing so as a result of IDHS educational efforts. Mrs. E and Mrs. F are among those who continue to drink their water unboiled.

Mrs. A, Who Obeys Custom

Mrs. A is about forty, a cholo and a native of Los Molinos. Her husband, who is fifty, came to Los Molinos as a child from his original home in the Andean highlands. He has lived in Los Molinos more than forty years, is ostensibly an accepted member of the community, and resembles native Los Molineros in appearance and actions. Yet behind his back, he is still referred to as "the highlander." He is the driver of the bus that makes two jarring round trips daily between Los Molinos and Ica. Besides the couple, there are two others in the house, a son and an unmarried sister of Mrs. A. Mrs. A used to teach in the community's public school but several years ago started a private school, which meets in her house. The A's are in the middle-income group and from bus and school enjoy a somewhat higher cash income than do most middle families.

Mrs. A suffers from what she says doctors in Ica have diagnosed as sinusitis. Although her sinus trouble is not incapacitating, the community perceives Mrs. A as one of the town's "sickly ones" by virtue of the chronic nature of the ailment. She likes to talk about her illness. The sinusitis came about, says Mrs. A, when "cold" entered her respiratory passages and lodged in her sinuses.

Every morning after breakfast she boils a potful of water. When it has had time to cool, she leaves her pupils to walk back to the kitchen and transfer the water to a fancy glass pitcher, covering it with a cloth. Mrs. A's daily habit of preparing and drinking boiled water is a practice she initiated prior to Nelida's arrival in Los Molinos and without understanding of the germ theory of disease. Her habit is linked to the local and complex system of hot and cold distinctions. The basic principle of the system is that many things in nature are inherently hot, cold, or something intermediate, quite apart from actual temperature. Things that can be so distinguished include foods, liquids, medicines, body states, illnesses, and even inanimate materials. In essence, hot-cold distinctions serve as a series of avoidances and prescriptions, important to such areas of belief and behavior as pregnancy and child rearing, food habits and work habits. They apply especially to the entire health-illness system, including prevention, diagnosis, prognosis, home medical care, convalescence. They also provide culturally plausible explanations for chronic illness and even death.

The hot or cold nature of most foods does not change regardless of temperature variation, cooking, or other processing. Water is one of the few exceptions. "Raw" water is cold; "cooked" water is hot. Cooked water in Los Molinos has become linked with illness. Through processes of association, Los Molineros learn from earliest childhood to loathe boiled water. Most residents can tolerate boiled water only if they add a flavoring—sugar, tea, lemon juice, cinnamon, onion, lemon peel, barley, corn, or herb. Mrs. A prefers a dash of cinnamon.

Once an individual is considered sick, whatever the specific diagnosis, he or his family invoke the avoidances and prescriptions of the system. Extremes of "hot" and "cold" are denied him; it would be unthinkable, for example, to let him eat pork, which is "very cold" or to drink brandy, which is "very hot." He must avoid extremes in general, but "cold" in particular. "Cold" is virtually an evil entity; it can be absorbed through "airs" or the ingestion of food, can take up lodgings within the body, and can wreak great harm even long after it has entered. The avoidance of "cold" is a must for the very young, the very old, the pregnant, the delicate, and the sick.

At no point does the notion of bacteriological contamination of water enter the scheme. By tradition, boiling is aimed at

eliminating not bacteria but the innate "cold" quality of unboiled water. Mrs. A's illness is chronic, but the same rules would
apply to an acute or a temporary illness. In obedience to custom,
one drinks boiled water during illness.

Mrs. A and others like her account for eight of the housewives
who were already boiling their drinking water when Nelida
arrived. All eight are sickly; only their ailments differ. Other than
Mrs. A, three complain of asthma, two have tuberculosis, one has
had typhoid fever, and one is just sick.

Mrs. B, Who Defies Custom

Mrs. B, like Mrs. A, is one of the 15 housewives who regularly
boiled water even before Nelida came to Los Molinos. But Mrs. B
does so for quite different reasons. She is about fifty-five and was
born and reared in Los Molinos. She and her family are cholos.
Mrs. B is a grandmother and the arbiter of domestic affairs in her
ten-person household. She lives with her husband, a grown son,
two married daughters and their spouses, and three grandchildren. Mr. B works on his small agricultural holdings and also
hires out occasionally as a plantation hand. The son and a son-in-
law work in the city of Ica, and one son-in-law is a plantation
laborer. Mrs. B and both married daughters are usually occupied
about the house. They keep one of the best-ordered houses of the
community, from tile-floored living room to dirt-floored kitchen.
Economically, they are in the community's middle group.

Mrs. B is the perennial butt of gossip, but her professed indifference blunts its bite. She is labeled a social climber, one who
is pretentious and apes her betters. According to gossip, Mrs. B is
no better than anyone else, "but doesn't she put on airs!" Mrs. B
puts it differently; she feels she is cleaner, more refined, and
generally superior to most of her neighbors. She says that Los
Molinos is really a dreary place, and its people are dull, backward,
and back-biting. As compared to her neighbors, she sees herself as
an island of high ideals and cleanliness in a sea of low ideals
and dirt.

An important event in Mrs. B's life, ultimately leading to daily
water boiling, was her brother's departure for the metropolis of
Lima many years ago. Starting as a poor but ambitious young

man, he apparently made good in the big city. As Mrs. B and Los Molinos now see him, he is a person of substance, worldly wisdom, and affluence. About twice a year, he visits Los Molinos for several days. Naturally, he is an authority on the current political situation, the price of cotton, and what one should do for a pain in the back. Everyone knows which parlor chair is his, and it gets dusted before he sits down. As they all sit in the parlor, Mrs. B listens attentively to her brother, while the barefoot and spectacularly dirty children of neighbors peek from the front door at the great man and the wonderful gleam of his gold teeth. When Mrs. B seats him at the head of the dining table, she gives his eating utensils another rub with the all-purpose cloth, dabs another dust speck off his plate. There is always some tension between him and the men of the household, and they rarely quote his opinions after he returns to Lima.

Why Mrs. B's brother began preferring boiled water during his sojourns in Los Molinos is unclear. At any rate, Mrs. B began to boil a daily drinking supply for him during his occasional visits. Whether because of direct suggestion or some indirect effect attached to his behavior and values, Mrs. B initiated water boiling as a daily year-round practice in her kitchen. Mrs. B herself drinks one liter of water daily and reproaches herself that she cannot get more down. "My brother says," confides Mrs. B, "that one should drink one and one-half to two liters of water a day."

Mrs. B apparently likes to talk with Nelida, perhaps in part because she has few friends. Mrs. B attended several of Dr. U's talks, including the one in which he demonstrated the microscope and emphasized the need to boil water. When Nelida visited her some days after his talk, Mrs. B was excited and quite proud of herself. "Imagine," she told Nelida in reference to her habit of boiling the water, "without even knowing, to be doing such a good thing!" In fact, a single talk by Dr. U was enough to convince her that microbes existed and that they could produce sickness. In essence, however, Mrs. B heard from Dr. U only what she wanted to hear. Microbes and dirt are identical for her; indeed, microbes is a more gratifyingly ominous synonym for plain dirtiness. To admit to "having" microbes is socially degrading;

therefore, enlightened people like Mrs. B use a duster on them, sweep them out, rub at them with a cloth.

To the community of Los Molinos, and particularly to the community of women, Mrs. B is a kind of cultural outlaw. What damns her as a deviant, in reference to water, is not simply that she boils water daily, but that she does so when no member of the family is sick. Los Molinos society exacts a price for water boiling. The price is "being sick," which involves both the right and obligation to depart from normal cultural standards. Mrs. A, we will recall, pays the price and thus is able to escape group censure.

Mrs. B, however, boils water without paying the price and thus becomes a target for semi-ostracism. Although healthy, in fact not even making a bow to cultural proprieties by pleading illness, she boils water. Of course, her repudiation of group expectations goes even further than boiling water while healthy. She also scorns local standards of cleanliness and in general flouts the values that promote group cohesiveness in Los Molinos. In rejecting local standards, Mrs. B is, of course, accepting others, the standards represented by her citified brother. She is a deviant by local norms, but according to her preferred standards is "progressive."

Mrs. B and four others like her account for five of the 15 housewives who began to boil water daily even before Nelida arrived. Of the five, three were swayed by relatives living in Lima and two by relatives in Ica. By simple arithmetic, we see that two diverging circumstances, enduring illness and the influence of a city relative, account for all but two of the 15 housewives whose water boiling antedated Nelida's arrival. The remaining two are special cases: one had worked as a cook for the mistress of a plantation and had boiled water for many years as part of her duties; the other worked with her as a laundress; and both now continue to boil their own water.

Mrs. C, Persuaded by Nelida

The C parents came originally from a valley in the Andes mountains that loom over Los Molinos to the east and north. Their home valley is "three days away" over steep animal trails. They are highlanders, but their children are accepted as coastal cholos. There are five adults in the household—Mr. and Mrs. C, two grown sons, and a grown daughter. There are also four children, a late child of the forty-five-year-old Mrs. C and her fifty-year-old husband, and three grandchildren, the daughter's offspring. The family belongs to the middle group. Mr. C uses Los Molinos as his base between trips to the highlands, where he goes to trade and to make sure that his highland relatives are taking care of his cattle and small landholdings back in his mountain valley. The parents moved to Los Molinos to secure an education for their children.

Like many highlanders, Mr. and Mrs. C have mixed attitudes toward the coast. In addition to its superior facilities for educating one's children, it has more goods of all kinds than the highlands, has superlative fruits, and, in general, is more prestigeful than the highlands. On the other hand, it has an unrelieved flatness and a desert monotony in color. Its heat and dryness are oppressive. Its people are disdainful of highlanders, even cruel to them. But perhaps worst of all, according to a deeply felt highland attitude dating back to pre-Columbian times, the coast is a miasma of disease and a potential deathtrap for highlanders. In particular, malaria and tuberculosis are feared. Within recent years the IDHS has practically eliminated malaria in the coastal area, but the fear of malaria still feeds on the terrible experiences of former years. Tuberculosis, too, is regarded by highlanders as a coastal disease, and one can collect many highland stories of individuals who have gone to the coast and even prospered, have been struck down with "the lungs," and have not even lived long enough to crawl back to their highland valleys to die. Mr. and Mrs. C, and particularly the latter, brought to Los Molinos their ambivalence toward the coast. It was a place of opportunity, wonders, good education for their children, but at the same time one of known dangers and unknown horrors.

Nelida does not patronize Mrs. C or treat her contemptuously but tries patiently to communicate with her, expresses interest in her opinions, and does not make fun of her poor Spanish. For Mrs. C, Nelida is a friendly authority who imparts "coastal" knowledge and brings protection against dangerous coastal diseases. Mrs. C now boils water regularly as a result of Nelida's efforts. She has also installed a privy and sent her youngest child to the hygiene center for examination and weight control, accompanied by her grown daughter. Mrs. C was too "ashamed" to bring him herself.

Mrs. C brightens when she talks about her highland village and at once saddens: "Three long days away." She still wears the twin braids of highland women, although she has long since abandoned the colorful waists and skirts of her home in favor of the plain cotton dresses of the Los Molinos mode. She converses in stumbling Spanish and speaks her native Quechua tongue only with recent arrivals from the highlands. Her sons and daughter would be "ashamed" to accompany her down the long street of Los Molinos, to ride with her on the bus, or to be seen with her in Ica. Her braids and speech and subtleties of gait and posture identify her as a member of a disparaged outgroup. She can never achieve more than marginal social acceptance in Los Molinos society.

However, being an outlander, her right to do certain outlandish things is tolerated. Hence, Mrs. C's practice of boiling water is not condemned by the community. It neither improves nor worsens her generally marginal position. Having nothing to lose socially, Mrs. C gains in personal security by heeding Nelida's friendly counsel. She is ready to grant that the water, like other things in Los Molinos, is dangerous. She is grateful to Nelida for teaching her the means to neutralize the danger of contaminated water.

Although Nelida's relations with housewives are generally informal and relaxed, some housewives have an especially keen need for a friendly confidante. They include women who are lonely or who lack close ties in the community—housewives without local kinswomen, newly married women who set up separate households, people like Mrs. B who have half alienated their neighbors, and some highlanders like Mrs. C. Responding positively to Nelida's friendly overtures, they are favorably disposed toward her health message.

Of the 11 new converts to water boiling, seven can be credited exclusively to Nelida's efforts. These seven tend to place high value on their social relationship with Nelida and look forward to her visits. Although the remaining four new boilers are on friendly terms with Nelida, friendship by itself was not enough to convert them. Mrs. D is an example.

Mrs. D, Persuaded by Dr. U

Mrs. D has been won over to water boiling but not for the same reasons as Mrs. C. Mrs. D lives in a small house. She and her husband are cholos and life-long residents of Los Molinos. Mrs. D is twenty-five, her husband about forty, and they have five children. He is a plantation field hand and she, as she says in a tone of resigned bitterness, is "always at home." They are poor.

Mrs. D receives Nelida well and enjoys talking with her. She envies Nelida's freedom to move around and talk to people about interesting things. She has responded well to the health department's program. Mrs. D and her husband are planning to install a privy. She obediently brought three of her infants to the hygiene center for examination and weight control and during her last pregnancy went to the center regularly for examinations. For this, both Nelida and Mrs. D deserve credit; extreme prudishness about exposure of the body prevents many women from submitting to prenatal examination by any person, male or female, other than one of the five local lay midwives. After her sixth visit, Nelida knew Mrs. D was convinced that local water was a potential source of disease and that boiling was an effective preventive measure. Nelida also knew that Mrs. D had both the time and facilities for boiling the water. Yet weeks and months went by and Mrs. D took no steps to put her new knowledge into practice.

After Nelida had visited Mrs. D for the twelfth time, Dr. U began his series of local talks, which were attended faithfully by Mr. and Mrs. D and all five children. On Nelida's thirteenth visit, Mrs. D announced she had already begun to boil a kettle of water after breakfast every morning. She related how Dr. U had said this and said that, and how he had recommended that everyone boil his drinking water. Nelida was pleased at the favorable turn of events. But she was also somewhat piqued; after all her patient explaining, helping Mrs. D understand the idea of contamination and providing strategic stimulation, Mrs. D ungratefully gave all the credit for her conversion to one talk by Dr. U. Mrs. D does not broadcast the fact that she boils water daily. To intimates, however, she explains that she does so because "the doctor recommended it." Nelida has heard this so often that she is tempted to retort, "Well, I recommended it first, you know."

In boiling her water and yet hoping to escape criticism, Mrs. D is trying to have her cake and eat it, too. Her group's standards, from which she wishes to depart without being penalized, hold it proper for healthy people to drink unboiled water and for sick people to drink boiled water. But the health department has other norms: boiling water for healthy people is right and necessary, while failure to do so shows lack of concern for safeguarding health. The two standards conflict. The people of Los Molinos equate health with unboiled water; the health department equates health with boiled water.

Mrs. D was caught in the middle of conflicting assumptions— until Dr. U entered the scene. Before that time the only available "authority" who could make a new set of water usages legitimate was Nelida. Unfortunately, she is not recognized as an authority by Mrs. D and by Los Molinos society in general. Traditional water habits are maintained by the weight of Los Molinos culture and society. This is a form of authority with teeth to penalize rule breakers; the derision directed against the pretentious Mrs. B has the added effect of forewarning other would-be deviants.

With Dr. U's public and official sponsorship of water boiling, Mrs. D gained a champion who could defend her new behavior. Physicians are recognized as authorities by Los Molinos society by virtue of their professional status and superior social rank. It is significant that almost at once following Dr. U's public endorsement of water boiling, Mrs. D adopted the new behavior.

Although it is possible that Dr. U added information not already imparted by Nelida and in this way helped to convince Mrs. D on logical grounds to boil her drinking water, it is highly probable that this rational appeal played only a minor role. More important than his facts and his logic was the sanction of an accepted and respected medical authority. As the IDHS and Dr. U himself see it, his principal job is to provide new knowledge and to appeal to reason. In this he is doubtlessly effective, but in the case of people like Mrs. D his primary contribution is to give socially acceptable authorization to a departure from local cultural norms.

Mrs. D wants a ticket to boil water without paying the traditional price of being sick. Mrs. A paid the customary price, got her ticket, and the cultural gatekeepers let her pass. Mrs. B appropriated the ticket without payment and aroused indignation. Mrs. C does not really need a ticket. It would do her little good; as an outsider, she is a gate crasher to begin with. But Mrs. D is an insider; she hopes that a free pass endorsed by medical authority will be culturally accepted.

Four of the 11 new boilers, including Mrs. D, found Nelida's patient persuasions insufficient, delaying action until listening to Dr. U at a public lecture. It is too soon to know whether Los Molinos society will continue to honor free passes to water boiling issued by the hygiene visitor or by the more respected IDHS physician. What will happen as still others take advantage of this free pass? Will sickness cease to be the price of water boiling in Los Molinos? Will free passes from IDHS representatives be declared invalid? Or will some compromise emerge?

Mrs. E, Who Would but Can't

Except for the fact that she does not boil water, Mrs. E is a living vindication of the IDHS philosophy that the hygiene visitor can help people help themselves to better health. Following the stimulation of Nelida's conversations and Dr. U's public talks, Mrs. E has initiated a number of ingenious changes in household routines and has been consistently receptive to IDHS ideas. She has had the men of the household install a privy and build pens for barnyard animals, and has made hygiene innovations in her impoverished kitchen. She is even convinced of the value of boiling the drinking water, yet does not do so.

The E family is poor and cholo with deep roots in Los Molinos and an impressive number of kinsmen. The titular heads of the household are the aged grandparents. Senile and ailing, the grandmother wields little authority in household affairs and leaves their effective management to a daughter, Mrs. E, who is in her early thirties. The latter has only a daughter and the title of "Señora" to show for a brief common-law union. Neither Mrs. E nor her child suffers any stigma within the family or in the community at large. In Los Molinos, unwed mothers and their chil-

dren are "more to be pitied than scorned." Mrs. E's resourcefulness and self-sufficiency, however, invite little pity. Three other
individuals complete the household of seven: Mrs. E's brother
and two teen-age nephews, offspring of a dead sister.

Mrs. E has learned the meaning of contamination and ac-
knowledges that water should be boiled, but she pleads lack of
time. Nelida knows she has made other changes despite shortage
of time and resources and cannot refrain from feeling, "If she
really wants to boil water, she can find the time." But can she?

Mrs. E rises at 5 a.m. and prepares breakfast, serving her
brother and nephews, who work as plantation field hands. She
bolts her own meal and then leaves the house to take breakfast to
her aged father, who has been working in the fields since 5:00 or
5:30. On her return route, she must collect fagots for the hearth
and fodder for fowl and animals. If her preschool child is awake
on her return, she slips a hand-me-down cotton dress over the
petticoat in which the child has slept, watches her slosh water
over hands and face, and sits her down for a morning piece of
bread, ripe olive or bit of cheese, and a cup of tea or, if Mrs. E has
dashed to the milk seller, coffee essence with boiled milk. At some
point, Mrs. E also manages to shepherd her ailing mother to the
breakfast table.

And now she shoos the child out of the way and really goes to
work. She must wash the breakfast utensils; feed chickens, pigs,
and a goat; take two or more trips to the well for water with a long
coil of rope over her shoulder, a filler pail, and two five-gallon
gasoline tins; wet down and sweep her hard-packed dirt floor and
the open sandy area in front of the house; slap and arrange the
bedding; check several times on why her daughter is so quiet or
why she is crying; listen to her mother complain of the heat as she
sits in the sun and hear her deplore the cold when moved into
the shade. Mrs. E also manages to visit the homemade privy in
the yard. And during the morning she has the almost daily little
argument with her mother, who refuses to use the privy, com-
plaining of the dangers of "evil odors" and "bad airs," and re-
marking that the fields were good enough for people in the old
days and, anyway, who ever heard of doing that sitting on a box
all penned up in a little enclosure of cane stalks.

Now the sun is climbing high, the day's terrible heat has begun, and Mrs. E thinks of the midday meal. She must shell corn or beans, grind peppers on a flat stone, pare potatoes, cut up squash, kindle the hearth fire, throw together a soup, and make one of the several daily premeal trips down the dusty road to the small general store. Not until all the others have been served their midday meal does Mrs. E sit down to eat.

During the baleful heat of the afternoon, all the dogs and some of the men take siestas, the children vanish, and only the flies and the women are awake. For an hour or more in the afternoon, Mrs. E relaxes. Nelida, who knows individual schedules well, may drop in, or the visitor may be one of Mrs. E's innumerable female relatives. Mrs. E may even do some visiting herself, to get away from her own kitchen and catch up on gossip.

Later in the afternoon, after one or more trips for additional water, fagots, or fodder, Mrs. E prepares the evening meal in time to serve it soon after sundown. She ends her day by crawling into the pallet beside her daughter once she has washed the meal's utensils, looked after her mother, prodded her daughter to bed, inspected the fowl and animals, and listened to her father's remarks on work and the hard life of the poor.

To generalize Mrs. E's daily schedule to other households in Los Molinos, one would subtract a little pressure for those with older daughters at home or smaller families, and would add proportionately for those with more small children or larger families. On Saturday or Sunday and on at least one weekday, she varies her routine and washes clothes. On those days, her nephews are obliged to relieve her of fetching fagots, although she compensates with more trips for water. Almost every Sunday she climbs the rickety bus for Ica and goes to the crowded Sunday market.

Nelida has visited Mrs. E more often than any other housewife in Los Molinos because they like each other and because of Mrs. E's eagerness to learn. Mrs. E has gained a workable grasp of the germ theory of disease from Nelida and from Dr. U's talks; she is one of the few members of the community who understand that houseflies are vectors rather than disease agents in themselves. Nelida is proud of Mrs. E, who does not "confuse hygiene with elegance" but uses her meager resources for health improvements. Mrs. E is admittedly very busy, but even so why doesn't she boil water? Let us look further into the daily schedule of housewives in Los Molinos, giving special heed to the hearth and the fuel supply.

Although a few households have kerosene stoves, the majority use wood-burning hearths, waist-high structures made of adobe bricks. The fagots which serve as fuel are abundant when vineyards are trimmed or old cotton plants destroyed and when irrigation ditches first fill and float wood down from upstream. During about half the year, however, people must scour the fields and the banks of dry waterways in search of fuel. Those who can afford it sometimes buy fagots from city wood sellers. Most housewives practice rather strict fuel economies. Fire is usually kindled but three times daily, in each case to prepare the family meal. Thus, the fuel situation and the three-meal pattern place a severe limit on water boiling: it can be done only during one of the three periods when fire is kindled.

A second limiting condition, of varying force from one household to another, relates to the hearth and cooking vessels. Most hearths can accommodate no more than two vessels at a time, and some hearths are so badly constructed that they can accommodate but one. This immediately rules out boiling while the meal is being prepared. Moreover, vessels are typically in short supply, most households possessing only a frying pan and two metal pots, supplemented with tin cans and other makeshift utensils. Hence, water can be boiled only *after* the meal is prepared, when the hearth has room and a vessel is free.

A third limiting condition is imposed by firm convictions relating to food and drink. Any prepared food or boiled water left overnight is "sleeping" food or "sleeping" water on the morrow. By virtue of having "slept," it becomes dangerously "cold" within the meaning of the pervasive system of hot-cold distinctions. To neutralize the danger of sleeping food or water, it must be re-cooked. Since it would have to be boiled all over again on the following day, it is useless to boil water after the evening meal. Thus, the possible boiling periods are now reduced to two, after breakfast and after the noon meal.

A fourth limiting condition concerns water-drinking habits and further reduces the possible boiling periods to one—after breakfast. Men, women, and children drink most of their daily water during the terrible heat of midday. Moreover, people prefer to drink boiled water only after it has cooled. Since the minimum time for cooling is about two hours, and since it should be drinkable by noon, there is no alternative but after-breakfast boiling. Although these limiting conditions—fuel scarcity, the crowded hearth, "sleeping" water, and drinking habits—may not seem entirely logical to the outsider, they are logical and forceful from the vantage point of a person reared in Los Molinos.

Mrs. E lacks time to boil water during the crucial after-breakfast interval; she has to leave the house to do essential chores. During the afternoon she has a little free time; even assuming her willingness to forgo part of her break, the afternoon is inappropriate as a time to boil water. It means kindling the hearth in the awful heat, using additional fuel, having the water ready too late to satisfy midday thirsts and, if she keeps it overnight, reboiling it to remove its "sleeping" quality. Without exception, every housewife who boils water in Los Molinos either does not have to leave the house after breakfast or has a household person to whom the chore can be delegated. On the other hand, among the group of ten who have not yielded to persuasion despite intensive efforts by Nelida and Dr. U, five simply have no time after breakfast. The other five apparently do have time but resist water boiling for other reasons. Mrs. F is an example.

Mrs. F, Who Could but Won't

Both Mrs. E and Mrs. F are poor, both have been exposed to Nelida's repeated visits and Dr. U's talks, and neither boils the drinking water. There the resemblances end. The F family is culturally conservative and unresponsive to the whole range of suggested health changes.

Twelve people live here; these include the sixty-year-old widow, Mrs. F; a daughter, her spouse, and a child; a widower son and his five children; and two other grandsons, children of a daughter working away from Los Molinos. The son and son-in-law both work as plantation field hands and are the economic mainstays of the household. Nelida visits with both Mrs. F and her daughter; one or both are invariably at home. The F family is Negro and deals with Nelida across ethnic barriers.

Although Nelida does not attempt to exercise authority, Mrs. F insists on setting her up as an expert in order to demolish her. When Nelida once discussed some safeguard to the health of infants and children, Mrs. F called to her cholo neighbor, "Come on over and listen to this young expert tell me how to take care of children." Mrs. F is locally renowned as a superb cook, and other families solicit her services to prepare feasts. Nelida usually avoids food topics with Mrs. F, except occasionally to ask for personal advice. On one occasion, however, the buoyant Mrs. F trapped Nelida into asserting that greens should not be boiled to death, and Mrs. F pounced. In a voice that carried far in the afternoon quiet, she called to her neighbor, "Come on over and listen to the expert tell me how to cook."

Mrs. F likes Nelida now, although at first she treated her with a coolness verging on hostility. During Nelida's first visits, Mrs. F let her carry the dead weight of a one-sided conversation. To Nelida's attempts to break conversational ground, Mrs. F returned, "Imagine," "humph," "really." On one occasion she flared up and said, "I know well enough my grandchildren aren't as healthy as the children of the whites and the rich. I don't need you to tell me that. How can we give them the right things to eat when our big worry is to give them something to eat?"

In her relationship with Mrs. F, Nelida is the victim of a cross-fire of ethnic differences. She is not a completely innocent victim, however, in that she shares prevailing cholo stereotypes about Negroes. Negroes have nicknames for cholos, referring to their "faded" skin, their attempts to mimic their rich betters, their insipid foods, and general lack of flavor in their stolid pleasures. Cholos also have nicknames for Negroes, which refer to relative darkness of skin color, hair type, assumed laziness, predilection for certain foods, and assumed possession of sorcery skills. Nelida is scrupulous about avoiding the use of all such derogatory terms.

Mrs. F is not only a Negro housewife but a representative of cultural conservatism. Hence for her, as for most residents whether cholo or Negro, beliefs in hot and cold distinctions dictate unboiled water for the healthy and boiled water only for the sick. Although Mrs. F and her daughter have attended several of Dr. U's talks, they remain unreceptive to the notion of bacteriological contamination and unconvinced of the need to boil their drinking water. Although accepting certain notions about germs, Mrs. F has effectively reinterpreted them to fit into the local theory of disease transmission, which is incompatible with the idea that germs may occur in water. Native theory holds, in part, that certain diseases are contagious in the sense that they can "stick to" people. Such diseases include syphilis, tuberculosis, and other respiratory disorders. They travel from the sick and "stick to" the well, crossing over by means of physical contact, the immediate air, and breath vapors. Mrs. F equates microbes with the "stick-to" quality of disease assumed in native theory.

Her understanding of microbes provides no directive for boiling water. How, she argues, can microbes fail to drown in water? Are they fish? If they are so small that they cannot be seen or felt, how can such delicate things survive in water? Even in the cleanest water, they would have no chance, let alone in dirty water. Furthermore, it is really a quality of the disease itself that brings sickness; if anything, it is the disease that produces the microbes and not the reverse. How can such minute animals, unescorted by the disease, hurt a grown person? How absurd and hypochrondriac can one get? There are enough *real* threats in the world to worry about—"cold" and "airs" and poverty and hunger—without bothering oneself about animals one cannot see, hear, touch, or smell.

Unlike the group represented by Mrs. E, Mrs. F is one of those who have time to boil water but whose allegiances to traditional standards are at odds with the notion of daily water boiling for the healthy. Between them, Mrs. E and Mrs. F stand for most of the 160-odd families in Los Molinos who still do not boil their drinking water.

Each of these types, from Mrs. A to Mrs F, represents social segments of varying sizes in the community. To shed more light on the problem of success and failure of water-boiling inducements, we must shift attention to the larger segments which the six housewives represent.

The Hygiene Worker and the Community

Nelida is very conscientious in her effort to carry out a hard job in a difficult situation. In some other aspects of her work—maximizing attendance of expectant mothers at the hygiene center, improving techniques of garbage disposal and house-fly control, serving as two-way liaison between the community and the several categories of IDHS personnel—Nelida secures results more positive than those in the household boiling of drinking water. Understandably, water-boiling efforts in Los Molinos produce slow and limited gains; they require behavioral changes which depart from prevailing patterns and are not answers to initially felt needs. This is not unusual in local health work. Although it is gratifying to tailor health work to felt needs, one must sometimes attempt to create new ones in order to bring felt needs into alignment with health requirements.

Nelida has made a good adjustment to trying circumstances. She conforms to local etiquette. She confines most of her interaction to women and is circumspect with men; defers to age seniors and is not overly intimate with juniors; accords to housewife, storekeeper, and town officers the respect, informality, or social distance due each. She knows more details of the town's life than even some of the native townspeople do. Nelida also possesses a kind of skill which virtually no amount of formal training could provide—an almost automatic understanding of the motivations of her people and the subtleties of their social structure. However, at least as important as the quality of Nelida's efforts in determining water-boiling results is the influence of factors relating to the town's social makeup and design of living.

Common to most residents are firm convictions about hot and cold distinctions, limitations of hearth and utensils, peak consumption of water during midday, the pressing fuel problem, and initial "misunderstandings" of Nelida's role. Yet there are differences between subgroups in Los Molinos which are critical for the water-boiling program.

The fuel problem is most severe for the poor, who cannot afford to buy wood when fagots are scarce; middle-level families can supplement the fagot search with wood purchased from wood sellers. During the dry-ditch season, many poor housewives take the long trek to the spring, an arduous and time-consuming chore; middle-rung housewives, on the other hand, can buy spring water from water sellers and are in a better position to devote the gained time to just such household chores as water boiling. Because they are poor, many women must do double duty as housewives and as field hands. These women must leave their houses early and do not have an unoccupied after-breakfast interval. In part, the community considers women middle level precisely because they need not perform the double role of housewife and field hand but can dedicate their full time and energy to the household.

As would be expected, there are more water boilers among middle-level than among poor housewives in Los Molinos. Of the 21 housewives who were exposed intensively and about equally to Nelida's and Dr. U's efforts, 10 were middle and 11 were poor; this intensive sample corresponds fairly well to the proportions of middle and poor families in the community at large. Of the 10 middle-group housewives, 8 initiated water boiling and only 2 did not. Of the 11 poor families, however, only 3 initiated water boiling and 8 did not. Moreover, it is not enough that housewives need time to boil water; they also must have time to receive Nelida's visits. As a rule, housewives in middle-level homes are simply more available to Nelida than are poor housewives, whether she schedules her visits in the morning or the afternoon.

The poor are also more insular, more bound to the horizons and values of Los Molinos. Holding more firmly to tradition, the poor tend to manifest greater resistance to new ways and to be more prone to regard innovations as threats to established custom. The instance of Mrs. F, typical of both cholo and Negro cultural conservatives, demonstrates how allegiance to tradition can block acceptance of water boiling.

Although she has not yet gained complete acceptance, Nelida is generally liked. Working for two years in a community that regards people born elsewhere but with forty years' residence as outsiders, Nelida has not done too badly. When she first arrived in Los Molinos, Nelida was perceived as a threat. She suddenly appeared, took up residence, and began to walk around and visit homes, ask questions, and try to make friends. Although an IDHS employee, she did not perform any tangible services such as examining children or giving immunizations. She was interested in one's children, animals, habits, and health. People who later grew to like Nelida were initially baffled that a stranger should want to learn about their health views and should be interested in helping them work out solutions to household problems of health and hygiene. Although it is likely that the entrance of any kind of health worker would have been regarded with suspicion, it is unfortunate that the IDHS did not hold an official ceremony to inaugurate the hygiene center and formally introduce Nelida to the community. As it was, some truly spectacular guesses were made as to what Nelida was *really* doing in town.

Where they stood in the social world of Los Molinos had much to do with the way individuals saw and evaluated Nelida and her program. Among the poor, Nelida had been cast as a dispenser of health department goods and also as a snooper. As an assumed dispenser of tangible health goods, she did not fulfill expectations; rather she proceeded to dispense quite intangible wares—attempted through tactful conversation to help people help themselves. For most poor families, she was a "dirt inspector," sent to Los Molinos to pry for dirt and to press already harassed housewives to keep cleaner houses. Their perceptions of Nelida in turn colored Nelida's perceptions of the poor. Aware of coolness toward her but unaware of its basis, she found herself responding with resentment. As she saw the situation in her first difficult months in Los Molinos, the more you try to help some people, the more they rebuff you.

Middle-group housewives perceived Nelida primarily as "dirt inspector," and still do to some extent. However, middle women have more time to set households in order; they feel more "inspectable" and resent Nelida's supposed snooping less than do the poor. Middle women also saw Nelida in a light that poor women did not: as an individual personality rather than a representative of a class. This is due to twin circumstances: middle-group housewives have more time to spend with Nelida, and Nelida herself is a middle-group person. Similarity of background promotes a feeling of identification and mutual sympathy between Nelida and middle-level housewives of Los Molinos.

We have said little about the few prosperous housewives. These have at least as much time and energy as the middle-group women to devote to things like boiling water. Yet Nelida has been unable to induce a single prosperous housewife to boil drinking water. These ten or so women cast Nelida in the role of "educator" or "civilizer" of the poor. When she first appeared they neither welcomed Nelida nor perceived her as a threat; in their opinion she and they obviously had nothing to do with each other. Moreover, they saw Nelida as a cholo of a lower social station than themselves. She succeeded in offending these housewives by merely visiting them and discussing the same topics she tried to cover with poor and middle families: house flies, exposed excrement, dangers of contaminated water, disposal of garbage. By attempting to "educate" them, she was perceived as equating them with the unwashed and uneducated poor, and by this token became a threat to their social position. Further, since she was tagged as belonging to a lower social level than theirs, their responses to her efforts were consistently indignant and hostile. They erected and still maintain barriers, not so much to specific water-boiling suggestions as to the socially degrading implication that their hygiene needs improving. Nelida's reception by prosperous housewives has been so cold that for practical purposes she has abandoned efforts to work with them.

Los Molinos has ethnic as well as social class differences, with a coastal cholo majority and minorities of highlanders and Negroes. We know that Nelida has achieved better results with middle-level than with poor families. We may now add that regardless of socioeconomic level she is more successful with native cholos than with the minority groups.

Among the 21 families that have been objects of Nelida's intensive efforts, 12 are cholos, 3 highlanders, and 6 Negroes; these figures correspond reasonably well to the total ethnic proportions in Los Molinos. Of the 12 cholos, 8 are now boiling water; but of the other 9, only 3—one highlander and two Negroes—have been won over. It is worth noting that the two Negroes who have been persuaded are in the middle group. Of the other four Negroes who are poor and include Mrs. F, none has begun to boil water. Expectably, Nelida's most discouraging results are with housewives who are both Negro and poor, and her most gratifying results are with those who are both cholo and middle class.

Attention to subgroup differences should not obscure the important similarities. There is no residential zoning by ethnic group, and people of diverse backgrounds get along fairly amicably as neighbors, intermarrying and sharing a great many traditions and common values.

However, relatively slight differences of degree become impressive differences of kind upon injection of the water-boiling issue. For example, small differences between housewives in economic standing and in disposition of the after-breakfast period create a clearcut dichotomy between those for whom the boiling of drinking water is possible and those for whom it is apparently not. In the same vein, slight differences between communities in the Ica valley lead to large differences in water-boiling results. Compared with other Ica communities in which hygiene visitors work, Los Molinos is somewhat more isolated from the city, has slightly poorer fuel resources, and has a higher proportion of women who must leave their homes early to work in the fields. The accumulation of differences which singly might be nonsignificant helps to explain why to date only about 5 per cent water-boiling success has been registered in Los Molinos, while as high as 15 or 20 per cent has been scored in some other towns.

Before proceeding to more general implications, it may be pertinent to mention the question of local leadership. The town's officers, a mayor and town council, are unconcerned either as officials or as men with women's household routines. Although the mayor's wife now boils a daily supply of drinking water owing to Nelida's influence, the mayor himself maintains an Olympian detachment as to what his wife does with water as long as it is there for him to drink. The local lay midwives do exercise informal leadership among women, but these part-time specialists have a stake in maintaining custom. Although they cooperate with the hygiene center on maternity issues, lay midwives tend to cast their weight against such innovations as domestic boiling of drinking water, taking a position on microbes akin to that of the conservative Mrs. F.

IMPLICATIONS

Native Auxiliaries in Public Health

An issue important in international public health concerns the place of native human resources in health work. Can a health team draw key workers from the towns and villages it serves and use them efficiently without sacrificing high standards of health work? In fact, the problem of whether and how to use native workers in regions like Ica has sometimes been phrased as a choice between high and low standards. In this view, one either uses the limited supply of highly trained personnel to do less work but of high standard, or one uses many Nelidas who are available in quantity to do more work but of lower standard.

The Los Molinos material seems to challenge the validity of this either-or question. It suggests rather the desirability of even more effective integration of the efforts of local workers such as Nelida with those of physicians (or other highly trained personnel). Thus, the Los Molinos team consists of a resident hygiene worker and a physician who comes on occasion. The particular health information disseminated and the cultural soil upon which it falls are both important in determining the outcome of an educational program. More than these are involved, however, in the process of communication. Critical, too, are such matters as the social standing of the communicating agent and the circumstances under which the message is conveyed. Unlike the physician, the hygiene worker is essentially an equal among equals, sharing many values and viewpoints with her public; the physician offsets this advantage by his higher standing in local estimation. The hygiene worker can communicate her message under more intimate interpersonal circumstances than can the physician; in compensation, the latter has opportunities to proclaim the health message publicly and thereby give it "official" warrant.

It is useless to debate whether the highly qualified professional or the native auxiliary is the more effective in rural hygiene work. Rather, the need is to combine the virtues of both in complementary team efforts; each performs well what the other can perform only imperfectly. To be sure, the Los Molinos evidence demonstrates the usefulness of the public health physician in regions marked by many health problems and few health experts; it also demonstrates that in such regions the local hygiene worker, operating as a team member at the grass-roots, can make a unique contribution to health work.

Reference Groups and Health Action

As we have seen, knowledge of the group affiliations of individuals helps one understand their responses to the water-boiling issue. Thus, by virtue of their common membership in the community as such, residents of Los Molinos share many customs and standards—including a core of common understandings about boiled and unboiled water. By providing its members with these and other standards, the community serves as a group to which individuals consciously or unconsciously refer in making judgments and decisions. In this sense, the community as a whole is a *reference group* for its component members.

However, individuals are also identified with one or another subgroup within the community. Despite its surface homogeneity, Los Molinos society constitutes a social checkerboard marked by cross-cutting distinctions of ethnic identification and relative socioeconomic standing. According to their particular subgroup allegiances within the community, individuals tend to be guided by subtly varying standards. Everyone "keeps up with the Joneses," although the relevant Joneses vary somewhat for the differing social segments.

For most individuals, the circles to which they belong are their *membership* groups as well as their *reference* groups. This is to be expected, since a self-reinforcing process is typically involved: one conforms to the standards of one's group in order to be socially accepted, and increasing acceptance in turn reinforces the drive to conform.

However, this is not always the case. Some individuals adopt reference groups other than those to which they apparently belong, sometimes even selecting groups that are totally outside the local community. Thus, the deviant Mrs. B adopts the standards of a social category beyond Los Molinos, an outgroup represented by her citified brother. For other individuals in Los Molinos, but not for all, the health department plays a role as an influential outside group, one to which they tend to look for certain standards of thought and behavior.

Acceptance of an outgroup's standards frequently involves defection from the standards of one's ingroup. It may be useful to view the IDHS as a reference group in competition with that of the community, and the health program as a set of standards alternative to those of the community. Health departments do more in communities like Los Molinos than promote the public health. They also, perhaps inadvertently, invite people to shift their group allegiances—to change their reference group.

New Health Habits and Cultural Integration

We have seen that a practice as mundane as the domestic boiling of water is arbitrated by local cultural standards and has an investigable sociology and psychology. This suggests that even the most taken-for-granted items of action programs may be found, on scrutiny, to have linkages with unexpected parts of culture and to carry meanings that have consequences for a program's career.

Even perceptions of so common an environmental object as water are culturally screened. A trained health worker can perceive "contamination" in water because his perceptions are linked to certain scientific understandings which permit him to view water in a specially conditioned way. A Los Molinos resident also views water in a specially conditioned way. Between him and the water he observes, his culture "filters out" bacteria and "filters in" cold, hot, or other qualities that are as meaningful to him as they are meaningless to the outsider.

It is axiomatic of all human culture that customs, like men, are not islands unto themselves. Beliefs and customs are parts of cultural systems; they relate to, support, and are enforced by other beliefs and customs. This principle, not so readily discernible when a society is "at rest," becomes more apparent when an action program "disturbs" the society. It is not enough that action workers know the items of custom that characterize the community's way of life; they must also understand how these customs are linked with one another. Otherwise, one may perceive strange, different, or "illogical" customs as fortuitous things or the vagaries of ignorance; one may also fallaciously assume that new health habits can be introduced by simply adding them to preexisting sequences, or that old habits can be "subtracted" and new ones "added" in their place. The attempt to introduce the use of boiled water for the healthy in Los Molinos represents a case in point.

The IDHS wants people to boil water before consuming it and construes the practice as essentially an *additive* thing: somewhere between the act of fetching water and that of consuming it, people should add a new act to the sequence, that of boiling. Surely this is not asking people to make grand changes in their way of life or to abandon deeply held beliefs, or even to spend any money; they are urged simply to boil water before consuming it. Yet, as we have seen, water boiling is not a simple or merely additive thing in Los Molinos, and the relatively meager response to the issue is not due simply to apathy, ignorance, or stubbornness. That housewives should boil drinking water and that healthy people should drink it are matters that run the gauntlet of many factors, including the group's ecology, its economy, social differentiations, and cultural convictions and behavior.

SUMMARY

A major concern of the Ica Departmental Health Service, a regional health department in Peru, is the attempt to introduce hygienic measures at family levels. A specific problem in the rural reaches of its jurisdiction is to induce people to boil their contaminated drinking water. After two years' effort in Los Molinos, a town of 200 families, a resident hygiene worker visiting individual homes has persuaded 11 housewives to boil water. In this she was aided by a physician, who gave occasional public talks. In addition, there were 15 housewives who were already in the habit of boiling their water prior to the hygiene worker's arrival in town.

A family-by-family investigation disclosed that housewives who decided to boil water did so for different and even opposing reasons. The diversity of motives also applied to the majority of residents who decided to continue consuming unboiled drinking water. Several boiled water because they were sickly, in conformity with pervasive theories about illness and its relation to the local dichotomy between "hot" and "cold" foods. Others boiled water because they rejected local cleanliness values and other standards. Of those who yielded to health department persuasions, some boiled their drinking water because the hygiene worker recommended it; others wanted to heed the hygiene worker but did not boil drinking water until the physician publicly "authorized" their departure from prevailing norms of water usage.

Among those who did not boil drinking water, as among those who did, motives differed. Some did not boil water because they did not have available an after-breakfast interval which, by virtue of local circumstance and belief, was the only possible and appropriate time to boil water. Included among those who decided not to do so were many whose allegiance to cultural values precluded acceptance of new and competing health values.

The hygiene worker was apparently able to secure more positive results with housewives whose economic level and cultural background were similar to her own. Her own background was middle class by Los Molinos standards, and she belonged to the majority cholo group. She was apparently unable to secure equally positive results when dealing with Negroes or with families of markedly different socioeconomic level from her own.

The Los Molinos experience supports the notion that action programs in regions like Ica can effectively supplement professional personnel with local people trained as auxiliary health workers. The study suggests that detailed knowledge of social and cultural factors of the community is vital to the efficiency of the water-boiling program. It also suggests that useful wisdom comes not simply from knowing the scattered items of cultural belief and practice but from the appreciation that they constitute a system in which the individual parts are linked to form a meaningful structure.

SELECTED REFERENCES

Foster, George M., "Relationships Between Spanish and Spanish-American Folk Medicine," *Journal of American Folklore*, vol. 66, July–September, 1953, pp. 201–219. The article includes an analysis of Hippocratic-Galenic "humoral" theory incorporated into Spanish-American folk medicine as sets of hot and cold distinctions. (See also Dr. Foster's "Relationships Between Theoretical and Applied Anthropology," *Human Organization*, vol. 11, Fall, 1952, pp. 5–16.)

Gillin, John, *Moche, A Peruvian Coastal Community*. Smithsonian Institution, Institute of Social Anthropology, Publication no. 3, Washington, D. C., 1947. An anthropological study of a north coastal community which, though unlike Los Molinos in many respects, shares many common features of culture and social organization. (Dr. Gillin also has written a more general article on "Mestizo America," drawing on Peruvian data, which appears in *Most of the World:* The Peoples of Africa, Latin America, and the East Today, edited by Ralph Linton, Columbia University Press, New York, 1949, pp. 156–212.)

Hydrick, John L., *Intensive Rural Hygiene Work in the Netherlands East Indies*. Public Health Service of the Netherlands East Indies, 1937. (Also The Netherlands Information Bureau, New York, 1942.) Exposition of Hydrick's principles of rural hygiene work in their first large-scale demonstration. With modifications, the principles are incorporated into the rural hygiene work carried out by the Ica Departmental Health Service.

James, Preston E., *Latin America*. Odyssey Press, New York, 1942. Chapter 5, Peru, is perhaps the best human geography source on Peru in general. A 1950 revised edition of this book is also available.

Merton, Robert K. and Alice S. Kitt, "Contributions to the Theory of Reference Group Behavior" in *Studies in the Scope and Method of "The American Soldier,"* edited by R. K. Merton and P. F. Lazersfeld. The Free Press, Glencoe, Ill., 1950. Two sociologists deal in detail with the concept of "reference group" briefly mentioned in the present case.

Simmons, Ozzie G., "The *Criollo* Outlook in the Mestizo Culture of Coastal Peru," *American Anthropologist*, vol. 57, February, 1955, pp. 107–118. A scholarly and very readable study, valuable for the understanding it provides of the changing culture of coastal Peru.

PART II
REACTION TO CRISES

Case 4

MEDICINE AND FAITH IN RURAL RAJASTHAN
by G. Morris Carstairs

To the people of rural India described by Dr. Carstairs sickness is as much a moral as a physical crisis. In their conception the roots of illness extend into the realm of human conduct and cosmic purpose. As a consequence they look for relief to ritual and reassurance, as well as to mundane medicines. "No matter how rare a medicine you give a patient," Dr. Carstairs was informed, "unless you and he have faith in it, he never will be cured." To set the patient right morally, as well as medically, the healer must serve as a link between mortal man and the purposeful cosmos. He can gain no grace for the afflicted nor can the sufferer receive it unless both are joined to each other and to the universe by a bond of faith.

The vivid episodes in this document dramatize the difficulties of achieving mutual understanding when doctor and patient behold each other through different kinds of cultural glasses. They also indicate, as do the preceding case studies, that culture is a connected system and not a mere summation of separate parts. To the western doctor complaints of physical weakness signified malnutrition and anemia and called for the prescription of iron tonics and vitamin concentrates. This was logical according to the premises of western culture. But according to the cultural system of the patient, symptoms of physical debility were connected to moral weakness by a chain of convictions involving nutrition, blood, semen, and transgressions of the ethical code. Ideal remedies therefore included pilgrimages and ritual baths to wash away one's sins—atonements rather than tonics.

*The role of the doctor in rural India is also the subject of the case study by Dr. Marriott, Case 9. For another instance of a cultural body image, the reader is referred to Dr. Cassel's observations in Case 1 on Zulu conceptions of digestion and fetal nourishment. Dr. Carstairs collected this material while conducting a medical clinic incidental to pursuing research on Indian culture and personality.—*EDITOR

THE PROBLEM
The Gulf of Misunderstanding Between the Western Doctor and the Indian Villager

In one of his many Indian short stories, Rudyard Kipling describes how a young district officer persuaded a frightened village community to submit to vaccination by reminding the people that its effectiveness derived from the sacred cow, and then by getting one or two of the leading men to be the first to undergo it. No doubt this story was founded on observation. Certainly it illustrated one way to make such a measure acceptable. Another method, adopted in the early years of this century by the chief health officer of Jodhpur State, turned upon a judicious use of showmanship. This doctor, an Irishman and a famous athlete, included in his retinue one of those emaciated beggars, blind and pock-marked who are still all too common a sight in India. When he came to a village he would summon everyone with his stentorian voice. "Take a good look at him," he would bellow, "that is what Mataji [the goddess of smallpox] does for you! And now look at this: this is what vaccination does to you!" He would then strip to the waist and display not only his vaccination scars but also his muscular torso. The demonstration was convincing.

In contrast, during my recent stay in the village of Delwara I witnessed a conspicuously less successful technique. The public vaccinator came to pay his annual visit of a few days. He was a supercilious young man from Udaipur city, who had passed a course in this specialty, and he regarded villagers as an inferior and stupid lot—especially when they refused to accept his scarifications. During his four-day stay in Delwara, the task degenerated into a hunt. I would see a herd of children and young mothers come bolting out of an alleyway with hilarity and panic mingled in their shrieks, while the vaccinator pursued them, brandishing the weapons of his trade.

It is not enough to bring new medical techniques to a community. No matter how well established these may be in Europe or America, they must be presented afresh to each new social group in a way that will command conviction and acceptance. In order to do this effectively, one has to understand the climate of ideas into which these new elements are to be introduced. A practitioner from another culture may find himself faced with situations that appear to him at first sight as incomprehensible.

For example, when I first practiced medicine in India, I found that in a case where I did nothing at all, except diagnose pregnancy, I was given great credit; in another where the patient died of diphtheria despite my treatment, I was lauded; and in a third, where I made an accurate diagnosis, I was held to blame. As a westerner, I was puzzled by these reactions. It was only gradually that I came to realize that they all made sense in the context of the villagers' own beliefs about sickness and its cure, and of their concept of the role of a physician. It was only after many months had passed and after numerous contretemps that I began to appreciate the reason for the misunderstandings between us. This process of learning can best be illustrated by describing some of the incidents during my apprenticeship as a country doctor in India.

THE SITUATION

Local Concepts of Disease and Modes of Treatment

Village Life in Rajasthan

In 1950 and 1951 I had the opportunity to spend a number of months in two different villages in Rajasthan, where until recently the maharajahs ruled with medieval splendor and unrestrained autocracy. It is a lovely country, although harsh to the eye like the Bad Lands of Wyoming, and the people are handsome in their bearing and in their bright peasant costumes; but still, I was rather disappointed at first that my sociological research should be carried out here. I had hoped to go and live among really primitive peoples—Sea Dayaks, perhaps, or Melanesians—whereas to my mind the people of Rajasthan were not at all primitive.

To begin with, I had been brought up among them. My earliest memories were of playing field hockey, marbles, and other local games with a pack of little Hindu boys; of riding through dusty villages on my shaggy country-bred pony; and of special occasions when we toured the countryside by bullock-cart, living under canvas. My father was a missionary, and there was nothing he liked better than these excursions away from the beaten track. At dusk or before sunrise he and I would scour the surrounding jungle for quail or duck or partridge for our next day's dinner. I well remember one such occasion when we saw from our bullock-cart a cavalcade of Rajput horsemen, lance in hand, galloping in chase of a wild boar. That night we camped beside the mud-walled fortress of the chief who had led the hunt and listened to his minstrels extemporizing songs in honor of the day's sport.

The Rajputs are far from being the only inhabitants of this region, but they do constitute its aristocracy and set standards of valor, self-respect, and pride of bearing to which many of the lowlier castes also aspire. The great historian of Rajasthan, Colonel James Tod (who was himself a Scot) was the first of many who have pointed out similarities between the clans of Scotland and the 36 principal lineages of the Rajputs, and in my first experience of life in a Rajput village I had many occasions to remember this. The village is called Sujarupa, and it is situated on the fringe of the jungle-covered slopes of the Aravli Mountains, in the extreme north of Udaipur State.

Sujarupa is a compact little hamlet of stone-walled cottages, each surrounded by a thorn fence that serves as a corral for the family herd of goats and one or two heads of cattle. The people are all farmers, cultivating fields that they or their immediate forebears have cleared from the jungle. Men and women work hard in these fields, the women covering their faces with a head cloth if a stranger approaches. The children work too; from the age of eight or nine they learn to drive the village flocks through the dry foothills. Like David, each carries a sling and practices throwing jagged stones that roar as they fly through the air, to scare off jackals, hyenas, and an occasional wolf. It is a hard-working community, accustomed to a minimum of comfort; and yet the people are usually sure of a meal twice a day. Except for years in which the rains fail—and this happens on an average every fourth year in Rajasthan—they are able to raise enough wheat to sell some for cash.

Nearly everything in the village is homemade. The plows and sickles that the villagers use are manufactured by artisans in the nearest large village, as are their cooking pots, their shoes, and their clothes. Their houses and their wells are made with their own hands. They are all Hindus, and on feast days some of them may visit a distant temple of Mahadev or Sri Krishna, but throughout the year they are more concerned with the local gods whom they regard as intermediaries between them and the remote Great Gods whom the Brahmans worship. It took me many weeks to distinguish the numerous stones and trees that were severally consecrated to these gods.

Almost all the farmers in Sujarupa, as well as those of the surrounding district, are Rawat Rajputs; and when we sat and talked together, or walked through their fields, or set off in a party to visit the nearest small township, I often thought how similar they were in many ways to the only other farming community that I knew at all well—my own kinsfolk, living in the Western Highlands of Scotland. Sometimes I used to think of those small clusters of houses, the hamlets of Clachan or Glenbreckrie, and wonder how those Highland farmers would react if a stranger with a different colored skin were to settle among them for a few months and presume to analyze their way of life. It was a profoundly discouraging reflection.

What Prognosis Meant to the Villagers

Fortunately, the farmers of Sujarupa were comparatively forthcoming. The very day after I had pitched my tent on some level ground near the village, a young man called Govind Singh came to summon me to his house. He had heard that I was a "Daktar Sahib" and he begged me to do something for his young wife, who was possessed by a devil and in great pain.

I found myself bitterly regretting the shortcomings of my training at Edinburgh University, which was all too light on exorcism; but bearing my stethoscope like a talisman, I followed him to his hut. Inside, a girl of seventeen was rolling about on the floor, wailing loudly. I examined her nervously at first but with more confidence as it dawned on me what was going on; and then I told Govind Singh that hers was a very healthy little devil, as he would soon see for himself. In fact, her first baby was born that evening, a lively boy. Govind Singh himself came to my tent with a present of milk and rich pudding to tell me the news. Afterward, he pretended that he had known all along what was the matter: "But these young women, you know, Sahib, they get frightened over nothing."

From that moment the people of Sujarupa were very cordial toward me. They said it must be drafty and uncomfortable out there in the tent, which was true, and invited me to live in the large *paul* or guestroom of their hamlet; and I received numerous requests to treat their children for sore eyes and their old people for chronic bronchitis. I was agreeably surprised at this welcome, but a little puzzled. It was only much later that I realized that although I had done nothing for the young mother, I had spoken the magic words: "She will be all right. She will have a healthy baby." And events had proved me right. In their opinion, pronouncing a prognosis is one of the most important functions of a healer, but with this difference: when their healers say, "He will recover," they are not expressing a personal opinion but are speaking with the authority of the supernatural power, which is. the real agent of their cure.

Curers and Treatment in Sujarupa

Throughout my five months' stay in Sujarupa, I carried on a small and intermittent dispensary practice; but I soon realized that my remedies were only one of several sorts of healing, and by no means the most popular. My village friends were not narrow-minded; they were willing to give my sort of medicine a trial, but they did expect immediate results. This did not mean that they always demanded immediate results from their own forms of cure—but that was a different matter, because they already had faith in these, and so once the condition was diagnosed and the prescription given, they felt assured that the correct steps had been taken and recovery was bound to follow. My sort of medicine carried no such aura of conviction, and therefore it was required to justify itself dramatically, and without delay.

I was naturally curious to hear about my rival practitioners, and to see their work; and I did not have long to wait. Within a week of my settling in Sujarupa village, my neighbors called me out one night to attend an open-air celebration of worship. A throng of men and boys sat around a great log fire beside a hill-top shrine and sang the praises of the god of that place, one Kagal-Devji, a black snake-god. Sometime after midnight, when the singing had worked up to a high pitch of excitement, an elderly man sitting at the side of the fire gave a loud cry and begin to dance and shake convulsively. It was whispered in my ear: "Look, he's begun to 'play.' The breath of Devji has come into him." Then the possessed individual, who was the priest of the shrine, ran indoors and saluted the idols; he then appeared in front of us still twitching and gasping for breath and called out a number of rather cryptic prophecies about the coming year. After this he sat trembling before the image, and people came before him one by one. They poured out small offerings of grain and begged the god to tell them the cause of their own, or their children's, or their cattle's illness; and what they must do to be well.

At this stage I knew too little of the local dialect to understand what was going on; one or other of my new friends had to keep prompting me in Hindustani. Several weeks later, however, I went with two families of Sujarupa to attend the weekly "possession" at a shrine which lay some seven miles off in the jungle. This was the shrine of Danaji, a local demon-god, who had acquired a special fame as a healer of all sorts of ills. It was generally conceded that it was better to go instead to Devji if one were bitten by a snake (cobras and kraits being the common local venomous varieties) because after all he was a snake-god himself. In such an emergency, the priest would invariably become possessed and then throw himself upon the patient, noisily sucking at the wound and supposedly drawing out the poison. For all other troubles, however, Danaji was regarded as the more reliable authority.

The importance of Danaji was brought home to me by an event in the hut next to the one which I came to occupy, in Sujarupa. This was the home of Nol Singh, his wife, and two sons, one of whom was a sturdy boy of twelve years, the other a sickly baby named Lum Singh. The father had served in the Indian Army, and hence was one of the three men in the village who had traveled far afield and who were literate. In keeping with his knowledge of the world, he professed to have great faith in "Sahibs' medicines" and called me in twice to attend to Lum Singh, first for acute conjunctivitis and next for dysentery. But Lum Singh fell sick again, and this time his father did not consult me but went to Danaji. Some days later, when there was a small waning moon, I saw Nol Singh enter the village carrying an all-black goat, which he had bought.

Two nights later, at the blackest of the moonless period, he came to ask for the loan of my sharp *kukri* knife. I was now sure that some curative rite was in progress, but he was very reluctant to talk about it, promising to tell me everything in due course. Next day he returned the knife and explained that the Danaji had diagnosed that a witch was eating Lum Singh's liver. In order to appease her, a black goat had to be killed at midnight, five men each putting a hand to the knife, and then the head and entrails were to be set in a broken pot at a place where three paths crossed. This was a striking demonstration of the parallels between folk beliefs about witchcraft in medieval Europe—the goat, the midnight sacrifice, the offering in the broken pot, and the place where three paths cross all are to be found in accounts of European witchcraft—but it had a tragic sequel.

Late one night a few days after the sacrifice, Nol Singh called me to his house. He was very anxious about his child's health, and with good reason, for I found him in a state of profound toxemia, suffering from diphtheria. There was nothing in my box of medicines that could meet the case, but I knew there was a government dispensary and a doctor in the large village a few miles off. So I set off by bicycle in the starlight and woke up the doctor. Unfortunately, he had no anti-diphtheritic serum in his stock, not even any penicillin. I cycled back and gave the child an injection of atropine, simply in order to let the distracted parents feel that something was being done. The boy died in a few hours, and I went with all the men of the village to his hurried burial, piling thorn branches and stones over the grave so that the hyenas could not dig up the body. Then we all went to bathe and wash our clothes at the well, to cleanse ourselves of the pollution of contact with death.

I thought that perhaps this time I would be blamed, because I had given Lum Singh an injection and he had shortly died; but I was wrong. Throughout the rest of my stay I had to listen again and again to Nol Singh's graphic account of my heroic ride on his son's behalf, braving countless ghosts, and twice crossing a stretch of the road which was known to be frequented by leopards. At the time, I was not aware that there were leopards about; and I am sure that I would not have enjoyed my ride so well had I known. In fact, neither I nor the Danaji was blamed. After the first outburst of grief, the family repeated the traditional formula: it was his fate; his day had come; he was a loan from God, to whom he had returned.

After this, I was curious to see the celebrated priest of Danaji at work. Accordingly, one Sunday night when two families of the village announced that they were going to his shrine to consult the oracle, I set out with them. The moon was big once more, and we enjoyed our seven-mile walk under the brilliant Indian night sky. The shrine was in an out-of-the-way little valley, and from some distance off we could see the flickering glow of a fire, and then as we drew nearer we could hear occasional loud cries from the priest, who was already in a state of possession. We removed our shoes and laid aside our swords and staves a little way from the sacred place, where many other visitors had already done the same, and then sat near the priest, who crouched, trembling violently, and now and again gave a sudden wild shout. The Spirit had come to him strongly this night.

There was something particularly dramatic in the way that he summoned certain of his supplicants. He would interrupt the series of patients who came before him with a cry: "A man and a woman of Kachabli," or "Three brothers from Taragarh!" and these would press forward from the waiting crowd. One of his summonses was for "Two men from Mandawar road!" and my companion of the walk nudged me, saying, "That means us, Sahib; we came by that road." He sat before the priest first and consulted him about his little boy, whom the Danaji had saved from witchcraft. He was told to perform certain offerings, and then to carry the child three times around the shrine. Then it was my turn. The priest gave me a pinch of grain. "How many?" he said. "Four grains." He gave me one more, to bring it up to the auspicious number, looked to the shrine for inspiration, and then shouted out his prophecies: "The British will return to rule again. You will get a promotion—a new post, with great power and much pay. When this happens, come back and honor the

Danaji." With this he gave me a small dried lemon, telling me to guard it carefully. Then he continued to attend a series of sick people and anxious parents, presenting their whimpering children for his advice. I watched about 30 of these consultations and noted his remedies, which all involved soliciting the help of the Danaji and other gods.

Late in the night the session came to an end. The priest raised his arms with a loud cry, and then became an ordinary villager once more as the Spirit left him. He came to talk with us, professing to recognize me for the first time. "I saw you once before, Sahib," he said. "Don't you remember I was lying sick in the government hospital, and you came and examined my chest with those tubes and said, 'It is all right; you will get well.' "

I did remember having seen him a month or so before, when he was acutely ill with pneumonia. Again I was reminded of the magic power ascribed to a confident prognosis. I replied, "You and I do the same work, helping the sick get well." But the priest replied at once, "It is not I, Sahib; God alone can do that,"—and I was reminded, as every practitioner must often be reminded, that our individual skill is only one part of the complex business of healing.

Village Concepts of Illness

It might be argued, by those who are accustomed to our pragmatic tests of the efficacy of treatment, that surely these magic prophecies must become discredited over and over again, and in time lose their efficacy. The answer to this is that these villagers do not, as we tend to do, believe that one can influence the course of events simply by the exercise of a technical skill. To them, the Supernatural is everywhere immanent, and events can be influenced only by enlisting supernatural aid. They naturally assume that there is a magic quality in the prescriptions of western medicine as well; and this is one reason why the administration of intramuscular injections, with its ritual of aseptic precautions and the dramatic quality of the act of acupuncture, is especially highly valued among those who have had some contact with allopathic doctors.

There was one young man in Sujarupa who, when he came home on leave from his work as a laborer in the distant city of Ahmedabad, used to beg me to give him just one very powerful "objection" in order to make him strong. He knew only two or three words of English, and this was one of them. I remember him particularly because he was a singularly robust man, and I used to tease him when he insisted that he felt weak, as though he were wasting away. During my few months' practice in this region, I frequently encountered patients who simply complained of weakness; and my head was so filled with anticipation of vitamin deficiency, of malnutrition, chronic malaria, dysentery, anemia, tuberculosis, and so on, that I sought and fancied that I had found one or another of these conditions in every case. It was not until the following year, in Delwara village, that I came to realize the true significance of this complaint.

In the meantime I gradually widened my circle of acquaintances in the nearby hamlets and encouraged some of the divinely inspired healers to share some of their secrets with me. One old man, who had recovered from an acute attack of dysentery after taking a course of sulfa drugs which I had sent him, was kind enough to explain to me how he could tell that a sick person was possessed by a witch or a demon, by feeling his pulse. What the old man actually did was to lay his forefinger gently across the patient's wrist and wait to see whether he could feel a tremor in one of the flexor tendons of the fingers. There was, however, no consistency in his interpretation of the sign; it served, rather, as the cue for an immediate intuition, as a clairvoyant will hold an object belonging to an absent person and then claim to have a direct awareness of details of his appearance and personality. The most important aspect of this procedure is that the patient and all the onlookers know what the healer expects to find. If there is deception, to our way of thinking, it is one in which they all participate; and one in which the western doctor can find himself unwittingly caught up. We take the act of feeling the pulse so much for granted that we can easily overlook the fact that this may have a quite different significance to the patient and to us.

Every practitioner is familiar with the misunderstandings that so readily occur in everyday practice. Patients and relatives, when keyed up with anxious fears, often place a wrong interpretation on their physician's smallest gesture, or his misheard remark. This is naturally still more likely to happen when patient and physician approach the illness with totally dissimilar systems of ideas. It is, of course, not only oriental peoples who have a non-scientific conception of their own bodily processes; one can find abundant instances much nearer home.

Elementary instruction in the physiology of reproduction is now recognized to be an essential part of prenatal care; and the experienced practitioner learns to elicit from his patients something of their own (often fantastic) beliefs about what is happening inside them to make them feel ill. Where the general level of formal education is low, an understanding of physiology can only grow slowly, in relation to what most intimately concerns the health of each particular community. For example, there are already many parts of India where the relationship between malaria, mosquitoes, and quinine has become part of everyday knowledge, whereas in less heavily endemic areas the onset of a malarial rigor is still believed to be the possession of the patient's body by a god. There is no propaganda agent so effective as a demonstrable cure; but it may take many years before conservative villagers are convinced that it is the western drug which has in fact effected the cure.

I remember one night when I was working with a neighbor (one of the priests of Devji) by the light of my pressure-lantern. We were interrupted by a young farmer who lived about a mile and a half away on the fringe of the jungle. He said that his wife was struck by a fierce witch, or so it seemed to him, and he came to ask the priest for help. They both invited me to accompany them, and so we set off in single file along a series of field paths. When we approached the house, we could hear loud moans and shrieks. The young woman crouched in the yard, giving full expression to the pain and terror she was suffering. A string bed was drawn forward to serve as a seat for the priest and myself, and then there followed a polite altercation: he urged me to attend to the patient, while I insisted that it was his help the family desired. Accordingly, he felt her pulse and confirmed the husband's diagnosis, then spoke a charm over a small brass pot of water and gave the woman a few drops of this sanctified water to drink. The pot was then placed on the roof-top, so that no one's shadow might fall across it and thus impair its virtue.

As soon as this was done, I was told that now it was my turn. With some difficulty, I managed to persuade the patient to calm down long enough to allow her to explain that she suffered from a severe pain in the chest, which had begun the day before; now it was much more severe, and she felt sure that her destruction was imminent. At the thought, she began to cry out once more. In the presence of her husband and strangers, it was impossible for her to unveil her face, but she was persuaded to reveal the side of her chest, where I found vesicles of herpes zoster. The husband led me back to Sujarupa, and I entrusted him with codeine tablets and with spirit for local application. He returned the next day for more, saying that his wife was very much better already.

In that instance everything was done so politely and with the exchange of so many flattering speeches that both the priest and I felt assured that we had made the significant contribution to the patient's recovery. The same was not the case, however, with another patient to whom I was summoned a few nights later. He was a merchant from a large village 20 miles away and lay on the bullock-cart on which he had made the journey. I examined him on the roadside by the light of my lantern and found him very ill indeed. He had had typhoid fever six weeks previously and now his heart was grossly enlarged and his pulse very rapid. On auscultation I could hear a gallop rhythm. He was extremely agitated and begged me to save his life. I felt doubtful of my ability to do this but encouraged him as best I could, and gave a heroic dose of digitalis. The cart took him to the nearest large village, where he stayed at a kinsman's house, and there I visited him daily. For the first two days he still looked and felt acutely ill, and his pulse did not fall below 120/minute; but on the third day there was a remarkable change. The pulse was 96, the patient sat up and talked cheerfully, and for the first time showed some desire to eat. I wondered if this was attributable to my therapy, and soon found that it was not. What he had omitted to tell me until then was the reason for his state of panic: he had become convinced that some enemy had caused fatal sorcery to be placed on him. Against this belief, neither my medicine nor my reassurances had been effective. He knew that Sahibs tend to make light of sorcery, and so he had not liked to discuss it with me. Instead, he had obtained the services of a local man who possessed a powerful charm, and on the previous night this man had brought it into play with a dramatic performance, at the end of which he branded the back of the patient's neck with a red-hot iron. This drove out the evil spell; and it was the relief that the patient experienced at his feeling of escape from mortal danger which had brought his pulse-rate down.

What Is Expected of a Healer

This case, and many others of my village cases, served to impress upon me that the expectation of my patients here was different from that to which I had been accustomed. There was not the same attribution of personal responsibility to the physician for the success or failure of his treatment, because a sovereign fatalism determined the patients' attitude to events; whatever happened was coming to one anyway. What was expected from the healer was reassurance. So long as the illness was nameless, patients felt desperately afraid, but once its magic origin had been defined and the appropriate measures taken, they could face the outcome calmly. The parallel with our own clinical experience is obvious.

The few months I had spent in Sujarupa gave me a little insight into local preconceptions about sickness and cure, and this proved invaluable next year when my wife and I made a ten months' stay in the larger, more sophisticated village of Delwara, which lay only 18 miles from Udaipur, the capital and indeed the only large town of this state. Delwara was almost a small town in itself, having 2,500 inhabitants and a row of merchants' shops in its central street. Unlike Sujarupa, but like most other large villages in India, it included households belonging to a wide variety of castes, both the upper crust of the "twice-born" (the landlord, priest, and merchant castes) and no fewer than 36 different groups of hereditary artisans, all interrelated in a complex pattern of traditional obligations and rewards. Besides their varied occupations, almost every family had a stake, however small, in the land. Until the recent change of government in India, Delwara had been the seat of authority of one of the powerful feudal landlords, the Raj Rana of Delwara. The former ruler's vast fortress-palace still towered above the village; and at a high window the Raj Rana himself sat every day, brooding over the slightest occurrences in the bazaar below. He generously put a section of his palace at our disposal for our kitchen and sleeping quarters, but in order to carry out my work I had to hire a room in the center of the village.

During my stay in Delwara I learned much more about village ideas concerning medicine; and some things I learned only slowly and painfully. In this category I should put my long and unsuccessful struggle to plan my day on western lines, by the clock. I tried to adhere to the rule that I would see patients only the first thing in the morning (this was at 6:30 a.m. in the hot weather) and again in the late afternoon, but it simply did not work. The villagers themselves preferred to wait until they saw me coming down their lane, and then would call me in with every sign of desperate urgency to see a patient who had been sick for days; and peasants from the surrounding countryside would just walk into my "office" and sit patiently on the floor until I attended to them. Often they would beg me to go with them to their hamlets to see a close relative who lay very sick, but after one or two such excursions I learned to harden my heart and stick to my rule of refusing these requests, the majority of which proved to be cases of advanced phthisis.

One day, however, during the first month of my stay, a powerfully built young farmer appealed to me with great earnestness to help his brother, who lay ill in a hamlet two miles off. He had a high fever and had coughed up a blood-stained sputum, which sounded ominous; but his brother insisted that the whole illness was of only a few days' duration. No doubt what finally persuaded me to go was that the young farmer had borrowed a horse from the palace and held it saddled for me to make the journey. I was very glad in the end that I did go, for the patient was suffering from double pneumonia and was acutely ill. I gave him a massive injection of penicillin and followed it up with sulfamerazine, and as I cantered home I wondered what his chances of survival were. He gave me the answer two weeks later by walking into my office with a *dali* (a ceremonial tray of gifts) of sweet corn and other produce of his fields.

At the time I thought that this might lead to my dispensary practice growing to uncomfortable proportions, but such was not the case. Throughout my stay both villagers and country folk remained very skeptical of the quality of my medicine. They had three grounds for distrusting it. First, I did not describe their illnesses in the terms they had come to expect from their own healers. Second, I failed to prescribe elaborate dietary restrictions as did the practitioners of classical Hindu medicine. Again and again my patients would pause after receiving their pills and say, "*Kattay parhez?*" which is the customary opening formula: "No bitter condiments, avoid this and this. . . ." In the end, I adopted a simple and familiar list which would do them no harm and seemed to make my treatment at once more comprehensible. Finally, they were dismayed to find that I did not invariably, and in dogmatic terms, assure them that my medicine would immediately cure them. In their eyes, my failure to do so amounted to malpractice. As many of them pointed out to me, it is not so much the ingredients of the prescription which effect the cure as the patient's unhesitating belief in its efficacy. For this reason, every homely recipe (of which everyone knew two or three) ended with the peroration: "Take that and you will *certainly* be cured of your fever within a day."

Near the end of my stay in Delwara I was called to a house to treat a merchant who seemed to be suffering from a cancer that obstructed the portal vein and gave rise to ascites. After we had tapped several pints of fluid from his abdomen, his son asked me how ill his father really was, and I told him the prognosis. That same evening a friend who had been present reminded me of this, with a smile; he found it simply incomprehensible that one could say a thing like that. "You know," he said, "our custom here is that even if a man is sure to die, we never say so. We always say something like 'If it is God's will, he will get better.' "

I realized that just as in the past I had been given credit for a decisive intervention simply because I had uttered a hopeful prognosis, now the reverse was the case. I had committed a serious impropriety in stating that the patient would not recover.

In Delwara I was able to keep a record of at least some of the new cases which I saw in my office. They are summarized below.

DIAGNOSES IN ORDER OF FREQUENCY

Malaria	44	Gonorrhea	10
Diarrhea	36	Severe anemia	7
"Spermatorrhea" as		Acute respiratory infections	6
presenting symptom	17	Syphilis	6
Scabies	16	Typhoid or paratyphoid	6
Chronic bronchitis	16	Cataract	5
Eye infections	15	Leukorrhea	3
Dermatitis (including		Chronic otitis media	2
leishmaniasis)	15	Chronic sinusitis	2
Tuberculosis	15	Rickets	2
Major involvement		Acute appendicitis	1
Chest	9	Leprosy	1
Other	6	Madura foot	1
Dyspepsia	13	Undiagnosed	5

Total new attendances recorded: 244

The list fails to include many patients whose arrival interrupted an interview with an informant and who were therefore seen and sent away as quickly as possible. It also omits a large number whom I was called in to see when I chanced to pass their doors; these were mostly cases of malaria, scabies, cutaneous leishmaniasis, septic eyes, and cataract.

A Cultural Body-Image

In Delwara, as previously in Sujarupa, I was frequently asked by apparently robust men to give them medicine—or better, an injection—to make them strong. At first, I continued to regard them as cases of anemia or malnutrition until my eyes were opened one day to the real condition by the interpolations of a bystander, who was watching me examine one of these patients: "Of course he's weak!" he said. "He was such a libertine when he was a young man that his semen got spoiled, and it's been leaving him ever since."

The patient seemed relieved to have it stated for him in this blunt manner. What he really wanted, he explained, was some medicine that would remedy this condition and cause his semen to stay inside his body instead of leaking away and making him feel weak. From that day on, whenever a man asked me for strength-giving medicine, I urged him to tell me more about his trouble, and once he realized that he and I "talked the same language" in terms of symptomatology, a similar story always came out. Perhaps it is important to mention that this preoccupation was quite independent of the recognition of venereal disease and the fear of having contracted it. Gonorrhea was specifically mentioned as being only one of many ways in which "spoiled semen" might leave the body.

I found that a consistent belief about the nature and functions of the semen was held by all these patients, in different degrees of complexity according to their education. They were all able to describe how blood is made by the digestion of good food in a sort of low fire contained in the stomach, from which comes the warmth of the body; and that from every 40 drops of blood one drop of semen is laboriously formed. This semen, in which lies the source of a man's strength and of his subjective sense of well-being, is stored in a reservoir in his skull, which has a capacity of about 20 fluid ounces. The amount of well-formed semen which a man carries in this hidden store is not merely an indication of his state of health; it is also a measure of his moral and religious status. This is made clear when one learns what factors are conducive to the increase of semen, and what detrimental. In the former category come "cool" foods, such as dairy products, wheat flour, sugar, some fruits, and a number of the milder spices; in the latter, the cheaper and heavier cereals, unrefined sugar, vegetable oil, strong spices, and some of the commonest fruits. An especial anathema is placed upon eating meat and eggs, and drinking all forms of alcohol.

The striking thing about these food preferences is that all the foods in the approved class are the more expensive ones, which only the wealthier members of the high castes can afford to eat regularly. The mass of low-caste peasants and artisans eat meat and cheap cereals and drink wine; it is only on feastdays that they

treat themselves to wheat cakes and pure sugar and dishes made
with milk.

Even more important than these dietary restrictions, however,
is the belief that the quality and amount of one's stored semen
can be diminished by a failure to observe "right behavior." Obviously, it will be dissipated by an excessive indulgence in sex; but
it will be lost more quickly and irretrievably if this indulgence is
extramarital, and the bad effect will be intensified if the sex
partner is of a low-caste community. Indeed, any act that incurs
the condemnation of the elders of one's caste is believed to mili-
tate against the formation of the "Royal Principle." For example, many people told me that the reason the present generation of young men is so puny is this: it is a consequence of the
growing habit of sitting in tea-shops, drinking "English tea"
(known in England as Indian tea). This habit is condemned, first,
because it implies a disregard for the serious, ritualistic practice
of eating the two meals of the day; second, because it is a frivolous
extravagance; and most important of all, because it exposes one
to the ritual pollution of sitting to drink in company with others
of lower caste. In general, it can be said that any violation of the
many strict rules of behavior which concern the orthodox Hindu
is regarded as detrimental to his store of semen, and thus to his
mental and physical well-being.

Now at last these reiterated complaints of weakness began to
make sense. They were the expression of chronic anxiety engendered by feelings of guilt. Small wonder, therefore, that my iron
tonics and vitamin concentrates had little effect; what these
people really wanted was a release from their burden of guilt, and
this release they could find only in their own traditional way, by
making a pilgrimage and bathing in one of the many sacred lakes
or rivers which have the property of washing away one's sins, or
by one of the elaborate and costly ceremonies of purification at
which the Brahman priest is always ready to preside. Actually,
these drastic measures are seldom taken; for the most part, they
seem content to go on worrying and resolving to do something
about it one day. There are even some who appear to derive a
certain pleasure in describing their impending physical decay, like
Calvinists who dwell lugubriously upon the prospect of hell-fire.

I have emphasized the element of guilt in this "general weakness" syndrome because there it was etiologically important. In time, however, I came to realize that it entered to some extent into every form of illness. The patient and his extended family always had the feeling that they were temporarily in a state of ill favor with some divine agency. One is reminded of the description of depression which is put forward by psychoanalysts of the Melanie Klein school as a phantasy of ingesting "bad objects" so that the whole self feels bad. Be that as it may, the village patient did not feel relieved of his illness unless he had the subjective assurance that the divine agent had been placated at the same time as his physical symptoms were relieved.

Sacred and Secular Diseases

This was dramatically shown in their treatment of snake-bites. All snakes, but especially the black cobras, were believed to be the embodiment of powerful godlings. For example, every plot of cultivated fields had a protector-god here known as Radaji, and in the form of a black snake the Radaji often patroled the fields entrusted to his care. Should anyone trespass or otherwise offend the god, he would get bitten. Here, as in Sujarupa, there were priests of the snake-god whom the sufferer might consult. They would become "possessed," suck out the poison, and be placated with an offering.

There was, however, another and more popular remedy. This was to consult one of the four elderly men in the village who were known to possess powerful charms against just such an occurrence. One of these, a handsome bearded Brahman called Nathu Lal, told me about an instance that occurred two years previously. A blacksmith called Partab had cut across a neighbor's cornfield and was bitten on the foot. One of the other healers was summoned, and a great crowd gathered in the yard of the blacksmith's house, Nathu Lal among them. It soon became clear to him that the other healer's charms were not strong enough to meet the case because this was evidently the work of a more than usually powerful god—probably the very Radaji whose shrine was set up to protect the main entrance of the village. At last, Nathu Lal himself decided to intervene. He took a pinch of dust between his fingers, whispered his strongest charm over it, and blew it toward the patient. "The dust did not touch him, Sahib, but the air of it was enough."

At once, compelled by the charm, the god entered the body of his victim, who shrieked with rage and flew at Nathu Lal, but he had anticipated this and dodged into a room, closing the door behind him, and calling out to the bystanders to tie Partab securely to a pillar. There then followed a heated discussion between him and the god speaking in the body of the patient. In the end, the Radaji promised to spare him if he made certain sacrifices before his shrine, and the "possession" came to an end. The case was not yet closed, however, because when Partab came to his senses, he maintained that the offering was more than he could afford and refused to make it. The onlookers were scandalized, but after he had had his face well slapped he did as he was told.

It was, of course, common knowledge that such possession might occur. Every adult villager has seen it happen many times; indeed, his familiarity with the expected behavior is presumably what causes the patient's trancelike state of dissociation to take this particular form. One patient of mine recalled how when he was a boy of five or six, both he and his mother were bitten by a snake. They went to an old man famous for his charms, and he took the precaution of tying them to a tree before magically summoning the snake's spirit. "My mother became possessed," said this young man, "I remember seeing her shake all over and cry out and struggle as she tried to attack the healer, but the Spirit did not come to me."

In later years, after he had seen two or three dramatic instances of possession and cure, suggestion would have told, and he too would be possessed—or so one might think. But actually the situation was quite different. This youth, whose name was Prithwi Singh, became a devoted worshiper of the Goddess Vijayshan-Mata, whose shrine stands just outside of Delwara. Like his soldier uncle before him, Prithwi Singh attended at all occasions of worship of this goddess, and it was he who performed the sacrifice of goats and sometimes young buffaloes in her name, decapitating them each with a single cut of his sword.

In the summer of 1950, Prithwi Singh was bitten on the finger by a cobra one afternoon as he was returning from his fields. This happened about a mile and a half from the village, and by the time he reached home, the poison was working in him. He felt thick-headed and confused, and could hardly drag his legs along.

"Sahib," he said, "at that time I really thought that I was about to die. But I managed to make my way to the shrine of Mataji, and I prayed to Her that if it was Her will, She should make me well. Then I went back to my house to an inner room where I have a little brass image of the Goddess, and I lay down below it on the floor, and at once I became unconscious. I lay there for some hours in a fever, and they said that I groaned in my sleep; and then I had a dream. In my dream I saw the Goddess come into the room and stand beside me. She lifted up my hand and sucked the poison from my finger, and then She turned and went away. I woke up, wet with perspiration and quite weak; but from that moment I began to get well."

Among my stock of medicines was a set of dried polyvalent antivenin serums for intravenous injection in cases of snake-bite. I let it be known that this was available, but although I heard in due course of several such cases, two of which were fatal, no one asked for this treatment. I believe now that this was on account of the close association of the illness and the god. A physician who was perversely insensible to the all-important divine agent could not inspire confidence in treating this condition.

In the same way there was bitter opposition to the efforts of governmental authorities to promote universal vaccination against smallpox. Here, as all over India, this disease is believed to be due to the wrath of the demon-goddess, locally known as Sitala-Mata. Epidemics always occur in the hot weather, when flies are most abundant. High fever is taken as a sign that the goddess is hot. She is angry. She devours children in her rage. For this reason at the beginning of the very hot season, there is a placatory ceremony at the goddess' shrine, and this is repeated should there be a spell of especially hot weather or should smallpox break out in the vicinity. On such occasions, the image of Sitala-Mata is bathed with cool water, and garlands and fruits are laid before her. "We are cooling her down," say the women.

In contrast, there were some afflictions that were less decidedly associated with divine intervention. For example, there was no talk of "possession" when one was stung by a scorpion, although every practitioner who had charms against snake-bite seemed also to know one of the lesser charms against such a sting. My local-analgesic oily preparation was in great demand during the hot weather nights, when stings were most frequent. On one occasion I came upon a group squatting in the dusty village lane. A young man had received a severe sting. His leg was swollen and very painful. My old friend Nathu Lal was engaged in exorcising the poison, stroking the leg over and over again with a twig of nimleaves and whispering the appropriate charm. When he saw me squat beside him, he paused and suggested that I should apply my medicine, but I knew that at this stage it could do nothing to relieve his pain, so I persuaded Nathu Lal to continue his good work.

The Role of Faith in Curing

There were so many lesser healers and magicians at work in Delwara that one tended to overlook the fact that there was also a government dispensary, with a doctor trained in Ayurvedic medicine, and a dispenser. Their services and their medicaments were available free; and yet strangely enough they found very few clients. In all the many conversations I had with them in their sparsely equipped premises, I can remember only thrice being interrupted by the arrival of a patient. This state of idleness, it must be confessed, was not uncongenial to the doctor's temperament; indeed, he tended to encourage it by maintaining that these free medicines provided by the government were not very good anyway—let people come to his house privately, and he would let them have others, which would cost a good deal and which were correspondingly effective. In this way, he carried on a desultory sort of practice among the better-off families but earned the resentment of the poorer majority.

In Delwara, as in Sujarupa, the chief resort of families afflicted with sickness (or indeed any other trouble) was to the priests of a number of shrines in the vicinity; and here, too, there was one shrine that enjoyed an outstanding reputation in this respect. It was the shrine of Vijayshan-Mata, of which Prithwi Singh was one of the attendants. Every Sunday night without fail the priest became possessed and sat quivering on the floor in front of the image of the goddess, while a long succession of patients and supplicants came before him to be diagnosed and treated. In time I got to know the priest quite well, and I could see that sometimes he seemed genuinely in trance, while at others he was wide awake and made only a pretense at still being "possessed." In fact, this was evident the first time I attended his ceremony, a few months after my wife and I had settled in the village. When the priest had worshiped Vijayshan-Mata to an accompaniment of gongs and conch-shell music, her spirit came to him and he flailed himself ecstatically with an iron chain, and then began to utter his divinations. At this point I found myself thrust forward to the door of the temple and voices said, "Go on, ask Mataji anything you want to know, and she will tell you the true answer."

After racking my brains for a moment, I asked a question which in fact had been exercising my wife and me for several weeks: "Mataji, this baby that we are going to have shortly, will it be a boy or a girl?" The quivering priest forgot himself for one moment and nearly burst out laughing. To conceal this, he turned toward the image as if seeking guidance, and then cried out, "*Choro vaygo!*" (village dialect for "It'll be a boy"). And for days everyone in the village made us repeat this prophecy and then congratulated us upon our coming good fortune; but the baby proved to be a girl after all.

I sat beside this priest for many hours watching villagers and peasants present their sickly children or themselves for the blessing of the goddess' treatment, and I became familiar with the small range of common complaints: fever, dysentery, tuberculosis, childlessness, and, above all, witchcraft, which covered a multitude of women's and children's illnesses. One thing impressed me especially: these patients did not give a history of their complaint in the way to which we are accustomed. They took it for granted that the divine healer would know at once what was wrong. (Here, as many times in these villages, one was reminded of analogies to the Gospel stories.) This observation reminded me of the many occasions when country people had come up to me and silently extended a hand for me to take their pulse. And when, after doing so, I asked, "What is troubling you?" they would answer, "Sahib, that is for you to say. We are only poor ignorant people; how should we know?"

This attitude bespoke their ready trust. It meant that, having once decided to believe in a certain healer, they would accept uncritically whatever he told them. It was an indication also of their faith in the physician's cure. And that faith was always absolute; they knew no half measure. My village informants were quite explicit on this point. "Medicines are all very well," they would say to me. "But really, Sahib, it is *tassili* (faith) that makes a sick man well. No matter how rare a medicine you give a patient, unless both you and he have faith in it, he never will be cured."

In the case of the priest's therapy, this was certainly true, because he seldom applied any physical treatment at all. Watching the scores of peasants who passed before him, I came to realize that what they asked from him (or rather, from the goddess) were two things: that the affliction should be given a name and so become less terrible, and that the priest should utter his prediction, "He will get well." It mattered not that this formula was repeated to every other patient, every night. To each one it was like a personal communication from the goddess herself and put new heart into him.

At first, I must confess, I was filled with scorn and hostility toward this charlatan; but in time I came to realize that he was no less convinced than all his patients of the worthwhileness of his work. After all, he was simply performing what is one of the most important functions of the general medical practitioner, by letting these sick people feel that they were not alone and helpless but part of a succoring community, both real and supernatural. In my boyhood in Scotland I knew an eccentric old country physician who was remarkable for two things: for his detestation of internal combustion engines ("Damn these motors! Damn these motors!" he would cry when an early Model-T Ford made him skip to the side of the road) and for his habit of falling to his knees and "putting up a prayer" whenever one of his patients chanced to die. Unkind critics pointed out that he had more scope for this exercise than had his younger competitors, but his practice remained a large one to the end of his days. Our Presbyterian neighbors felt that in him they had a guide through life and the hereafter.

IMPLICATIONS

Nowadays simple piety is at a discount in the western world. In its place we offer the assurance of a securely based scientific training, which enables us to treat our patients and utter our prognosis with a sincere, if measured, confidence. It will be a long time before the scientific approach to the understanding and treatment of disease reaches remoter villages such as Sujarupa and Delwara. Until the material resources and the educational level of the public permit us to give them something demonstrably better, it would be a disservice to these people to try to undermine the chief solace they have in time of trouble.

By this I do not mean that we are justified in adopting a defeatist attitude toward the problem, but simply that we have to work from below upward. There were evidences of such new ideas in Delwara in 1951. Young men who had left the village to work in the city or to serve in the army came home with a smattering of new ideas about hygiene and sanitation. They spoke up at the village council in favor of cleaning up the lanes and building proper city-style latrines. A young Congress-party worker read in the newspaper about infections spread by water and persuaded the council to disinfect the main well of drinking water during the fly-infested season. It was here, I felt, at the village level itself, that the new ideas must take root if they were ever to command the confidence, the all-important "tassili" of the village people, which alone could make them work.

Perhaps the most significant lesson of my stay in these two villages was the realization that it was not enough to bring good medicines and efficient hygienic techniques to these country people. Before they can take effect, they must be *accepted*, and this will never come about so long as a wide gulf separates the thinking and the experience of western doctors from that of their village patients. There are three ways in which this gulf can be bridged: by the slow diffusion of information about sepsis and infection; by a better understanding of the expectations with which the people approach the doctor; and by presenting new techniques in a way which will link them up with what they are expected to supersede. Just as the earliest "horseless carriages" evolved only slowly and as if reluctantly toward the streamlined efficiency of a modern roadster, so we must expect new ideas in medicine to take root, at first by emphasizing their continuity with old traditions. To confront the villager with radically new departures from all that is familiar in the domain of health and sickness will only alarm and bewilder him and forfeit his coopera- tion, as has so frequently happened.

SUMMARY

This paper has been devoted to the recording of a number of lessons that I learned in the course of my attempts to practice medicine in two country villages of northern India. I was forced to recognize the seriousness of certain obstacles to the acceptance of western medicine, obstacles whose true nature could be under- stood only when I had learned a good deal about the villagers' own beliefs concerning sickness and cure. Misunderstandings were found to arise from false expectations on both sides, based on different theories of etiology, different techniques of cure, and different conceptions of the role of the physician.

After a period of practical experience, I realized that one can scarcely expect village people to change their whole cosmology simply to accord with the outlook of a western-trained doctor. Scientific knowledge seems likely to be disseminated throughout India as education becomes widespread and the products of western technology become a part of everyone's environment— but one cannot afford to wait for this to happen. In the immediate future, it devolves upon those who are introducing western tech- niques in public health and medicine to study how best they can adapt the roles of the doctor, the pharmacist, and the public hygienist to fit into the existing cultural expectations. In the process, they may have to consent to assume the mantle of the priest or the magician. This does not mean, of course, that they will themselves subscribe to nonrational beliefs, but simply that they will accept the inevitable fact that their own techniques of healing will be accepted "irrationally," as indeed they are for the most part in the West. Western health personnel can, however, turn this fact to advantage by dramatizing the concepts of infection, sterilization, and chemotherapy for all they are worth and by accepting as an asset the quite unscientific awe which the ritual of even minor surgery can inspire.

Public health workers will have to formulate their measures so that they can be linked with the old teachings, and above all must aim to enlist the support of the leaders of village opinion. These considerations may sound devious and Machiavellian, but so long as western-trained workers remain clear in their own minds about the worth of the contribution they have to make to the community's well-being, they will be able to play their roles with that conviction and assurance of ultimate success which the villagers themselves recognize as the hallmark of truly potent therapy.

SELECTED REFERENCES

Carstairs, G. Morris, "The Case of Thakur Khuman Singh: A Culture-conditioned Crime," *British Journal of Delinquency*, vol. 4, 1953–1954, pp. 14–25; and "Daru and Bhang: Cultural Factors in the Choice of Intoxicants," *Quarterly Journal of Studies in Alcohol*, vol. 15, June, 1954, pp. 220–237. These two papers describe characteristic caste-specific attitudes to two items of behavior observed in a Rajasthan village. One paper concerns reactions to a violent double murder; the second, reactions to intoxicating drugs.

The Psychology of High-Caste Hindus. (In preparation for publication.) This volume is based on observations in Rajasthan made by the writer in 1951–1952.

Fuchs, Stephen, *The Children of Hari.* Verlag Herold, Vienna, 1950. This social-anthropological study of a low-caste community in a village of central India contains an interesting chapter on "Disease and Its Cure."

Taylor, W. S., "Basic Personality in Orthodox Hindu Culture Patterns," *Journal of Abnormal and Social Psychology*, vol. 43, 1948, pp. 3–12. A study of the influence exercised by conscious ideal values upon Indian villagers' behavior and personality.

Wiser, Charlotte, and W. H. Wiser, *Behind Mud Walls.* Friendship Press, New York, 1946. (Previously published as *Behind Mud Walls in India.* Geo. Allen, London, 1934.) A pioneer example of observations of Indian village life from within, written by two missionaries who were also sociologists.

Zimmer, Henry R., *Hindu Medicine.* Johns Hopkins Press, Baltimore, 1948. This volume examines the conceptions of the body, medicine, and the traditional Hindu physician that emerge from analysis of Vedic and classical Hindu texts.

Case 5

A CHOLERA EPIDEMIC IN A CHINESE TOWN
by Francis L. K. Hsu

To gain perspective on one's own culture, it is often useful to view it from the vantage point of another culture. As an American who was once a member of Chinese society, Dr. Hsu can appraise either western or Chinese culture from the standpoint of the other. His observations of group behavior during a cholera epidemic in a southwestern Chinese town afford a springboard for comparing Chinese and American worldviews. The common man in China, he indicates, will accept science if it is disguised as magic, whereas the common man in America will accept magic if it is disguised as science.

The Chinese in the stricken community preferred their native "fairy water" to western anticholera injections. At the time, western-trained health personnel assumed the injections were effective; retrospectively the vaccine appears to have been just another kind of fairy water, an unwitting instance of magic offered in a scientific package. This ironic development is somewhat beside the main point of the case, however, since it appears that the people preferred other methods of control for reasons unrelated to considerations of technical efficiency. They placed primary reliance on elaborate and costly prayer meetings in order to please the gods, in accordance with their traditional view of the world as a moral rather than a mechanistic order. This view is comparable to the Indian outlook depicted in the previous case study by Dr. Carstairs.

In a concluding section, Dr. Hsu reviews some of the general circumstances under which communities will accept or reject new ideas or techniques of foreign origin. The South African study by Dr. Cassel is similarly concerned with the problem of differential acceptance and resistance. — EDITOR

THE PROBLEM

The Community Ignores Western Medicine in Fighting Cholera

In the spring of 1942 a serious cholera epidemic struck the community of Hsi-ch'eng, a rural market town of 8,000 inhabitants in Yunnan Province, southwestern China. Unlike many similar communities in this area, Hsi-ch'eng lacked neither the facilities nor the trained personnel that would make possible the use of the best techniques known to western medical science for fighting the disease. Some years prior to the epidemic several of the wealthiest families had supported the establishment in the community of a hospital and three modern schools. The hospital had about 20 beds, one graduate nurse, two fully qualified medical doctors, a number of assistant nurses, and a nursing training class. The three schools, two of which were coeducational, had a total enrollment of approximately 1,400 from Hsi-ch'eng and other communities. In addition, there was a missionary college, with a Chinese and western faculty, which had moved to this area from a part of China devastated by the war with Japan.

Immediately after the first cases of cholera were detected, these agencies went into action. The schools made up and distributed posters and other informational material detailing measures for limiting spread of the disease. The hospital offered its facilities to all stricken inhabitants, and announced that bed space would be free for those too poor to pay.

The inhabitants were deeply disturbed by the epidemic and expended a tremendous amount of energy in measures to fight it. Nevertheless, practically no one took advantage of the modern services freely offered by the hospital. Nurses even went out into the streets urging people to adopt certain preventive and curative measures; yet they found few people willing to follow these measures. Meanwhile the death rate mounted. Between the tenth of May and the tenth of June, when the epidemic abated, nearly two hundred men, women, and children died of the disease in Hsi-ch'eng—an alarming fatality figure.

Why did the people of Hsi-ch'eng fail to avail themselves of medical services that were readily available and freely offered, in the face of so dire a threat to their lives and health? What measures did they adopt? What does their choice of methods reveal about the role of culture in affecting a population's response to a crisis?

THE SITUATION

Hsi-ch'eng Combats a Cholera Epidemic[1]

The Town of Hsi-ch'eng

Hsi-ch'eng is located within a day's journey on foot or horse-back from the Burma Road and lies about 6,700 feet above sea level. It is bordered by a lake on one side and a mountain rising to 14,000 feet on the other. The general occupation of the entire area is agriculture, rice being the staple crop. However, trading in various forms is also very common; it represents the backbone of Hsi-ch'eng economy. Trading in this community includes both local exchanges in periodic markets and large-scale commercial adventures into the outer world.

The town of Hsi-ch'eng proper is not walled. There is only one continuous thoroughfare, which leads from the north to the south. Into it at irregular intervals run other streets in east-west direction. Some years ago four gates were erected, one at each end of the main thoroughfare, one at the end of a street running into it from the east, and one at the end of a street from the west. In this way a large section of the town is shut off from the outlying areas at night, when a town watchman patrols the streets with a gang. However, Hsi-ch'eng's population is not confined within these gates. Outside are at least nine clearly marked clusters of houses, each called a village. Within the four gates, each street, or each section of a street, is also designated a village.

The racial origin of the inhabitants is open to question. Both the town and the district seat as well as their satellite villages have legends about the migration of their ancestors from some central provinces into Yunnan. The place most frequently given for the original habitat is "Nanking," a place which bears, however, little semblance to the former national capital. A few genealogical records indicate that their ancestors were from Anwhei Province. However this may be, the inhabitants today are proud of their claimed Chinese origin.

---

[1] The factual material in this case study is extracted from Hsu, F. L. K., *Religion, Science, and Human Crises:* A Study of China in Transition and Its Implications for the West. Routledge and Kegan Paul, Ltd., London, 1952.

The people of Hsi-ch'eng emphasize the difference between the sexes. They zealously guard the virginity of unmarried women and the chastity of married women. The cult of ancestors is deeply institutionalized. Not only the very powerful and wealthy clans but also some ordinary ones establish a separate clan temple. Every family tries hard to assure good sites for its graveyards according to geomancy, a system of divination to determine whether a burial site is favorable or not. The nature of the site is supposed to affect the rise or fall of future descendants of the family group. Old imperial honors granted from Peking continue to be highly valued. When real honors are lacking, imaginary ones are often substituted. By these and other tokens the people of Hsi-ch'eng are not only Chinese in culture but also, by their own insistence, more Chinese in some ways than the residents of many other parts of China.

Hsi-ch'eng is distinguished from most rural Chinese towns in having a disproportionately large number of wealthy families. Some of these families are outstanding not merely locally but even in the larger provincial cities and in Kunming. Thus, Hsi-ch'eng includes the three usual social classes of China, a small upper crust, a somewhat larger middle group, and a rather large lower class. But class distinctions are blurred. For one thing, the rich and the poor meet and join in conversation as a matter of course at community functions. For another, many poor people claim remote common ancestry with some of the rich. The importance of the cult of ancestors overshadows the significance of the class difference.

How the People Dealt with Cholera

Cholera is known and dreaded in all parts of China. When the disease struck Hsi-ch'eng in the spring of 1942, the face of the village was profoundly changed. Funeral processions became a common sight. At first, some processions were as elaborate as the families of the dead could afford. Later, all processions became hasty and comparatively simple. During the evenings the streets, crowded before the onset of the epidemic, were virtually empty. Except for the carpenters' shops, darkness and silence prevailed. Even during the day the streets were nearly deserted. Men and women became reticent and gloomy. There is no question that all were deeply disturbed by the epidemic and would do nearly anything to eliminate it.

Cholera is a disease for which western medicine has at its command fairly effective methods of diagnosis and prevention. The etiological agent, *vibrio comma*, is known. The primary source of infection is fecal contamination; diagnosis can be made by direct microscopic examination. The mode of transmission, the incubation period, and the period of communicability are known. Methods of control center on instituting stringent sanitary measures to prevent communication of the disease and involve detection and isolation of carriers and thorough disinfection of all contaminated materials.

Western methods for combating cholera were at the disposal of the people of Hsi-ch'eng through its modern hospital and schools. At the onset of the epidemic, the physician in charge of the college infirmary, who was an American missionary and a graduate of Harvard Medical School, gave a special lecture to the entire student body on the cause, prevention, and treatment of cholera. The college authorities advised the students to take stringent sanitary precautions and to refrain from eating raw food or food exposed to flies, and from drinking unboiled water. In addition, arrangements were made to have students and faculty receive injections, a measure generally believed at that time to be effective.

The hospital and the local schools also went into action. At first, the hospital administered injections on the premises. Later, nurses were sent into the streets to give free injections. Hospital beds were made available for stricken patients, free of charge for those too poor to pay. The number of beds was limited, but even these were not used to capacity.

The local schools did things in a much more dramatic manner. They exhibited large posters everywhere in town. One poster displayed pictures of several food peddlers with their retailing stands of sweets, pea-curd, and the like. These stands were covered with flies. Several customers were pictured eating the food. Another poster pictured an open-air toilet in use. Several people were seen in the act of vomiting. Flies swarmed on their stools and on the material ejected from their mouths. The caption below the picture read: "The flies in both places are the same and carry cholera germs from the one to the other." A third poster showed in enlarged form the structure of a fly and of some cholera germs, with detailed scientific explanatory notes on how these germs could be communicated and by what means such communication could be prevented.

The inhabitants of Hsi-ch'eng reacted vigorously to the cholera threat, but they responded according to their own ideas of its cause and of effective countermeasures, and not the ideas of the school and hospital authorities. The popular explanation of cholera was that it was brought by epidemic-carrying spirits sent by the gods and might be withdrawn by the gods, provided they were propitiated by moral behavior and prayer. The spirits, meanwhile, could be kept off by charms. The first and most important measure the people undertook was to stage prayer meetings, one after another. These prayer meetings were elaborate and costly. They were staged in different neighborhoods and were primarily the work of hired priests and other religious specialists. The shortest one lasted one day and one night, and the longest, six days and seven nights. Thousands of gods were invoked. During the course of the epidemic, 19 such prayer meetings took place. Money for the prayer meetings came from a multitude of small donors as well as from the leading families.

The prayer meetings, though most colorful and certainly occupying the central place in Hsi-ch'eng's mode of dealing with the epidemic, were not the only steps taken. Along with the prayer meetings, in which the priests prayed to the gods to forgive misconduct and exhorted the populace to be moral, the inhabitants also resorted to a number of other measures designed to protect the individual or the community from the ailment.

Native cures and prescriptions were offered by individuals as a public service by means of handwritten or printed posters displayed in various parts of the town. Some of the prescriptions consisted of herbs cited in *The Codex of Chinese Drugs*, a volume prepared by Chinese doctors with western training. Other prescriptions advised the consumption of certain ready-made drugs in pill or powder form as well as acupunctural practices. These public notices were signed by actual names or by such designations as "a retired oldster" or "a famous physician in the army."

Moral injunctions from priests and others, exhorting the populace to abstain from sex and otherwise purge themselves of evil thoughts and deeds, were posted throughout the town. These posters emphasized the need for keeping streets and alleys free from animal droppings and household refuse. The bases for the exhortations were made explicit: "What you see means more to the gods than what you hear; what you think means more to the gods than what you eat." People were reminded: "Flat earth has no waves; all trouble begins with the human heart." But the inhabitants did not limit themselves to words. In conjunction with the local police, leaders made strong efforts to bring about general cleanliness in the community so as to please the gods. Taboos were placed on many varieties of food, from pea-curd and potatoes to meat and fish.

Palm-shaped cacti were hung on gates, lime powder lines were drawn on walls to connect the lintels of the family portal, and amulets of yellow paper with drawings were carried around by individuals. The Chinese name for palm-shaped cactus is Fairy-Palm, and since the epidemic was believed to be caused by evil spirits, the sign of hands of fairies or of superior deities would ward off the disease-making spirits. The drawing of lime powder lines was a recent innovation. Residents had observed people of the missionary college and hospital spread lime powder on the floor to disinfect wards and outhouses and had adopted this practice without much knowledge of its practical function. Amulets have been used by the inhabitants of Hsi-ch'eng and all China since time beyond memory.

People secured medicine from the gods and drank what they described as "fairy water" for prevention or cure. The medicine was generally a package of sandy material composed of ashes of burned incense sticks obtained in a shrine after a request for help made by an applicant or by the priest acting on his behalf. The contents of the package were then taken home and administered with water. The bulk of Hsi-ch'eng's fairy water came from a rock located about ten miles south of the community. The rock, known as Nine Goddesses Spring, was said to gush water only when an epidemic struck and to remain dry at all other times. All during the cholera epidemic this water was carried to Hsi-ch'eng on pack horses and sold at 50 cents a cup. Not all fairy water came from that particular rock. Residents also drank water from a fountain-like arrangement in an incense burner located in front of a temporary shrine. This was also considered fairy water by virtue of its association with the abode of the gods.

From a western viewpoint, the effectiveness of indigenous methods for coping with the epidemic varied greatly. For example, the taboos on a large number of foods, though imposed for supernatural reasons, might actually have restricted the spread of the epidemic. The taboo on fresh fruits and vegetables was helpful because fruits were usually eaten unwashed and unpeeled, while vegetables were as a rule cleaned in the contaminated public streams before cooking, and sometimes were consumed raw. The taboo on meat and fish can be seen in a similar light, especially because meat, broth, and potato are all suitable media for the growth of cholera bacteria.

Other indigenous measures such as the prayers, the various rituals, and the moral injunctions, while they might have helped to reassure and stabilize the disturbed community, had no demonstrable effect on the epidemic. Furthermore, some measures might actually have led to effects diametrically opposed to the desired ones. For example, one of the indigenous cures for cholera directed the victim to open up his finger tips to let out blood. This could lead to serious infection and complicate later treatment. Drinking fairy water from unclean containers might have resulted in increasing the rate of infection to a considerable extent.

The indigenous practices for dealing with the epidemic can be grouped into three categories: those which could have beneficial effects, those which could produce results with no direct bearing on the epidemic, and those which tended to be harmful. Below are classified the various measures according to these categories.

There is no doubt that some of the local practices were based on valid knowledge. However, since people indiscriminately employed the three kinds of measures and resorted to some of them under what medical science would regard as false assumptions, it

MEASURES TAKEN AND THEIR RESULTS

Measures taken	Local rationale	Effects according to western medical theory
Taboos on eating potatoes, string beans, turnips, all sour fruits, confections, new wheat flour, fresh meat, fish, pumpkin, egg plant, etc.	To please the gods To avoid making the abdomen cold	Taboos on meat and potatoes would limit the growth and spread of the bacillus; other food taboos neither harmful nor beneficial
Taboo on dirt and on animal and human soil in streets	To make the air and ground clean for gods	Improvement in general sanitation, which might mitigate the epidemic
Emphasis on morals	To purify the heart and thus please the gods	Without demonstrable connection with the epidemic
Prayer meetings and scripture - elaboration sessions	To beg forgiveness of the gods through a collective appeal	Congregating might contribute to spreading the disease
Hanging cactus stalks on gates; making hand prints on walls and doors; drawing lime powder arcs in front of house gates, etc.	To ward off epidemic-giving spirits	Without demonstrable connection with the epidemic
Medicinal prescriptions	To cure cholera To prevent cholera	Some prescriptions harmful, some good, others indifferent
Drinking fairy water	To cure and prevent cholera	Possible increase in the incidence of infection

is clear that they made no distinction in their own minds between "nonscientific" and "scientific" practices. This conclusion is further underlined by the attitude of Hsi-ch'eng toward the modern measures. For example, local police made sure that the inhabitants kept the streets much cleaner than before, but they also enforced the taboo on meat as well as taking part in the prayer meetings. Similarly, some of the prescriptions offered by local people as a public service were evidently compounded of both western and indigenous specifics, mixed together. But most of the local people either failed to utilize modern precautions and remedies or used them concurrently with all the indigenous practices for the same purpose.

The People Explain Their Actions

Following the epidemic, the writer, at that time an instructor in the local college, interviewed 31 residents of Hsi-ch'eng in an effort to discover the reasons behind the pattern of response to the epidemic. The basic idea shared by all informants was that modern measures were evidently useful in fighting the epidemic but that they were neither the only devices nor the most important ones. A majority of those questioned had contributed substantial sums to the prayer meetings; several were important officers at these meetings; and many had also employed amulets, indigenous prescriptions, and other traditional devices. One man who had received an injection and required all his children and grandchildren to be immunized also served as an official at a prayer meeting, explaining: "After all, nobody knows which spirit he might have offended unintentionally." Another man who received injections explained that he also served as an officer in a prayer meeting because his parents wanted him to be there. One man who took his son for an injection after the youngster became ill claimed that the boy got well as a result. On the other hand, scores of men and women, whether or not they were parents of school children, refused the injections and paid virtually no attention to the other modern measures available to them.

Some men and women refused injections on the ground that it was "too painful." In fact, this was the most frequently used reason for refusing an injection. This reason was apparently a polite excuse for avoiding something which did not appeal to them, for most local men and women, when seriously ill, would not hesitate to allow native acupuncture practitioners to insert long silver pins deep into their bodies. These pins were not sharp and certainly not disinfected. Other reasons given for not taking the injections were that the informant had "no time," or that the injections were inconvenient.

Limited Appeal of Western Techniques

Why did the inhabitants of Hsi-ch'eng mix modern measures with ancient practices or even refuse the newer methods outright? It is not an adequate answer simply to say that these Chinese farmers were "unreasonable" or "prelogical" as is sometimes asserted. In Hsi-ch'eng, as in all societies, the individual's perception is guided by the traditional tenets of his culture. As the average individual in Hsi-ch'eng grows up, he learns to view the world as it is seen by the people around him. In the minds of most of these people, no clear separation is made between that which is "natural" and that which is "supernatural." Supernatural forces are seen as operating in everything; it is only in certain segments of western or westernized society that people consistently call one kind of cause "natural" or "scientific" and another kind "supernatural" or "magic."

This does not mean that the people in Hsi-ch'eng possess a different order of mentality from people in societies that do make a distinction between these two kinds of causality—that they are "illogical" while people in western societies are "logical." In both cases an individual will judge any practice to be reasonable or "logical" not on the basis of his own pure, abstract "rational" analysis, but on the basis of the fundamental premises about the nature of cause and effect provided for him by his culture. If his culture stresses the "scientific" nature of cause and effect, he will tend to judge things by this standard; if his culture assumes that there are supernatural forces at work in all happenings, he will inevitably see things in this way. In either case it is the culture and not the individual that plays the determining part.

The residents of Hsi-ch'eng, in dealing with the cholera epidemic, relied but little on injections and other scientific measures because they were reared in a cultural milieu to which the western practices were totally alien. Under such circumstances, even the select few who might have been skeptical of indigenous usages because of western education and contact had to follow suit, or at least not be drastically different, in order to maintain their status and respectability in their community. This was why those who sponsored and supported the modern institutions also contributed much to the indigenous practices.

Thus, to the man of Hsi-ch'eng, in dealing with the cholera epidemic, the taboos and prayers were as logical in terms of his own culture as injections and hospitalization would be to one whose outlook had been conditioned by modern science. In either case the diagnosis made and the means resorted to are culturally given. Brought up in their cultural setting, the people of Hsi-ch'eng had acquired ideas about ghosts, epidemic-giving spirits, gods, punishment, and personal fate. They left the bulk of the work of prevention and cure to the specialists of their culture—the priests. The Euro-American and western-trained personnel in Hsi-ch'eng had also acquired, under similar circumstances but in a different cultural environment, ideas about bacteria, hospitals, medicine, and injection. They felt that the burden of cure and prevention should rightfully fall upon those designated by their culture as specialists—doctors and public health officers.

In each case it was the culture and not the individual that had a magico-religious bias, or a leaning toward the scientific. In each case individuals acted according to their cultural conditioning. The fact that many western medical personnel in 1942 believed implicitly in the efficacy of anticholera injections—a measure which today is considered of little value—documents the determining quality of culturally reinforced beliefs, independent of their ultimate objective validity.

Neither the people of Hsi-ch'eng nor any other population invariably reject all new elements. But whenever people borrow from other cultures they tend to reinterpret the new elements and to alter them to fit their own framework of expectations. This was why the villagers either refused modern scientific measures or mixed them with indigenous practices. Modern medicine and its practitioners had no definite place in their own cultural tradition —a tradition in which a cholera epidemic or any other emergency, such as a drought, was dealt with by using *all* available measures. Taboos on fruits, meat, and fish were maintained during the epidemic, not out of consideration for the preventive measures of modern science, but as a means of pleasing the gods. The lines drawn with lime powder on the walls of family homes and semicircles drawn in front of the lintels of others may be seen in the same light. Elders of Hsi-ch'eng had noted the first appearance of such designs some ten years before, after residents saw lime powder used as a disinfectant. It was only natural for a spirit-wary people who had been using cactus leaves to ward off cholera-giving spirits to turn this new product to a similar purpose.

IMPLICATIONS

Science in Chinese Life and Magic in American Life

It is widely held that western societies put a high premium on "rational" explanations and behavior. A little reflection will show that magic in its various forms is still prevalent in many parts of the western world. Even in contemporary American life "scientific" thinking characterizes the thought-processes of only a small minority. Peasant peoples in Europe and rural American communities still maintain practices and beliefs properly called "magical." The prevalence of magical thinking is attested by the tremendous circulation of horoscope magazines, the prosperity of the Spiritualist churches here and in Europe, and the utilitarian expectations of church-goers in Mexico and other Latin countries.

However, the relative importance of magic or science, especially on a conscious level, differs widely from culture to culture. In this, Hsi-ch'eng and the cities of America contrast sharply. In Hsi-ch'eng the place of honor is reserved for spirits and priests, benevolent or malicious, and for traditional prescriptions and herbs. In such a culture, modern medicine, to enter into local consideration, has to compete with spirits, fairy water, and herbs.

On the other hand, the culture of America is one in which scientists and technicians are believed to provide answers for everything. In America these occupy the place of honor enjoyed by supernatural forces and priests in Hsi-ch'eng. Consequently, Americans who believe in luck, charms, talismans, and horo-scopes have to do so apologetically. They will either announce that they do it for fun, dismiss these things as insignificant, or use them with great discretion. But Americans who work with science are under no such handicap regarding their work.

In the light of this picture, it is understandable why so many advertisements in America, offering toothbrushes with a curvature resembling that of the dentist's mirror or cigarettes that have been endorsed by "doctors in a nationwide survey," and so on, try to cash in on the name of science. While some of these advertising offerings are undoubtedly honest and sound, many are not. For example, the Vrilium Products Company in Chicago in 1948 sold about 5,000 of their "healing pencils" at about $300 each. According to the company's literature, each pencil contained "vrilium catalytic barium chloride," guaranteed to "emit healing rays for the relief of burns, sprains, aches, sinus trouble, blood disturbances and a number of other ailments." Among the customers were many prominent people. During the trial of the company's officials in 1950 under the Pure Food and Drug Act, about 70 witnesses from many walks of life were willing to testify for the defense. After the company's officials were convicted, an entrepreneur offered the sum of $10,000 to purchase the firm's name and stock.

To most Americans, mysterious phenomena must be given acceptable explanations in terms of atoms, neutrons, magnetic power, or other concepts of modern science. In contrast, when flying machines first passed over my native village at night in north China, the villagers concluded that these represented terrible appearances of the gods, and they prostrated themselves in worship. This is not to deny that Chinese even in the old days had empirical knowledge, nor that many modern Americans still maintain belief in the occult. An example of an American counterpart of Hsi-ch'eng's appeal to the supernatural was found in the continued and concentrated prayer meetings held by Texans during a recent drought. But such efforts are no longer a nationwide matter in America, while resort to western science continues to concern only a few Chinese.

The basic similarity between Hsi-ch'eng in China and a town in the United States, along with the basic contrast between them, is thus obvious. Their similarity comes from the fact that both peoples react to new stimuli by reinterpreting them or altering them to conform with known practices. Their difference is in what constitutes the "known practices." In Hsi-ch'eng, scientific measures must be put in harmony with local notions about spirits, taboos, and herb doctors which customarily figure in healing and prevention of diseases. In America, on the other hand, chemical compounds, healers, and new ideas and goods, whether sound or otherwise, become most marketable when put forward as the brain child of "scientists," or as products of some laboratory where accuracy is allegedly measured in one millionth of an inch. It is thus not too far-fetched to say that to achieve popular acceptance, magic has to be dressed like science in America, while science has to be cloaked as magic in Hsi-ch'eng.

Introducing Western Techniques to Nonwestern Peoples

The magico-religious way of coping with disease is as firmly entrenched in the culture of Hsi-ch'eng as is the scientific way in the culture of Americans. In the face of this how and under what circumstances can we expect communities to be receptive to new medical techniques or other ideas of foreign origin?

The possibility of such changes seems to depend upon a variety of circumstances. In the first place, there is no doubt that an individual separated from his native society can change much more readily than a community. A native of Hsi-ch'eng, if removed to an American metropolitan center, will tend to fall in line with the ideas held by the Americans about the nature and cure of disease. He will not change all of his previous ideas and customs in this area, but he will be more receptive than his people at home to ideas about the effectiveness of scientific precautions against disease. And as soon as he is convinced, he can go ahead and act in accordance with these new beliefs without fear of losing the respect of his neighbors.

In the second place, products of science which do not involve vital matters tend to be more readily accepted, on a trial basis, than others. For example, Chinese peasants definitely prefer trains or buses, when available, to horsecarts, or the telephone and post office to divination as a means of communication. On the other hand, a new and scientifically developed agricultural technique will not be readily trusted by farmers whose entire livelihood depends upon the success of next year's crop. The smaller the economic margin, the smaller will be the desire to experiment with new techniques.

In the third place, new elements which do not interfere with the existing social organization, or can be easily fitted into the framework of existing practices will generally encounter little resistance. Thus, articles of ornamentation go freely from one culture to another, and few peoples have been known to prefer their native weapons to western firearms once the latter are made available to them. On the other hand, mechanized pumps did not make any headway in Chinese villages principally because their use would have necessitated a type of cooperation to which Chinese farmers are not accustomed.

In the fourth place, some western technological improvements require organized enterprise and operation on a scale that is beyond the capacity of individuals or even a number of communities. The droughts and famines that periodically plague the Chinese could no more be controlled by a few Chinese communities than the Mississippi River rampages can be remedied by any single county or even state in the United States. In such a connection a strong central government, capable of coordinating and cementing local differences, can be a positive factor. Past differences between China and Japan in the pace of industrialization are certainly related to the existence, in the latter country, of a strong centralized government, as contrasted with its much weaker counterpart in China.

In the fifth place, it makes a good deal of difference whether a people have been exposed to foreign contact voluntarily or as the result of political pressure or military conquest. In the latter case, the impact of contact may be very different from any instance thus far discussed, because the "selectivity" of the people is affected. This may happen within a society, when an autocratic government is bent on forcing westernization, or between two societies where one is under the thumb of the other. At one time the Board of Health of the Yunnan provincial government in China compelled all individuals seen in the streets to be inoculated against typhoid and cholera. In this case the villagers evaded the order by staying away from all markets. These strong-arm tactics were later abandoned because they had failed. By contrast, the British authorities in Africa have frequently required that bushes be cleared by compulsory labor or that whole villages in the tsetse fly area be moved, so as to eliminate the sickness which the fly causes. In this case the method is still being used because it has apparently succeeded.

However, the differences in ultimate outcome may not be so great as the immediate success or failure would seem to indicate. The immediate results may have been brought about with such brutality or such total disregard for indigenous culture patterns, that the changes themselves, though apparently beneficial, may have produced emotionally disturbing effects. Then, later, when voluntary action becomes possible, even beneficial changes may be psychologically identified with the disturbing and unpleasant aspects of the former contact situation, and negated. Changes undertaken voluntarily have a better chance to persist than forced changes.

This brings us to two considerations concerning the relationship between change and emotional factors. No human behavior is free from emotional content and all cultural practices are invested with emotional significance. It follows that changes tend to be easier to introduce where the emotions of the recipients are least disturbed. On the other hand, where strong emotional involvement is inevitable, change may be expedited if these emotions can be mobilized for and not against the program.

The second consideration follows the first. Although positive emotions may be helpful when they support desired changes, they may ruin the chances of successful change when those who urge change are overexuberant, overmilitant, or extreme in their expectations. People all over the world find changes distasteful or, at the least, troublesome. Urban westerners are no exception. It is true that most westerners consciously seek change in science and industry. But attempts to bring about changes in family life, religious institutions, patterns of government, or even their recreational and dietary habits, would encounter considerable lack of enthusiasm, if not firm resistance. The desire for change in science and industry is part of their way of life, deeply rooted in the very social, religious, political, and personal habits which they would be highly reluctant to change.

Westerners who are engaged in effecting changes in the nonwestern world must remember that a reluctance to accept changes even in cases of severe problems of economic underdevelopment, malnutrition, and famine, or disease and epidemics, is also deeply rooted in local social, religious, political, and personal habits. In such circumstances any frontal attack on traditional usages, or an insistence that the native peoples give up their accustomed practices and champion only the new technique, tool, or idea, is doomed to failure.

While serving as a medical social worker in the Peking Union Medical College Hospital between the years 1934 and 1937, the writer observed many instances of such failure in respect to medicine. This college has produced some of the best medical technicians trained in the western tradition that China has ever known. But it failed to train its men to be aware of their patients as human beings with a given way of life which could be upset by the ideas and procedures of the foreign treatments the doctors tried to introduce. In Chinese tradition, and in the traditions of a vast majority of mankind, a sick individual will try any and all cures. If he cannot do so himself, it will be the duty of his kin to do so on his behalf. It is not at all unusual for a Chinese to consult three or four doctors simultaneously, while at the same time petitioning several gods. Consequently, when patients were persuaded to come to a western-trained doctor or to a modern hospital, they did not feel bound to that doctor or hospital in the same way as western patients would be. If the modern clinic could clear away their ailment in one visit, fine. If not, they had no compunction about seeing another man or visiting a temple, with the full intention of trying the western-trained doctor again, later on. However, the American-trained Chinese doctors often got furious with such patients, giving them a severe scolding, or even refusing to see them again. The doctors failed to realize that their job was to employ western modes of treatment insofar as possible, but not to convert the patients to a western outlook. Such an outlook would involve a drastic reorganization of the patient's social and psychological orientation that could not possibly be achieved in short order, nor within the context of the doctor-patient relationship.

People who are used to resorting to a variety of practitioners or sources of help in any emergency, medical or otherwise, will find the idea of concentrating on one doctor or one type of cure strange and disturbing. By insisting on all or none, modern medical workers do a disservice to their own cause, inducing social and ideological conflict. When this happens, people will either withdraw altogether or fight back with determination. In either case, the effort to introduce something new has backfired.

What is true with reference to the acceptance or rejection of western medicine by individual patients is equally true in a situation which involves favorable or unfavorable reactions to new public health measures by whole communities. If the innovators will promote their cause with a degree of modesty and humility, and present their ideas to the natives as one of the alternatives but not as the only true road to salvation, they will find their chances of success materially improved.

SUMMARY

When a serious cholera epidemic struck the rural Chinese market town of Hsi-ch'eng in 1942, the inhabitants expended most of their efforts to combat the disease in measures based on their traditional understandings of the nature of disease and the methods of cure. Western medical facilities available in the town were for the most part ignored or utilized inconsistently. The behavior of the residents becomes comprehensible if we realize that the distinction made by westerners between "magical" and "scientific" practices is not relevant to rural Chinese. Their culture has taught them that supernatural and moral considerations play an intimate part in cause and effect, and they trust this belief. The average American, on the other hand, has been taught to have an equally strong and implicit faith in science, and will subscribe to nearly any sort of idea or technique so long as it is represented as scientific. Any attempt to introduce new knowledge or new techniques in a foreign setting will benefit from the realization that all communities respond to these attempts according to premises implicit in their own cultural traditions.

SELECTED REFERENCES

Fei, H. T., and T. Y. Chang, *Earthbound China*. University of Chicago Press, 1945. This is a study of land, economy, and basic social structure in two Chinese communities not too far from the town that has here been called "Hsi-ch'eng"; the life of the people in all three communities was basically similar.

Hsu, F. L. K., *Under the Ancestor's Shadow*. Columbia University Press, New York, 1948. This is a study of the family, religion, and psychology of Hsi-ch'eng; the book contains a general description of the town.

Americans and Chinese: Two Ways of Life. Abelard-Schuman, New York, 1953. This is an intensive comparative analysis of the two ways of life. It is not confined to any local community, although specific field results are used. It attempts to synthesize the intellectual currents and the daily routines in the lives of the two peoples; it covers subjects ranging from art and literature to government, economy, and science.

"Cultural Factors" in *Economic Development, Principles and Patterns*, edited by Harold F. Williamson and John A. Buttrick, Prentice Hall, Inc., New York, 1954, pp. 318–364. This is an attempt to apply the theory outlined in the preceding reference to the problem of industrializing the technologically undeveloped areas of the world.

Wright, Arthur F., editor, *Studies in Chinese Thought*. University of Chicago Press, 1953. This volume contains ten scholarly essays by Sinologues, philosophers, and social scientists on Chinese religion, philosophy, ideas, values, art, and language.

Yang, Martin C., *A Chinese Village*. Columbia University Press, New York, 1945. This is a personal account of a village in Shantung, North China, written by a native from memory.

Case 6

DIPHTHERIA IMMUNIZATION IN A THAI COMMUNITY

by L. M. Hanks, Jr., and Jane R. Hanks

with the assistance of Kamol Janlekha, Aram Emarun,

Jadun Kongsa, and Saowanni Sudsaneh

Under the auspices of Cornell University, a team of American and Thai research workers has been making a detailed social and cultural study of a rural area near Bangkok in preparation for the experimental introduction of new techniques in health and agriculture. While working on this baseline study before any public health program was initiated, Dr. Hanks and his colleagues were drawn into community action by a medical emergency involving the children of two local residents with whom they had established close relationships. The influential position of the research team stimulated the district officer to issue a directive that led to the immunization of several hundred children. Unintentionally the authors thus became agents as well as observers of change.

But an even greater number of children failed to appear for antidiphtheria injections despite orders and publicity. Curious to know why some responded and others did not, the researchers embarked on a program of inquiry. The particular combination of factors uncovered by their investigation was peculiar to the local situation, but every health officer confronts a similar order of circumstances in trying to mobilize mass response to a community emergency—season of the year, settlement pattern, cultural orientations, attitudes toward authority, and the customary chain of command.

*This study traces the attenuation of a message as it travels from its source to the receivers. As such the case documents an important aspect of the process of communication and therefore has a kinship to the case studies in Part I.—*EDITOR

THE PROBLEM

An Urgent Health Message Fails to Arouse Bang Chan

The "dramatic incident" is frequently cited by health workers as an effective opening wedge in bringing about acceptance of modern medical ideas. On the basis of the principle that nothing succeeds like success, health workers can occasionally capitalize on a dramatic situation, ready-made or arranged, where modern medicine proves its effectiveness or superiority in a striking way. Such an incident occurred·in the Thai community of Bang Chan in the summer of 1953.

Bang Chan comprises an area of scattered hamlets on the central plains of Thailand. Most of the residents appear healthy; one seldom encounters anyone whose plight might arouse pity. Malaria, tuberculosis, and intestinal diseases are fairly prevalent but cause death only rarely. People do not consider themselves sick if they are able to work.

Occasionally, however, epidemics do strike. In 1910 cholera broke out, and the disease ran its course uncontrolled. In 1940 the same disease broke out again. But this time, with the services of a health officer available, only five persons died. A little later, smallpox took a heavy toll, since few had been immunized. The resultant deaths and painful memories of personal agony vividly impressed the people with the idea of contagion and spurred the acceptance of immunization. Thus, in 1948 when disease struck the water buffalo, the people of Bang Chan hastened to have their beloved beasts inoculated.

In 1953 a three-year-old girl contracted diphtheria. Her parents, after an initial period of apparent unconcern, brought her to a local traditional practitioner for treatment. A week later, the small son of a neighboring family contracted the same disease. His parents brought him to a modern hospital in the nearby market center of Minburi. The child treated by the traditional practitioner died; the child who went to the hospital was cured.

Local administrative and health officials, influenced in part by members of an anthropological research team who were in the community, arranged an emergency immunization program. They were motivated first and foremost by the desire to protect the children of Bang Chan from the imminent threat of a contagious disease. Less urgent but also important, at least in the estimation of the research team, was the desire to utilize the occasion for demonstrating the effectiveness of modern medical techniques.

The message sent out to the community was originally formulated so as to include two principal elements: an item of information and an order. The information included the fact that diphtheria was in the community, that it was dangerous and contagious, and that modern methods of control had been proved eminently effective. The order advised the parents of Bang Chan to bring their children to be immunized at a given place and time.

The response to the order was spotty and patently inconsistent. About one-third of the children in the community appeared for immunization, some reappearing for a second inoculation and others failing to come. The response to the informational part of the message was apparently negligible. Practically no one seemed to have acquired any better understanding of the nature of contagion or the relation between diphtheria and modern methods of control. Even more impressive was the fact that few considered the information a logical basis for issuing the order.

Why did the people of Bang Chan fail to perceive a possible diphtheria epidemic as a crisis? What was behind the uneven response to the call for immunization? Why did the demonstrated contrast between modern and traditional medical methods fail to have much educational impact? Why did so few people connect the information about diphtheria with the immunization order? The community of Bang Chan, with its own local characteristics and its own culture, lay between the issuance of the message and its reception. A more detailed picture of the nature of that community and the events leading up to the immunization campaign will help us understand the community's response to the immunization message.

THE SITUATION

Community Response to a Call for Immunization

Contagious Disease Threatens Bang Chan

Rim and Sawang were Buddhist rice farmers who had lived in Bang Chan all their lives. Rim had married Sawang's sister, and their houses stood side by side. They helped each other with plowing and seeding, kept their buffalo together in the same area in front of their houses, and borrowed each other's boats to paddle to the local temple or to the store. Fortune had treated

Rim kindly. His crops had been good. His four sons were living. The oldest, aged fourteen, was able to help with the farm work. Fortune had dealt more severely with Sawang. Whenever he seemed about to get ahead, something came along to interfere. His mother gave all the family land to his younger sister instead of dividing it among the five children. Shortly after he started out on rented land, one of his buffalo died. His older daughter died at the age of four, and the family was left with only one child, a baby girl. When things went badly, Sawang drank a bit to console himself.

Diphtheria Strikes. In 1953 things began to look a little brighter for Sawang. A son was born and survived. The rain came early so that Sawang could plant his seed bed sooner than expected. And as a result he paid little attention when Prang, his little daughter now aged three, contracted a fever one evening just as transplanting was about to begin. She would be all right, he thought, and he quieted her with aspirin borrowed from Rim's house next door. But Prang did not recover on the second day, nor on the third. Rim and his wife both advised going to a doctor at the nearby market center of Minburi, three kilometers away. So Sawang paddled his daughter to Awn's store at the junction of the Bang Chan Canal and the highway between Bangkok and Minburi, and caught the bus for Minburi.

At the house of the doctor, Prang, still feverish, complained of a sore throat. The so-called doctor had been trained only as an army medical orderly but had gained a local reputation through many years of practice. He said Prang had typhoid fever, gave her an injection, and told Sawang to bring her back in a day or two. That evening she seemed no better; in fact, she could scarcely eat, and little white blisters appeared in her throat. Sawang felt anxious and took her back to the doctor in Minburi, but the servant said he had gone to Bangkok. On the way home Sawang asked a Chinese druggist in the market place to look at Prang and bought some white pills.

During the night Prang became still more fretful. She could eat nothing; she could not even swallow the little white pills. The next day friends advised Sawang to consult old Dr. Maw, a traditional practitioner living in the village. He would come when needed, and being an uncle of Sawang, would take a real interest in Prang. That evening Dr. Maw diagnosed the malady as "sang," a type of children's disease caused by a temporary loss of soul. Prang was afflicted by red sang and elephant sang combined. He made holy water and blew it at her as he uttered a magic formula. This would cool the fever. He painted her throat with lime and a little powdered betel nut to reduce the swelling. Then he sent the two home, advising their return if there was no improvement soon.

A week from the time Prang became sick, Rim's youngest boy who often played with Prang became feverish and had a sore throat, too. When Dr. Maw came to see Prang at Sawang's house, Rim's wife brought in her son for him to examine. Dr. Maw made some black paste and painted the boy's throat where it hurt, but the boy showed no improvement the next day. Rim talked the situation over with Awn, proprietor of the store. Both Awn and his wife recommended going to see the doctor in Minburi. The following day Rim visited the same doctor Sawang had consulted. He said the little boy had typhoid fever and he gave him an injection. Rim brought his son for an injection every day for three days. On the fourth day when the boy could no longer eat, the doctor told Rim that the symptoms had changed. It was no longer typhoid but diphtheria. The boy should be taken to the hospital in Bangkok as soon as possible. At Awn's store, Rim learned that the research staff was taking a man to the hospital in the morning; Rim and his son might come, too, instead of bumping along on the bus.

All assembled in the early morning for the trip, and soon they had passed through the clogged streets of Bangkok to the river where a ferryman rowed them across to the big hospital. In the waiting room Rim waited quietly for his turn with his son in his lap. The child was breathing with difficulty and gasped a bit. A passing doctor happened to hear the gasp, glanced at the child, snatched him into her arms, and rushed to the operating room. She plunged a knife into his windpipe, and the child took his first easy breath. A few minutes later she inserted a tube, administered an injection, and the patient was wheeled off to a bed in the ward.

Meanwhile, old Dr. Maw had taken Prang, her baby brother, and her mother to his home for closer care. In addition to sang, he felt Prang's case may have been aggravated by a spirit who was lingering near the house and had even attacked the doctor. The child would be safer under Dr. Maw's roof where his teacher's aegis protected the occupants. After a few days she could now eat a little boiled rice. So when Rim's son was taken to the hospital, Sawang felt optimistic enough to tell the critical gossips at Awn's store that Prang was better and did not have to be taken to Bangkok. Awn and his wife, however, counseled against waiting; they said that Prang had diphtheria, which was fatal unless the child received injections, but Sawang did not heed their advice.

Two days later Prang took a turn for the worse. She was listless and weak. Something new was attacking, for there was pronounced swelling in her lower abdomen and legs. Dr. Maw felt discouraged and recommended taking her to the hospital; in fact, he would take her there himself if Sawang would arrange transportation. Sawang met the research team the next morning as it came to the village. A few minutes later Sawang, Dr. Maw, and Prang were on their way to the hospital, but Prang died en route. The group turned back to Bang Chan with Prang on her father's lap. A few relatives were quickly summoned to help bring the little body to the temple for rites for the dead.

Prang's death crystallized the sentiments of the child's immediate relatives. Protagonists of traditional medicine may still have doubted the value of the new, but with Prang's death and the recovery of Rim's son as dramatic evidence, they could at least admit the possibility of an alternative. Before Prang's body had been placed in a coffin, people were worrying about the safety of the remaining members of the family, apparently accepting certain aspects of the modern concept of diphtheria. It was a disease recognizable by its symptoms; it was contagious; there were remedies. They eagerly sought information from the research team. The latter explained diphtheria as a child's disease and offered to take any child for injection to Minburi, where there was a government Health Center with a modern staff. The team was eager to introduce all to the Health Center under circumstances that might overcome their reluctance to utilize its facilities. Plans were laid to meet interested persons the following morning at Awn's store.

The turnout was disappointing, and the party waited for an hour hoping for latecomers. Sawang's wife came with two other sons of Rim, and an older sister of Sawang brought her daughter who had a sore throat. At the Center a researcher described the symptoms of the dead girl to the chief doctor, who agreed on the diagnosis and consented to inject the exposed children. A few minutes later the doctor returned from the storeroom and announced that the serum on hand was out of date. If the research group would buy some new serum in Bangkok, he would inject it at the Center.

An occidental member of the team then paid a call on the governmental district officer at Minburi. After hearing about the foregoing incidents, the district officer immediately assured his visitor that it would be unnecessary to purchase the serum; he would have it ordered from Bangkok. Furthermore, if the researchers would collect the children of Bang Chan, he would order enough serum to immunize them all as soon as the public health officer attached to the district office returned from a training course he was attending. He then apologized for the inefficiency of the Health Center, explaining that the chief doctor was very old and about to retire; that the district public health officer, however, was young, energetic, and able.

Events had taken an unexpected turn. Instead of the limited neighborhood immunization program visualized by the researchers, a communitywide program under official auspices was now planned. This new situation appeared to offer the opportunity not only to protect threatened lives but at the same time to disseminate certain important concepts about health and disease. The immediate job was that of arranging the time with the public health officer and spreading the word in Bang Chan.

The Immunization Campaign. The district office took immediate action. An order was sent to the Division of Communicable Disease in Bangkok for twenty 50 cc vials of diphtheria toxoid. The serum came from the laboratories of the Red Cross and was paid for by the district office making the request. The district officer himself visited the appropriate office in Bangkok and reported the negligence of the chief doctor at the center in not having fresh serum. On the following day this doctor came to Bangkok to fetch the supply of serum.

Within a few days the public health officer returned to find an immunization campaign waiting on his desk. A member of the research team offered to take him to Bang Chan. At Awn's store the public health officer doubted whether he was authorized to immunize children in all the surrounding hamlets, some of which were outside his jurisdiction. But Awn observed that germs know no boundaries; why should the doctor? The officer yielded and wrote letters to four headmen, three of whom were within, and one outside, his jurisdiction. A fifth, the headman of hamlet KY-5 (see sketch map), also outside the health office jurisdiction but a brother of Sawang, happened to witness the conversation. He said an official letter to him would be unnecessary; he would get out word anyway.

A researcher asked Awn to help spread the word, too, and during the coming days Awn busied himself speaking to people as they got on and off the buses in front of his store. Others who passed in their boats were hailed. The highway gang heard him as they picked up their boats to go home. There was no time for explanations; he just told them to bring their children the next Saturday for injections. Meanwhile, the headmen of the five hamlets sent out word. Some visited all the homes personally; others sent out word as people passed their house. Ordinarily the two local schools, one Thai and one Moslem, would have been alerted, but they were still closed for vacation.

On August 22 the public health officer began injections at Awn's store. The officer chose the store through considerations of accessibility and personal convenience. He had come alone, but a member of the research team volunteered to assist him. Boatloads of children had already arrived, even from hamlets that were not notified. Because this was the extremely busy season of rice transplanting, no one had time to come just to see the show. Many a preschool tot paddled his own boat to the scene, bringing a still younger brother or sister, although adults escorted them if they could. In describing the scene, Awn said that the first child grew frightened and began to cry before receiving his injection, with the result that all children cried, and his store rang with wails until the last child was injected. But mothers and aunts tried to soothe the little ones, and candy sold well that day. All were told to return the following week for a second injection.

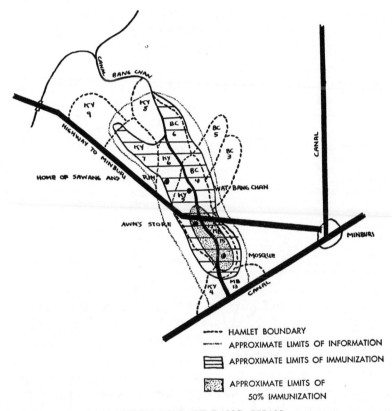

- - - - HAMLET BOUNDARY
- - - - APPROXIMATE LIMITS OF INFORMATION
▤ APPROXIMATE LIMITS OF IMMUNIZATION
▦ APPROXIMATE LIMITS OF
50% IMMUNIZATION

SKETCH MAP OF BANG CHAN
and neighboring hamlets showing effects of immunization announcement

Word was circulated again, and on August 29 even more children appeared. Since the schools had meanwhile opened, the headman of the Moslem hamlet (MB–15) directed the teacher to send all the school children. New children came to Awn's store, but many of the preceding week's children did not reappear. The public health officer announced that those who had not received a second injection should meet at the Minburi Health Center in a week for the final injection. At the Center one week later, although some children appeared, none came from Bang Chan.

Table 1 shows the number of children who came for injection on the two dates of immunization. The base population would ideally include all hamlets that received information. Since census data are not available for all 12 hamlets in the area, the data are grouped under two headings: eight hamlets for which census data are available and four for which they are not.

TABLE 1. CHILDREN APPEARING FOR IMMUNIZATION IN 12 BANG CHAN HAMLETS

Number of hamlets	Children injected				Population under age 15	
	August 22 only	August 29 only	Both times	Total	Number	Per cent immunized
Eight—Census data available	28	63	113	204	601	34
Four—Census data not available	3	8	8	19	19+	?
Total	31	71	121	223	620+	Under 36

Following the immunization, the research workers conducted a brief survey to uncover some of the factors underlying the pattern of community response to the immunization message. They had been struck by the limited and uneven response to what they had perceived as a dangerous crisis, and decided to take advantage of the unanticipated immunization program to further their research into the nature of community processes.

From the point of view of the research team, the immunization message was a rational communication that carried a compelling quality through its appeal both to logic and self-interest. Events had made it clear, however, that the message signified something else to the community. The survey undertook to uncover the factors that gave the original message a different coloration in the eyes of the community. For any such message to be effective, it must be received, understood, and acted on. These three factors

—reception, understanding, and compliance—depend in turn on certain characteristics of the community itself.

For a message to be adequately understood, it must correspond to a significant extent to the basic assumptions, attitudes, and values of the community. A Bang Chan farmer might react to a message in accordance with what he was doing when it arrived and the value he placed on that activity. For a message to be received, it must traverse available channels of communication. As sound travels farther through the earth than through the air, so a message may go different distances, depending on whether it is routed through children or adults, roads or canals, formal channels or word of mouth. For a message to be acted on, it has to carry the weight of respected and accepted authority. Different sources of a given message may have varying effects in producing action.

The Cultural Matrix of the Immunization Message

The Community of Bang Chan. On a map of Thailand, one cannot find Bang Chan. It is neither a unitary village nor a landmark, but an area of about three square miles in the flat central plain of Thailand. This area straddles the Bangkok-Minburi highway about 20 miles east of Bangkok and two miles west of Minburi, the regional market center and seat of the district government. The population of 1,700 is largely Buddhist. One hamlet, MB–15, with a small mosque contains only Moslem inhabitants, although a few Moslem families are scattered through other hamlets as well.

Practically everyone in the area is a rice farmer or laborer. About half the rice producers own their own land, and the rest rent, usually from landholders of the village. The bulk of the rice is sold to the Minburi mills for cash, but each grower holds enough for his own consumption. Fish caught in the canals and vegetables or fruits from the garden patch provide the additional necessary food. Although the community is largely self-sufficient, commodities such as cloth, kerosene, sugar, household utensils, roofing thatch, and lumber must be brought from outside the village.

From an airplane, the area of Bang Chan looks like an endlessly flat expanse of neatly diked paddy fields. Scattered throughout like islands in a sea are man-made groves of trees which shade from one to five houses. Next, one may notice a tiny canal leading between these groves, and if one follows its course, it may be seen to connect with others, which in turn connect with still others to form part of a vast network covering the whole central plain with waterways that are used for transport, for irrigation, and for domestic purposes.

Along one of the bigger canals one can distinguish taller trees, a kind of larch that towers above all the others, and one or two larger buildings with brightly colored roofs. This grove marks the Buddhist temple compound, or wat, which contains a school, a building for the sacred images, a meeting hall, accommodations for the priests, and an occasional store. To this temple as a center, people come paddling their skittish boats a mile or two with offerings for the priests. Here the children, three or four in their own boats, come to school, and adults pull up alongside the store to chat over a glass of coffee or to buy a few areca nuts on their way home. To the temple they bring their sons for ordination into the priesthood and their dead for cremation.

In this sense, the temple compound furnishes a center for community living, but it is a community with no fixed boundaries. As a center, it fades in importance as one passes toward other temples, schools, or stores. Perhaps the nearest American equivalent is the vanishing rural church, school, and general store at the crossroads.

Family Individualism. Like the American farmer, these people esteem the ideal of self-sufficiency of family units. In theory, each family provides entirely for its own members and cares for its own needs only. Because of the demands of rice farming, however, more hands are needed than on an American farm. Thus, the larger extended family living in its own compound offers a larger labor force than the single family unit, but even within a compound, land, houses, and tools may be owned individually. When labor demands exceed the supply, as in building a house, transplanting the rice seedlings to the field, or preparing for a large celebration, extra hands are brought in on a reciprocal basis. This picture of self-sufficiency often means that little is undertaken in the public interest.

Considerable contrast to this pattern of family individualism is found in the single Moslem hamlet, which in addition to the mosque contains a school for the children of the area. Intercourse with neighboring Buddhist hamlets proceeds in a friendly fashion with little self-consciousness, but the Moslem community has a tighter organization with its headmen and elders of the mosque than the Buddhist hamlets. A casual observer would note the better repaired bridges, the well-trimmed pathways, and above all, a new schoolhouse, recently built by concerted volunteer labor. This hamlet has recognized public responsibility and possesses some techniques to meet it on a local level. As noted, there are a few Moslem families in every hamlet. They keep in touch with each other through Friday meetings at the mosque.

Children are regarded as potential rather than immediate assets. Although loved, young children are considered difficult to handle; the completely obedient child stands as the ideal. Not until children are old enough to help with farming is their value partly recognized; in addition, sons may bring merit to the parents by becoming priests, daughters bring "milk money" at the time of marriage. By means of rites, exhortations, punishments, and material care, the Thai make sure that the infant will survive, the child remain uninjured, and the adolescent will not wander from home. After the first two or three years, sickness no longer signifies an important threat. At the same time, when a child dies despite all precautions, people do not bemoan their misfortune.

Sickness and Health in Bang Chan. The concepts of sickness and its treatment in Bang Chan reflect the wide cultural diversity of southeastern Asia, where influences from China, India, and the Indies converge. Both traditional and modern concepts are used to combat ill health. One may look in vain for an active quest of "good health" in the occidental sense. Sicknesses range from a vague series of essentially undiagnosed maladies to those whose symptoms are fairly well defined. Some diseases are attributed to malevolent spirits which attack unexpectedly for no particular reason or because taboos have been transgressed. In another group of sicknesses, attributed to sorcery, foreign objects are thought to enter the body by accident or malicious design. They cause intense abdominal pain which, under proper treatment, is relieved by passage of a foreign body with the feces.

Imbalance of the four basic elements—earth, wind, fire, and water—also produces disorder. The elements may get out of proportion so that fire dominates, producing fever; or winds may blow upward instead of in a circle through the body, producing belching, headaches, and dizziness. Some diseases, characterized by inflammation and swelling in the head and neck region, afflict children only; these are called "sang" and are associated with temporary loss of soul or with astral confluences, so that a child born on Sunday, for instance, is more susceptible to red inflammation. Village practitioners also speak of malaria, typhoid, cholera, and smallpox, although the symptoms would probably be recognized only in the more advanced stages and certainly not be understood in western terms.

Distress due to organic disturbance is not clearly distinguished from other kinds of human misfortunes. Traditional doctors may use some of the same general cures for a woman suffering as a result of the disappearance of her husband as one suffering from rheumatism or spirit possession. A man who is the victim of false accusations from his neighbors may be doused with holy water much as if he were afflicted by pains in the legs; holy water cools the heat of emotional as well as organic upset. Indeed, a person with sufficient merit from good deeds in present and past existences is likely to avoid misfortune, so that moral considerations enter the picture as well.

Yet the near-Buddha is rare whose virtue will protect him from all misfortune. Most people must depend on foreknowledge, protective devices, or curing after the damage has occurred. Individuals facing a critical period heed the advice of astrology and the portent of omens. Others fearing attack by man or beast wear amulets or have protective insignia tattooed on their chests; needles inserted under the skin offer permanent protection from wounds; some women seek to minimize labor pains by a small tattooed device; but against those things where man is powerless, he can only repair the damage.

When misfortune strikes in Bang Chan, the people initially posit a mundane cause; only when difficulties become aggravated are more cosmic and less optimistic explanations invoked. Colds, coughs, constipation, and diarrhea may strike even the most virtuous; these ailments generally pass unnoticed. If symptoms persist, however, family members may recommend an all-purpose tonic from the Chinese pharmacist. In certain children's diseases, parents may decide to let a top knot grow on the child's head by leaving an island of untrimmed hair on its scalp. For continuous crying or brief losses of consciousness, ritual techniques may be used to induce return of the soul stuff. More disturbing symptoms, however, call for help from either a traditional or modern practitioner, depending on the presumed nature of the sickness. By and large, people go first to their own local doctors rather than to the more expensive modern doctors.

How long a patient will remain under the care of a given doctor varies. Optimally, cure occurs in a day or two, but confidence does not necessarily diminish if progress is slow. Except where cutting or injecting is deemed necessary by preliminary diagnosis, people tend to view modern doctors as a secondary recourse, perhaps to be sought out after two or three traditional doctors have been tried. As symptoms persist and anxiety grows, people solicit the advice of other friends who may have had satisfactory experience with another doctor. Rarely does the traditional doctor consult another traditional doctor of his own accord, although sometimes he may recommend visiting a modern doctor. These in turn may invoke other recourses such as the modern hospitals of Bangkok. Then those who have submitted to some or all of these treatments without improvement or alleviation may blame sorcery or ponder the teachings of religion for consolation.

In Bang Chan approximately eight traditional doctors and about 15 traditional midwives practice their skills but earn their living primarily as farmers. In the Minburi market center live the four persons the villagers call doctors. Only one has received a complete medical training and can be considered a first-class doctor. The other three have had less formal training. The first-class doctor, a nurse-midwife, and a dentist form the staff of the Minburi Health Center. Under the Ministry of Public Health, this organization makes diagnoses and referrals but treats only the less acute illnesses. One or two beds serve the critically ill until they can be transported to a Bangkok hospital. Fees are low, and treatment can be free. Despite its official status, the Health Center is less popular than the more friendly second-class doctors of the market place. These men diagnose and treat freely the less critical cases, although they, too, refer patients with serious complaints to the Bangkok hospitals. Frequently they state their diagnoses in terms familiar to the farmers; they administer injections wherever possible and tend to ask relatively high fees for their services.

On the side of prevention, one sanitarian is attached to the district office as public health officer. He is particularly on the alert for communicable diseases, conducting regular immunizations in the schools of the district and taking such measures as are necessary to combat a particular threat. A single death due to plague recently brought him and a special staff from Bangkok into action to exterminate rats and fleas in the market place. There are government programs for improving sanitation, but since he is a lone worker in the district, his time for health education is necessarily limited.

The Standing of Modern Medicine. Concepts of modern medicine such as deficiencies, infection, and disturbances of growth are little understood in Bang Chan. The idea that drinking water may contain potentially harmful substances is foreign. Yet there is little active antagonism to modern medicine as such. For many years the people of Thailand have accepted ideas and practices from different cultures; resistance to western medicine does not arise from its foreign origin. Some regard surgery with apprehension because Buddhism forbids activities which threaten human life, but even this antagonism is disappearing as surgery continues to prove successful. Farmers go readily to hospitals to have lumps and growths removed. Stories are told in Bangkok of both patients and physicians who combine traditional and modern medical techniques.

The spread of modern medicine is slow because its ideas are strange and because people are slow to become alerted to the dangers of certain diseases. They have learned to fear cholera and typhoid, but not diphtheria. Moreover, children's sicknesses in general cause little alarm. The danger of diphtheria was recognized only by the families of the afflicted children. Nevertheless, previous contact with modern medicine facilitates acceptance of new ideas. The government immunization program in the schools plus the century-long activities of Christian missionaries equipped with Bible and smallpox vaccine have helped to implant the idea of preventive medicine. The people of Bang Chan have also accepted injections as beneficial. Indeed, a patient often visits a modern doctor anticipating an injection. But the farmers of Bang Chan do not yet distinguish between different kinds of injections; antibiotics and antitoxins are all the same as long as they come through syringe and needle.

Religious beliefs and attitudes also influenced response to the call for immunization. The Islamic hamlet responded more fully to the announcement than the Buddhist hamlets. In addition to this hamlet's greater integration, it is possible that Islam may offer a more favorable climate than Buddhism for the acceptance of modern medicine. Interview evidence indicates that Moslems make more frequent use of modern doctors than do the Buddhists.

For Islam the physical body contains both good and evil. Great stress is laid on purifying the body, and salvation consists in removing the corruption from both body and spirit. Buddhism, on the other hand, considers the body a source of contamination for the soul. One may purify the soul by prayer and discipline, but the body remains a continuous handicap. Thus, Islam not only heeds the body, but in its concept of corruption possesses ideas congenial to modern theories of disease. In both religions, pain is a lesser evil than it is for occidentals, but Islam links pain with sin, which may be overcome by prayer, pilgrimage, or other means. For Buddhism, pain is in part the inevitable product of cosmic retribution for past misconduct.

Like the West, Islam distinguishes more clearly between the moral order and natural order of the cosmos, while Buddhism perceives a greater interdependence of the two. Furthermore, in Islam as well as in the West, man appears to be granted greater freedom to act upon his world. On the basis of such considerations, we would expect Islam to present a more fertile basis than Buddhism for the acceptance of modern medicine.

All the foregoing facets of Bang Chan culture combined to form the backdrop against which the call for immunization was seen by local people and to set the attitudes of the farmer who was suddenly told to have his children report for immunization. He was hard at work at rice planting during the critical transplanting phase of the community's basic subsistence activity. Sending children off in a boat meant cessation of work in the fields; it also meant disrupting a laboriously arranged cooperative work party. The Bang Chan farmer was heir to a tradition of individualistic rather than collective methods for coping with disease; diseases of childhood were customarily regarded with relatively little concern, and his children were neither sick nor visibly threatened. His attitude to disease in general was essentially more passive than active, with Buddhism fostering a relatively fatalistic attitude toward the outcome of illness. He was unfamiliar with diphtheria and what it meant and not well informed on general concepts of contagion and immunization.

In addition to these aspects of Bang Chan culture that influenced the reception of the immunization call, immunizations were customarily given in school by a public health officer, not at a store, and information involving health programs for children was generally disseminated via the school system. The practical matter of how and through what channels information could and did reach people also contributed to the pattern of response.

Channels of Communication

When the rains come to Bang Chan, the canals fill with water. From the dyked fields travel turns to the canals. Every morning priests glide to the households and wait silently for offerings. Men, women, and children pole their boats with bundles of seedlings to be planted. Along these same routes come vendors from the market center in Minburi to hawk their wares.

These geographical channels of communication may be seen on the map. As the dotted line indicates, information about immunization moved up the side canals from the main canal. In this boating community, canals provide better avenues of information than highways. The map also shows that the political divisions between hamlets scarcely impeded the flow of information; gaps between clusters of houses are probably more effective barriers.

There are social as well as geographical channels. The Buddhist temple is such a channel. During most of the year the priests go out into the area to collect alms, and people come to the temple with holiday offerings. But at transplanting time, only a few old people visit the temple. At such times the mosque is a better channel than the temple, since Moslems take time off to attend services regardless of season. The schools, too, provide a channel for reaching the community, especially the families of school children. Within the hamlet, the headman is expected to pass on official communications from the district officer to all households. The stores also spread information, despite the fact that business decreases during the planting season. Lastly, a message given to any one of a group of kinsmen or neighbors will reach most members of that group.

Several of these social channels were utilized to convey the announcement of immunization. Some of the headmen had been officially reached by the district health officer. Schools resumed during the second week of immunization, and the Moslem school (in MB–15) was notified by the hamlet headman. Finally Awn, from his store at the junction of the highway and the main canal, hailed passersby who in turn carried the message to kinsmen and neighbors. Neither the temple nor the mosque was utilized to spread information.

Can the relative effectiveness of these channels be compared? One might assume that the number of children coming for immunization reflected the effectiveness of the particular channel used. Such an assumption needs strong qualification, particularly in view of the distinction between receiving information and acting upon it. However, if the strength of motivation to respond to the message is held relatively constant, the effectiveness of the different channels of information may be compared. The distance of any area from Awn's store provides a rough index of motivation, for the time and pains required to paddle children by boat to Awn's store was one important deterrent to heeding the announcement.

TABLE 2. NUMBER OF IMMUNIZED CHILDREN LIVING AT VARYING
DISTANCES FROM AWN'S STORE

Distance from Awn's store to center of hamlet	Hamlets	Children injected	Children in hamlets	Per cent injected	Per cent range by hamlet
0 to 1 km	2	87	181	48	37–59
1 to 2 km	3	87	173	50	19–92
2 to 3 km	3	30	247	12	0–20

The foregoing table shows that distance from place of immunization does not correlate well with response to the announcement. The wide range of percentages from the various hamlets, particularly those lying at the middle distances, suggests that other factors were involved in the response. By holding distance constant, however, we may be able to isolate some of the features influencing the effectiveness of communication.

Table 3 indicates the effectiveness of the headmen as agents of communication by comparing the response in hamlets where headmen announced the immunization with response in hamlets where they did not announce it. In the latter hamlets, those responding to the call received the news directly from Awn or from a neighbor or kinsman. Distance is held constant in the two groups of hamlets.

TABLE 3. PERCENTAGE IMMUNIZED IN HAMLETS AT VARYING DIS-
TANCES FROM AWN'S STORE ACCORDING TO WHETHER
NOTIFIED BY HEADMAN OR NOT

Distance of hamlet from Awn's store	Per cent immunized in hamlets notified by headmen	Per cent immunized in hamlets not notified by headmen
0 to 1 km	48 (KY–5, BC–4)	—
1 to 2 km	66 (MB–15, KY–6)	19 (BC–5)
2 to 3 km	20 (BC–6)	8 (KY–7, KY–8)

Although the percentages should not be taken too literally, they suggest that headmen were more effective as channels of communication than informal circulation of information through neighbors.

Some evidence is available for comparing the relative effectiveness of headmen and schools. It will be recalled that the headman of one hamlet notified the Moslem school after the first immunization on August 22. By comparing the number of children immunized from this hamlet on the two occasions (Table 4), one gets some indication of the comparative strength of these two channels.

TABLE 4. NUMBER AND PERCENTAGE OF CHILDREN FROM HAM-
LET MB–15 DURING TWO IMMUNIZATION SESSIONS

Immunization date	Children immunized	Per cent of all children in hamlet
August 22	34	58
August 29	53	92

The comparison suggests that teachers were more effective than headmen in conveying this kind of information. Such a conclusion is in agreement with the fact that child immunization was associated, in the minds of the people, with the schools. Circumstances did not permit similar comparison in the larger school at the Buddhist temple, since the teachers were not asked to announce the immunization.

We may conclude that the schools of Bang Chan provided the best potential channels for disseminating health information involving children; they were better than the headmen and certainly better than Awn's persistent personal efforts.

Weight of the Message

Previous sections have reviewed factors obstructing reception of the immunization message. We have seen, however, that a rough third of the children in Bang Chan did appear for immunization, and that in one hamlet as many as 92 per cent of the children were immunized. How are we to account for the children that did respond to the call? If we return again to the content of the message, we will recall that it contained several items of information and an implied order.

It could be said that the diphtheria immunization message was fully communicated if the following information were conveyed: Rim's son had been afflicted by a contagious disease known to modern medicine and had been cured with the aid of modern

medicine; Prang, without the aid of modern medicine, had died
of the same disease; this disease could attack other children and
cause them to die; a specific medicine to prevent this disease
would be available at a certain time and place at no cost to the
recipient.

As already indicated, this entire message was transmitted to the
district officer at Minburi and relayed by him to the district
public health officer. But the letters which the public health
officer sent to the hamlet headmen contained only the bald instruction to announce the time and place of immunization without further explanation. Thus, only the bare announcement came
through official channels, and Awn, too, only shouted what he
could to passing boatmen.

Who, then, heard of the recovery of Rim's son, of Prang's
death, and of the contagious character of the disease? The survey
showed that this information remained within the group of relatives and neighbors of Rim and Sawang. To be sure, there were
others who heard this news if they happened to stop at Awn's
store long enough for a chat. But these were few, and they remembered only fragments of what they heard: "Yes, I did hear
that Sawang's child died. . . . No, I didn't hear what caused
it," or "No, no one said anything about Rim's boy; was he sick?"
This kind of information failed to circulate widely; it lacked news
interest. The death of a child is not a rare event.

Obviously, few gained a sense of urgency from the information
they received, and so far as the survey could discover, no one
undertook to inquire the reasons for the immunization announcement. What then was the weight of an announcement stemming
from the district office? By what kinds of authority and under
what conditions are the people of Bang Chan induced to act?

For most Thai, the government appears as a remote and powerful agency symbolized by the revered figure of the king. Although absolute monarchy was replaced in 1932 by a constitu-
tionally limited monarchy, decisions are still made at the top
level without consulting the ruled. Government with its police,
conscription, registration, and collection of taxes has intruded
increasingly into the life of the farmers, but the idea of social
services or of governmental agencies aiding the individual is thus

far weakly developed. Certainly the idea of the rights and privileges of citizenship has yet to come to Bang Chan.

The district officer at Minburi is the nearest representative of this government, and in the past few decades, district officers have helped to introduce elementary education, water control, immunization against epidemic disease, and other programs. At monthly meetings district officers may direct people through their headmen to register their children's names, to plant gardens, or to send their sons to the recruiting office. Although the farmers have generally approved the agricultural aid programs, orders imposing taxes and conscription have made them wary. They have learned to scrutinize orders carefully, to inquire about penalties and govern their conduct accordingly.

Over the years the district office has increased its authority considerably. This expansion has been effected largely at the expense of the headmen. Formerly headmen kept the peace and arbitrated quarrels, but the police have now taken over this job. People know the headman to be the lowest member of the governmental hierarchy with little power to communicate popular desires upward, and the headman recognizes that he lacks authority to implement orders from above. As a result, his personality and local reputation largely determine his efficacy in performing his official duties.

Now in fact, the immunization announcement came not from the district officer, but from the public health officer. The headmen have had far less contact with him than with the district officer, and certainly recognize fewer bonds of personal attachment. Although the health officer's official status and relation to the district officer gave some weight to the announcement, the immunization order he issued was backed by little personal authority. Hence, some headmen executed their orders perfunctorily.

In the two hamlets nearest Awn's store, 59 per cent and 37 per cent, respectively, of the children were immunized. The headman in the former hamlet, a kinsman of Rim and Sawang, personally visited all homes in his hamlet. He knew the full tale of the diphtheria incident and was personally esteemed as genial, industrious, and responsible. The headman in the other hamlet, preoccupied with his own affairs, delegated the announcement to a boy. Only in one hamlet did the headman succeed in bettering the figure of 59 per cent, namely, the more tightly organized Moslem hamlet where the schools gave additional weight to the order. In other hamlets where headmen did not receive official orders, persons questioned stated that since no official order was received, it was assumed that participation by that particular hamlet was not necessary.

In some respects, Awn's position was stronger than that of the headmen. His age and past experience as a successful farmer, as well as his present position as a successful storekeeper and amiable host, gave him considerable influence. With broad patronage in the hamlets, he could grant favors as well as solicit them. Yet he lacked official authority to issue orders, and some people may have suspected he was drumming up business for his own store. For whatever reason, his influence contributed little to the attendance of those beyond the circle of his own kinsmen.

The majority of farmers regarded the message as an official order, but one more like an exhortation to plant pineapples than a command to report for registration. The message lacked teeth, so that its imperative resounded gently. Further, with most of its informational substance stripped away, little sense of urgency was communicated. Since children were ordinarily injected at school, parents may have wondered why the public health officer did not wait a few days and go to the school instead of suddenly asking everyone to bring the children to Awn's store. It was a long way to travel during a season of rice transplanting. Yet like any response to a request, if it were not too troublesome, if a boat could be borrowed in which grandmother could take the children, it would be better to go, particularly so if neighbors sent their children.

It is thus evident that the pattern of response to the immunization announcement was determined primarily by the pattern of response to authority. The immunization message had become translated into a routine order whose weight depended largely on the personal position and energy of the headman. Where no direct order was issued, the message itself had little capacity to impel compliance. Where orders were issued, compliance depended on a complex of factors, including the influence of the headman who issued the order.

The reasons behind Bang Chan's pattern of response to the immunization message may now be summarized. (1) Prevailing attitudes toward the health of children, especially during the season of heavy agricultural work, predisposed the majority of farmers to disregard the announcement of immunization. (2) The officially notified headmen spread the news fairly effectively, but a school announcement of immunization was more effective. (3) The weight of the announcement was greater: (a) when the school circulated the information, since schools customarily oversee affairs of children and have a routine immunization program for certain diseases; (b) where the population was better acquainted with the threat of an epidemic; (c) where headmen responded more energetically to the notification by the district health officer; (d) where there was greater inclination to obey official orders from the district office. (4) Except for the kinsmen of the two children afflicted with diphtheria, the events described had little or no effect on popular attitudes toward modern medicine.

IMPLICATIONS

Health Information and the Communication Process

The history of Bang Chan's immunization message focuses attention on a number of salient aspects of the communication process. It will be recalled that the research staff felt that an unexpected tragedy—the death of Prang—could be turned to advantage if wisely handled. A child treated by traditional methods had died of diphtheria; another treated by modern methods had been saved. This story with its dramatic contrast, if made known, could serve two useful purposes. First, it could underscore the danger of a contagious disease and heighten interest in bringing children for immunization. Second, it could increase familiarity with modern medicine and thus have a lasting educational effect.

As it developed, however, neither of these two objectives was attained. Although a substantial number of parents did send their children to be immunized, investigation showed that they did so mainly because they had been told to send them. The hoped-for educational impact of the incident proved to be negligible: the incident failed to convey new knowledge about modern medicine or to induce compliance with a simple order. How was an apparently excellent opportunity for getting across an important message converted into a virtual failure? Part of the answer may be found in the complexities of the communication process.

For a message to have any real effect, as we have seen, it must be received, it must be understood, and it must be perceived as cogent and reasonable. For each of these aspects of communication, the nature of the community and of its culture can be of critical importance. The community and its culture act as a series of filters through which any communicated message must pass if it is to be received and understood.

As shown by the fate of Bang Chan's immunization message, the reception of a health message is significantly influenced by prevailing attitudes, beliefs, and cultural predispositions. To most Americans—and to the members of the research team as well—the terms "diphtheria," "contagion," "exposed children" signaled an emergency. To the residents of Bang Chan, none of these words signaled danger, since disease in general does not provoke comparable alarm. These attitudes are related to the widely held view that disease is controlled in part by cosmic forces which ordain cure or continuing illness. Human action can be effective only within given limits. Children's diseases are not regarded with particular concern, in contrast to the attitudes of most American parents. Although the ideas of contagion and immunization had gained some currency in Bang Chan as a result of past experience, neither of these ideas had become associated with the idea of diphtheria, which remained a new and unfamiliar concept. The climate of receptivity in Bang Chan was very different from that which would prevail in a typical American community.

Although the particular features of the cultural predisposition cited above are peculiar to Bang Chan and to much of Thailand, the same principle prevails in any community. No message falls on the unsullied ear of logic. In all societies it must pass through a series of cultural screens—attitudes, assumptions, beliefs—from which it emerges in a form often unrecognizable to those who originated it. In Bang Chan a major effect of this system of screens was to strip away portions of the message which appeared crucial to its originators, but which the cultural climate of Bang Chan apparently defined as insignificant or of negligible import. In another situation, prevailing attitudes might add to a message new content that would inaccurately augment or entirely distort its meaning.

A consideration more tangible than the general state of cultural receptivity to a communicated message is the set of physical channels of communication available in any given community. By what medium or media will word reach people most quickly and most effectively? The answer to this question can only be found in the set of conditions found in a particular community. In Bang Chan word passed more effectively along the canals than over the roads, and a message transmitted through official channels penetrated farther and more convincingly than information disseminated by word of mouth. Elsewhere, other channels may serve better to spread a similar message. Modern media of communication such as the newspaper, radio, or telephone were not available in Bang Chan, but even in communities where such facilities are available, more traditional methods may still be superior. In each community the adequacy of a communication channel can be discovered only by systematic local investigation.

Many health messages aim, directly or indirectly, to arouse some sort of action. The source of the message and the route it travels can be of great importance in influencing compliance. The Bang Chan experience showed that the official transmission of a message can involve hidden pitfalls. Although the health officer was the logical official to originate the immunization order, his authority was not nearly so well established as that of the district officer, whose domain, however, did not officially and directly involve health. While the message was routed through the health officer, compliance would in all likelihood have been greater had the district officer assumed direct responsibility. In addition, a message involving the health of children would have been more effectively communicated if transmitted by the teachers. This might not have held true, for example, in the case of a message involving the inoculation of cattle.

In addition, it is important to be apprised of possible discontinuities in the chain of command or weaknesses in a system of authority. The health officer passed the immunization message through the headmen, but these local officers, once influential, now constitute a weak appendage to the growing system of governmental officials. Because the headmen's authority has been weakened by new trends, the force of the message depended in large part on the degree of respect commanded by the headmen as individuals rather than as officials.

The reception given to a health message may thus be influenced by the position of officials who transmit it and popular attitudes toward them. A good working knowledge of the channels of communication and the system of authority in any particular community is an important prerequisite to the successful communication of health information.

"Felt Needs" in a Crisis Situation

The Bang Chan immunization incident, in addition to raising problems concerning the mechanics of communication and the execution of an emergency program, also raised some rather difficult policy questions. Insofar as our research staff functioned in an action capacity, we were committed on principle to a policy involving the concept of "felt needs." In brief, we believed that no measure should be imposed on the people of a community unless they themselves requested it or were able to recognize its desirability. If a community were unable to see the wisdom of a measure we regarded as beneficial, our aim would be to help the people, by slow and careful educational methods, to realize the value of the measure.

The outbreak of diphtheria faced us with a dilemma. There was little "felt need" for diphtheria immunization. The disease did not signal danger to the parents, immunization was not seen by them as an appropriate preventive measure, and the community in general was not very receptive to any widescale cooperative program involving the children. However, since we perceived in the situation a danger not recognized by the community, we relaxed our self-imposed limitation of acting only in response to popular demand. Had we adhered strictly to our limitation, we might have considered our duty discharged when injections had been received by the children of those families actually wishing to have their children immunized. As it was, we exceeded our limitation only to the extent of activating the machinery of district and local government by calling attention to the emergency. Moreover, if we regard the official system of authority as falling within the framework of the local community, it becomes difficult to say whether or not we were responding to the felt needs of the community. In any case, we did not relax our limitations sufficiently to conduct an educational program which might both have immunized more children and left behind an understanding of diphtheria for the future. Did we go too far, or did we not go far enough?

We faced but did not solve an issue that must frequently confront health workers. Should a health worker strive primarily to ameliorate a situation that appears to him as urgent or dangerous —but does not appear so to the people—at the expense of violating the ideals of voluntary consent and free choice? Or should he rather strive first and foremost to realize these ideals, on the assumption that no end, however humanitarian, justifies coercive methods? When humanitarianism dictates firmness, should democratic ideals be sacrificed? Or should a prime regard for the expressed needs and wishes of the people take precedence over considerations of expediency?

SUMMARY

In a rice-farming community on the central plains of Thailand, two children were stricken with diphtheria. One died; the other was saved by modern doctors. When this information was conveyed to the district office, a day was set for the immunization of children and announced to their parents. About one-third of the available children were immunized by the public health officer. What factors determined the pattern of response to the call for immunization?

Answers to this query were discussed in terms of the social and cultural milieu of the community. By and large, the farmers of the community are individualists who usually pay little attention to disease in general, and to children's diseases in particular. There are no modern doctors in the immediate area, and people utilize their services only when traditional medicine has failed. They were not alarmed by the appearance of the disease. It was the rice-planting season, and they were exceedingly busy.

With this background, few were disposed to send children for immunization even though they knew of the opportunity. Information on diphtheria and the immunization announcement were transformed into bald official directives and circulated through the headmen rather than the more customary channel for dealing with child health offered by the schools. Few learned of the death of a child or understood the danger of possible contagion from the disease. Most parents who did have their children immunized responded largely to the authority of the headmen, public health officer, and other governmental officials; they did not act out of a sense of danger.

In such a setting, it is the task of health education to increase understanding of modern medical concepts and not just to show how modern medicine may satisfy the expressed wants of the people.

SELECTED REFERENCES

Benedict, Ruth, *Thai Culture and Behavior*. Cornell University Southeast Asia Program, Data Paper no. 4, Ithaca, 1952. Thai family life, child-rearing, and value structure are interpreted on the basis of interviews with educated Thai.

Crosby, Josiah, *Siam: The Crossroads*. Hollis and Carter, London, 1945. These memoirs and interpretations of events witnessed during a lifetime with the British foreign service reveal some changes during the present century up to World War II. The book richly characterizes state affairs and leading personalities of the day.

DuBois, Cora, *Social Forces in Southeast Asia*. University of Minnesota, Minneapolis, 1949. Chapters 2 and 3 succinctly and panoramically depict the operation of republicanism, population changes, western technology, and economic weakness in altering the countries of southeast Asia.

Embree, John F., "Thailand—A Loosely Structured Social System," *American Anthropologist*, vol. 52, April–June, 1950, pp. 181–193. This description of individual goals, social duties, and obligations draws particularly on experiences in Bangkok. The author is struck by discrepancies between stated rule and behavior, between expressed obligation and its fulfillment.

Landon, Kenneth P., *Siam in Transition*. University of Chicago Press, 1939. Although not a current publication, this book remains one of the finest all-round sources on Thailand.

Sharp, Lauriston, Hazel M. Hauck, Kamol Janlekha, Robert B. Textor, *Siamese Rice Village:* A Preliminary Study of Bang Chan, 1948–1949. Cornell University Southeast Asia Program, Bangkok and Ithaca, N. Y., 1953. The community where the diphtheria immunization occurred is broadly described. Section III considerably amplifies the health data briefly mentioned in the present essay.

Zimmerman, Carle C., *Siam:* Rural Economic Survey, 1930–31. Ministry of Commerce and Communications, Bangkok, 1931. Along with the economic conclusions from a survey for improving rural conditions are chapters on health and diet.

PART III

SEX PATTERNS
AND POPULATION PROBLEMS

Case 7

BIRTH CONTROL CLINICS IN CROWDED PUERTO RICO

by J. Mayone Stycos

During the past few centuries a technological revolution has trans-formed the western world. In much of Europe and North America three linked consequences of this transformation have emerged: an increase in the material standards of living, a sharp decrease in infant mortality, and an ethic justifying the limitation of family size. It has been easier to export to other nations the technical means for reducing infant mortality rates than to export either the means for elevating living standards or the practice of controlling births. The resulting population imbalance in various parts of the world may be only a transitional phase, but in the meantime govern-ments are under pressure to do something concrete about bringing resources and population into better alignment. Puerto Rico is trying out all the means at its disposal, including the dissemination of birth control methods.

*Built into the cultural systems of all societies are sets of values aimed directly or indirectly at encouraging human reproduction and discouraging unnecessary death. No society could long survive without these values. Hence, technical assistance to save lives tends to run with the cultural grain, while efforts to restrict reproduction often run against it. As one of the directors of the Family Life Project in Puerto Rico, Dr. Stycos con-ducted a survey among members of the lower-income group to discover what values, motives, and communication barriers impeded the success of the birth control campaign. This case is not intended to pass judgment on the propriety of birth control; its objective is to disclose processes of family life and draw attention to the system of cultural checks and balances by which societies attempt to regulate their fertility rates.—*EDITOR

THE PROBLEM

The Ineffectiveness of a Population Control Program

To the student of population, the field of public health presents a curious paradox; its very successes, in some parts of the world, have been self-defeating. In those areas where high death rates have for centuries reduced the number of people competing for scarce goods, public health measures, by reducing these death rates, have vastly multiplied social problems by creating new mouths to feed, new organisms to care for, new demands on struggling economies. Wherever a population grows much faster than its economy—and this is frequently the case in the present-day world—starvation, ill health, and political unrest are specters on the horizon.

Puerto Rico is a good case in point, for it illustrates how effective public health measures can create dangerous problems in a short span of time. In many ways Puerto Rico is subject to less drastic effects than other areas, for it has a very advantageous position politically, geographically, and economically in reference to the United States. However, if we can understand what is happening in Puerto Rico, despite its many advantages, we will have a good idea of how easily even greater problems can occur in other underdeveloped areas of the world.

When the United States took possession of Puerto Rico at the turn of this century, the island had fewer than a million inhabitants; at the present time, with scant natural resources and a per capita income half that of Mississippi, its population has increased to more than two and a quarter millions, despite heavy emigration. Only about half the land is arable, and the present number of people per square mile is roughly 15 times that of the United States.

This amazing increase in population has been brought about by spectacular declines in mortality, largely as a result of effective public health work. At the turn of the century, births were occurring annually at the rate of 40 per thousand, and deaths at the rate of about 25 per thousand, creating a relatively modest rate of increase. The birth rate is still around 40—twice that of the United States—but the death rate has dropped to 10, roughly that of the continental United States. At this rate of increase, assuming no migration, the island would have approximately nine million inhabitants in another fifty years! The sharp drop in mortality has been largely accomplished in the short span of two decades and is not hard to explain. Deaths due to diseases such as diarrhea, enteritis, pneumonia, tuberculosis, and malaria have been greatly and rapidly reduced, as a result of improvements in sanitation, transportation, and public health.[1]

[1] These data have been drawn from Davis, Kingsley, "Puerto Rico: A Crowded Island," *Annals of the American Academy of Political and Social Science*, vol. 285, January, 1953, pp. 116–122.

But population increase is not inherently detrimental and must be judged in relation to a nation's resources. If the economy can expand as rapidly as the population, the nation will at least be no worse off than previously. How has Puerto Rico fared? Favored by United States federal benefits, American military installations, American citizenship, which facilitates emigration, American capital and know-how, it is also blessed by a stable government and far-sighted leadership. The government has invested its revenues in a broad program of industrialization aimed at providing more nonagricultural jobs for the population. These efforts have added 80 new industries with 14,000 employees to the economy within the past decade. But the impact of this formidable accomplishment is largely vitiated by the fact that *every year* there are 16,000 new entrants into the labor force. Thus, the gains of industrialization have largely been eaten up by a growing population. This is not to mention the strains placed on the educational and health facilities of the island, which cannot keep pace with the snowballing population.

Very much aware that the island's program of development and industrialization was being undermined by a too rapidly expanding population, the government of Puerto Rico set up, in 1939, a network of 160 birth control clinics. Part of the extensive facilities of insular public health, these clinics are staffed by regular members of public health units, provided with contraceptives, and empowered to provide both information and free materials to all individuals who meet broadly interpreted medical criteria. The clinics carry condoms, diaphragms, creams, jellies, and sponges; are open for an afternoon or two a week; and are well located in both rural and urban areas of the small island. Despite this seemingly ideal setup, the clinics have as yet had no significant effect on the birth rate. In the first place, they are not used by most of the population—in 1950 the clinics showed 15,410 active cases—nor do the statistics over the past decade indicate any strong trend toward increasing use. Second, as we will explain, even those who acquire materials from the clinics do not use them systematically and carefully.

Why do the Puerto Ricans fail to take advantage of these readily available services, in light of the fact that more effective birth control would help substantially to relieve evident and pressing difficulties?

THE SITUATION

The Human Factors Behind Resistance to Birth Control

A research project designed in part to discover the reasons for the ineffectiveness of the clinics was set up in 1951, under the auspices of the Family Life Project, Social Science Research Center, University of Puerto Rico. Seventy-two couples in the lower-income groups were interviewed on courtship, marriage, child-rearing, and birth control. Husband interviews consumed about two hours, and wife interviews about four. Interviews were conducted by Puerto Rican personnel with academic and professional backgrounds in the social sciences and social work. Four women and two men were intensively trained in depth interviewing techniques for two weeks prior to field work. Using a flexible interview form, the team took verbatim notes in the presence of the respondents.[1] A full report of this study is contained in the author's forthcoming book, *Family and Fertility in Puerto Rico*.

The following sections will summarize the factors found to underlie the Puerto Ricans' reluctance to use the services of the birth control clinics. The findings fall into three general categories: attitudes toward family size, explicit and implicit objections to birth control practice, and the communication of birth control information.

Large Families or Small

An obvious reason for the Puerto Ricans' failure to use birth control would be that they are not interested in small families. If this were so, the public health program would have little effect unless accompanied by an educational campaign to stir up interest in smaller families. There is, however, evidence that some interest in reducing family size does exist. In a 1948 poll of 13,000 randomly selected Puerto Ricans, over three-quarters of

[1] For detailed accounts of interviewer training, see Stycos, J. Mayone, "Interviewer Training in Another Culture," *Public Opinion Quarterly*, vol. 16, Summer, 1952, pp. 236–246.

those interviewed stated that a family of three or fewer children is ideal.[1] The writer's own case studies of 72 lower-class families reveal a similar interest in small families. Here are the remarks of a mother with two years of schooling:

> If one is poor he shouldn't have more than two children. The rich can have more because they have money to educate them and do not sacrifice or even kill themselves working as the poor do. For the rich, they are even a recreation; for the poor man they are always a burden. The rich care better for the children, but it's a great task for the poor; and the wife of the poor man gets sick with many children, because she can't feed herself well nor have the proper medicines if she needs them. So two is enough.

Such attitudes are common. Parents feel that it is a burden to have many children; it requires hard work; it is a drain on family finances; and it is felt to be detrimental to health. This is not to say that children are not appreciated, for in general they are regarded with affection. It indicates rather that there is a growing awareness of the disadvantages of having a large number of children.

Evidently, then, there does exist sentiment in favor of small families. However, other motivations serve to foster the continuance of large families. For example, Puerto Ricans still say that children can help them in their old age, and that having a lot of children is a kind of social security that will pay dividends in later years. There is much less basis for this belief today than formerly, but many Puerto Ricans continue to believe it, or want to believe it—and the belief runs counter to the expressed desire for small families.

Again, while nearly everyone claims to want a small family, hardly anyone thinks of delaying the first pregnancy. One reason for this is the male fear of sterility. Lower-class Puerto Rican men are very conscious of their virility, and try to manifest it in different ways. One way is having children, and a married man without children is laughed at. Although men ordinarily have sexual experiences before marriage, these encounters are usually with prostitutes. Only by marrying and having children can men

[1] Hatt, Paul K., *Backgrounds of Human Fertility in Puerto Rico*. University Press, Princeton, 1952, Table 37, p. 53.

give manifest "proof" of virility. Most of the men in our sample said they were eager to have their first child. These are some of their explanations:

> A man feels more man when he knows he can make a child.
>
> I was anxious to have my first child to see if I was sterile or not, because one has to avoid children with other women before marriage.
>
> This business of being married and having no children looks bad. One likes to have them to prove he is not barren.

Having a child is also a kind of initiation into the community of adults. Without children, a man is still a youth, or worse, only half a man.

> My brother-in-law, who is only sixteen, got married, had a child, and his wife is now pregnant again. When he fights with other men people tell him he is not a man, he is only sixteen. But he tells them, "Well, I have children, I am a complete man."

In the Puerto Rican lower classes there are very few ways in which a man can "show off." It is almost impossible for him to accumulate capital or to buy those luxuries that would prove him to be better off than his fellows. Annual per capita income is about $400. In 1951–1952 approximately 15 per cent of the total labor force was unemployed each month, and for most agricultural workers, who represent about a third of the labor force, employment is obtainable only during harvest periods. Perhaps as a consequence of this scarcity of material goods, men put high emphasis on having children as a sign of superiority. Once a man has proved that he is not sterile, he may go on to show that he is "more man" than his neighbors by producing more children than they. Thus, keeping up with the Joneses may mean having as many children as they, and being able to keep them alive.

> My husband likes it when another baby is coming, for he feels more male if he has many.
>
> A large family helps to prove the manliness of a person. It takes a real man to maintain and educate a large family.

There is still another factor that encourages large families. As in many cultures where the double standard of sexual behavior prevails, men are extremely jealous of their wives, and wives are very unsure and suspicious of their husbands. There is some realistic justification for these feelings, for there is in fact a great deal of desertion and extramarital activity. Even so, the emotional reaction to such occurrences is unusually intense. These strong sentiments have an effect on attitudes toward family size. Both men and women feel that having a large number of children ties down their spouses and helps to keep them faithful. This technique works better for holding a woman than a man, but the illustrations below show that women as well as men are well aware of it.

> He told me the more kids I have the more tied to him I was . . . that with so many kids I could not abandon him to go with another man or return to my family.
> By having children they know that their wives are obliged to stay at home while they can go out after other women.

In one case this policy was carried out quite methodically. The story was told independently by both husband and wife. The husband told the interviewer that he had wanted no children at all and was then asked why he had just had one.

> Because I got angry with my wife. Her mother took her to town and got her work as a servant. Later she came back to me full of love, and I forgave her so she stopped working. I had that child so that she couldn't go away any more. Having a child she was bound to stay.

Thus, even though individuals say they prefer small families, there are other forces operative in Puerto Rican culture that work at cross-purposes. Along with the expressed preference for small families one finds attitudes, beliefs, and practices that support the traditional custom of having large families.

Objection to Birth Control

Birth Control and the Church. As in other Catholic countries, the church in Puerto Rico officially opposes birth control. However, most people do not regard church opposition as a reason for not controlling family size. In the extensive survey conducted by Paul Hatt, 87 per cent of those interviewed claimed the right to limit family size if they so wished; other studies in Puerto Rico showed that specifically religious reasons for not practicing birth control are those least frequently cited. For the Puerto Rican lower classes Catholicism is in considerable part a series of rituals that are combined with social festivals, and a cult of saints to bring good fortune. People are aware of the attitude of the church, but many tend to disregard it.

> The Catholic religion says it's a sin to use birth control, but I think it's a greater sin if (the children) don't eat.
>
> The church forbids birth control, but if one has many children the church is not going to support them.

Our own survey showed that the few respondents who did cite church opposition as a reason for objecting to birth control were those with the smallest families; they had not yet felt any real need for birth control practice. Church opposition has even served to foster interest in birth control:

> A pastoral letter, read in all the churches in one region, denouncing a newly established mountain clinic which had performed a number of sterilizations, generated most effective word-of-mouth advertising. . . . The clinic was swamped with demands for information concerning the operation which the Bishop had denounced.[1]

If most lower-class Puerto Ricans do not regard church opposition as a deterrent, they do raise other serious objections to birth control: it undermines male authority; it promotes infidelity; it is detrimental to health; it inhibits pleasure.

Male Authority. Some men object to their wives' using contraceptives because they feel it robs them of rightful male authority. They hold that control in the sexual sphere belongs exclusively to the husband. This means that the husband may have extramarital sexual contacts, but can forbid these to his wife; and that he and not his wife will determine the time, form, and frequency of sexual relations. Birth control, then, is just one aspect of the sexual relationship which he feels is his domain.

> I don't like to be governed by my wife. If she tries to use birth control I will leave her.

[1] Cook, Robert C., *Human Fertility:* The Modern Dilemma. William Sloane Associates, New York, 1951, p. 338.

I am the one who avoids them (contraceptives). She doesn't know the secret of birth control. The woman gets pregnant if the man wants her to.

Fear of Infidelity. Closely related to this point is the man's fear that allowing the wife to control conception will give her freedom to have sexual relations with other men. As mentioned previously, a man is extremely jealous and suspicious of his wife. At the same time, he tends to consider her naïve, lightheaded, and unable to reason as well as a man. He holds contrary views of men. Men are clever, wise, on the lookout for sexual relationships; and can easily win women over. Consequently, granting any freedom to the wife only makes it easier for some clever male to conquer her.

The husband assumes that fear of pregnancy is a deterrent to infidelity on the part of the wife. If she were to have a child while her husband was using birth control, he would then have positive proof that she was having an affair. If, on the other hand, the wife uses birth control, the husband cannot detect her illicit relations. A number of women in our sample expressed fear at suggesting female methods of birth control to their husbands:

> If the woman is sterilized, the husband mistrusts her. He thinks the wife is unfaithful. You must keep all those things in mind.

> I wanted to be sterilized but I didn't dare to tell him. Many men don't like their wives to be operated on because they think the women want this in order to have relations with other men.

This suspicion is a barrier to free communication between wives and husbands, a subject to be discussed later. It also leads to anxiety by women in whose families birth control is used, for if the method fails, there is always the danger that the husband will attribute pregnancy to illicit relations. Two clear examples of such anxiety are given below.

> I heard of a woman here who used the diaphragm. Later she became pregnant, and the husband said the child was not his. They almost separated because, inasmuch as they were using birth control, the husband thought she was pregnant by another man.

> (After I had nine children) I brought condoms home from the health center and he used them for about two years. Since I had my

last child four months ago I haven't asked him to use them yet because I haven't menstruated. If he uses them and then finds out I am pregnant again, my husband might think I was having relations with other men; so I can't ask him to use them until I know whether I am pregnant or not.

Men may also, because of jealousy, forbid their wives to be examined by a male physician, thus keeping them from learning about contraception.

Health. The most frequently cited objection to the program is that it might impair one's health. Both men and women fear that birth control methods cause cancer and other dread diseases in women; that diaphragms get trapped in the vagina and require extraordinary measures to remove; and that sterilization may cause a woman to be chronically ill and "useless." While public health physicians in Puerto Rico are not subject to such misgivings, there is evidence that certain private physicians, either as a result of ignorance or religious fervor, do propagate such beliefs; and at least one religious organization is known to use such propaganda. In the absence of authoritative information to the contrary, it is not surprising that such beliefs are strong and tenacious.

I don't know any (birth control) methods. At the Public Health Unit they give instructions, but I fear them because people say it causes cancer.

I have never used prophylactics with my wife nor will I. That is dangerous because if it breaks the woman may die if that stays inside her womb.

Pleasure. The previous discussion has concentrated mainly on female contraceptives, suggesting that men preferred to control conception. While this is true, it does not mean that men have no objections to the condom. Nine out of every ten men in our sample objected to it, giving as their most frequent reason that it destroys the pleasure of the sexual act. It is true that rubber is a poor conductor of body warmth, and this may be what was meant. Other comments, however, suggest that for some, the diminished pleasure is a result of psychological as well as physical factors. To understand the psychological aspect it is necessary to know something about sexual relations in Puerto Rico.

As in other societies with a double standard of sexual morality, Puerto Rican men feel that there are two classes of women, "good" and "bad." Bad women are the prostitutes with whom one can really enjoy oneself sexually—but good women are the kind of girl whom one can marry. They are pure and good just as one's mother or sister and must be treated with courtesy, respect, and reserve. To some extent this attitude is maintained even in marriage. Sexual relations may become somewhat mechanical and nonerotic, both because the husband cannot get over the idea that his wife is a good and pure woman, and because his wife, brought up to regard sex as ugly and unladylike, may encourage this attitude by her own passivity or frigidity. For variety, or for a more sensual kind of sexual relationship, a man turns to the prostitute. To protect himself from venereal disease, he usually uses a contraceptive. He then comes to feel that the condom is part of the world of evil, and has no place in relationships with his wife. Using it at home would degrade a pure and sacred relationship.

> Those things I don't use with my wife, because it debases my wife to use something that is used with prostitutes.
>
> Those are used only with prostitutes, and my wife is an honest woman.
>
> My husband says, "I am clean and my wife is clean, so we don't need to use those."

Perhaps it is for this reason that so many men speak of the condom as something dirty, and regard it as revolting and loathsome.

> They are filthy . . . repulsive . . . I feel sick to my stomach.
>
> I consider them filthy because of the disgust they give after one finishes the sexual act.

The complaint that the condom is less pleasurable thus appears to be based not only on purely physical factors, but also on other considerations that reduce the psychological pleasure of the sexual act.

Barriers to Communication of Birth Control Information

To be successful, a birth control program should provide for effective publicity and easily available information about aims and methods of birth control. In this matter Puerto Rico would appear to be in a favorable position. The birth control clinics have been in existence for over a decade; the newspapers have been full of arguments for and against birth control; and, as already indicated, the pulpit itself has inadvertently contributed to awareness of means for limiting births.

In nearly every family in our sample, both husbands and wives knew about sterilization, and in every family the husband knew about the condom. However, we discovered that frequently one spouse knew of methods which the other did not know. A similar pattern was discovered with respect to motivation. While both spouses might have had identical ideas about family size, one spouse frequently either did not know what the other spouse wanted, or assumed that more children were wanted than actually were. The explanation of these findings is that sexual matters are not a common topic of discussion between husband and wife. Women are brought up with great prudishness, are often ignorant of sex upon marriage, and are taught that modesty and reticence on sexual matters are important attributes of the good woman. At the same time, the male learns that it is not fitting to discuss such matters with a "good" woman—and by definition his wife is always a good woman. As stated earlier, a woman is very reluctant to suggest to her husband that she use contraceptive methods, lest he suspect her of wanting to engage in extramarital sexual activity without being detected. These are typical comments:

> I have heard some of my friends talking about condoms, and I liked the idea. (Did you tell your husband?) No. I did not dare to. I never speak of those things with him. I get ashamed.
>
> I don't know how he feels about that. I don't like to talk about certain things. I don't speak of those things with my husband. I feel ashamed.
>
> To my wife? Me talk about these things? Look man, I couldn't even try . . . I am not accustomed to talk about such things with my wife.

The wife would be offended if one used the condom. (Have you ever talked it over with her?) No, never. I would not dare to do it.

The decision to use birth control is usually a mutual one. Even if both partners have knowledge of birth control methods little action can occur unless this knowledge is communicated by discussion. This is also true in the matter of motivation. If each partner thinks that the other wants a large family, little action will be taken. The couple will consider contraception only if both become aware that their wishes are identical.

Also important to know is which spouse is more influential in family decision-making. Where the man feels that it is his exclusive prerogative to initiate birth control, the wife's knowledge or attitudes may be irrelevant. A few men in the sample were surprised at the idea that women might have anything to say about this matter, and would consider it impertinent of them to suggest something that is obviously the man's business. When such a situation exists, it is a waste of effort to concentrate on the women in public health clinics. Since men are usually the least interested in birth control, appeals to them must be much more forceful if they are to be effective.

Modesty in women also impedes knowledge-seeking. Puerto Rican women are usually ashamed to ask for birth control information and materials. They are also ashamed to be examined by a male physician (many are ashamed at being seen by their own husbands), and some are even ashamed of being seen in a birth control clinic. Thus, modesty is one of the major stumbling blocks to the program, for it obstructs both the seeking and sharing of information.

The preceding sections have described a number of cultural factors seriously hampering the effectiveness of the birth control program. Ambivalence about family size; fears that contraception will foster infidelity, undermine male authority, produce illness or diminish pleasure; and barriers to communication of birth control information have all contributed to reluctance to use contraception. This does not mean, however, that birth control has been completely rejected. Of the 72 families studied by the Family Life Project, over two-thirds reported having some experience with contraception. This is probably higher than the percentage for the population as a whole, but other studies indicate that a substantial proportion of lower-class families have at some time practiced birth control. Interviews with 2,125 women who attended the public health clinics in 1948 disclosed that 34 per cent had already tried some method of birth control.[1] Although many of these families discontinued birth control or use it ineffectively, we must account for their attempts.

It should be pointed out that cultural factors influence motivation not only where contraceptive methods are used but also where they are not practiced. The one method that has proved increasingly attractive in Puerto Rico is sterilization. A review of the reasons will illustrate the interplay of culture, motivation, and the decision to accept or reject methods of controlling birth.

In 1950 close to one out of every five deliveries in Puerto Rican hospitals was followed by sterilization. Between four and five thousand sterilizations occur every year. This has not, however, produced any appreciable reduction in fertility as yet for several reasons; most deliveries do not occur in hospitals, the popularity of sterilization is relatively recent, and the operation is generally performed only after several pregnancies. But the demand for sterilizations continues to grow. Physicians turn down many women because of insufficient hospital bed space, or because they feel these particular women have not had enough children to merit the operation. Sterilization is so popular that local politicians dispense the necessary bed space in return for political allegiance. What explains this phenomenal popularity?

Sterilization is effective and relatively easy. As one woman put it, "It is only once, sure, and then you forget about it and don't have to use those dirty things." Another reason is that sterilization is usually performed in the hospital, postpartum, thus removing some of the onus and embarrassment of a special trip and a special examination. Yet by at least two criteria the measure is drastic. It requires an operation and it is irreversible; one cannot later change one's mind about wanting more children. Nevertheless, some families experiment with less drastic methods and

[1] Cofresi, Emilio, *Realidad Poblacional de Puerto Rico*. San Juan, 1951, Table 33, p. 88.

switch later to sterilization; others try only this method. Our study showed that few people in the sample continued to use chemical or mechanical contraceptives, and either moved to sterilization, or stopped birth control altogether.

This trend away from birth "control" and toward sterilization can be explained by describing a pattern characteristic of many families whose case histories were collected.

In the early years of marriage little thought is given to fertility control. For various reasons, some of which we have indicated, the couple is eager to start a family, but reluctant to discuss matters pertaining to sex and childbearing. Consequently, when thought of family limitation occurs, it is usually the wife who feels concern. Too modest or fearful to seek information or discuss the matter with her husband, she cannot implement her desire to limit the size of her family, and no positive steps are taken. As a result, the Puerto Rican woman finds herself with as many children as she ever wants while she is still very young. By age twenty-five, for example, "more second births have occurred per 1,000 women on the island than occur in the United States by age 35."[1]

With three or four children, motivation for some kind of action becomes stronger. The family may begin to feel desperate—the average per capita income is only $400—and decide that something must be done that is swift and sure. The course of action chosen depends largely on the couple's knowledge of, and attitudes toward, birth control. If there is little knowledge or attitudes are strongly prejudicial, one or more children may be given away; the husband may desert the family; or sterilization, which is apparently known to everyone, will be sought. If knowledge and attitudes are different, ordinary birth control methods may be tried. At this point of high motivation, the availability of competent advice may be the deciding factor. Advice from a midwife, a public health nurse, or a physician is very likely to touch off action on birth control. Under such circumstances, the wife frequently breaks through the communication barrier, discusses the matter with her husband, gets his permission, and takes action.

[1] Combs, J. W., Jr., and Kingsley Davis, "The Pattern of Puerto Rican Fertility," *Population Studies*, vol. 4, March, 1951, p. 371.

By now, however, the couple is used to intercourse without mechanical devices and finds the prescribed techniques burdensome. Moreover, having conquered some of her modesty, the woman may discuss the matter with a married friend, who may tell her of the danger of contracting cancer. The husband may find the prescribed method tiresome, "unclean," or unpleasurable. Consequently, it is either discontinued or used erratically. Another pregnancy ensues. The family now feels that contraception is ineffective or impracticable and that something must be done once and for all. Sterilization provides an answer.

IMPLICATIONS

Possible Program Modifications

How can knowledge of the cultural influences at work in Puerto Rico help in planning a more effective birth control program? Such planning should take into account those cultural factors that bear most directly on public acceptance of the program, as well as taking into account what is realistically possible.[1] Methods of contraception other than those mentioned here might provide a solution to the problem, and in this case it might be advisable to encourage intensified medical research for new techniques. A safe and effective contraceptive pill might minimize many of the objections currently encountered.

From the standpoint of sheer technical expediency and in view of existing preferences in rural Puerto Rico, increased sterilization might provide the answer. It is already the most popular and widely known method of birth control; it does not interfere with sexual pleasure; and it requires that the family take action only once. But other considerations cannot be overlooked. Many Puerto Rican medical men feel that sterilization is too drastic a measure. By its very nature the policy is susceptible to attack; one of the political parties now out of power has charged that sterilization would lead to genocide and mass elimination of the poor.

[1] Solutions to this problem will, of course, vary from society to society. In the British West Indies, for example, questions of modesty and communication between spouses appear to be of lesser importance, and a different kind of program would be indicated for this area.

Ruling out pills as unavailable and sterilization as undesirable, much could be done to increase the effectiveness of existing facilities, in light of known cultural factors. It is of prime importance to improve methods of disseminating birth control information. If one were operating in a political vacuum, a public campaign with posters, leaflets, motion pictures, broadcasts, and mobile units might be the most effective method of spreading knowledge of contraception. However, the delicate nature of the subject makes it advisable to disseminate the information in quieter ways.[1]

At the present time, the clinics are passive repositories of birth control materials. Even without a public campaign, greater efforts could be made to attract women to these clinics. These clinics are only one of about a dozen kinds of public health clinics. In all these others, physicians and nurses could influence their patients by stressing the bearing of excessive fertility on tuberculosis, malnutrition, and so on. The importance of the health and psychological well-being of *every child* could be stressed in children's clinics. Wherever possible, women could be referred to the prematernal birth control clinics.

Another aid to spreading knowledge of birth control practice would be premarital and marital counseling. Newlyweds could be apprised of the heavy responsibilities of parenthood *before* such status is achieved, thus stimulating early interest in birth control. If the public health agencies could not do this directly, they could at least encourage other agencies to do so. Moreover, since the communication block between husband and wife appears to be a crucial barrier to action, and since the Puerto Rican husband is the key figure in decision-making, every effort should be made to reach men. If husbands and wives are able to express themselves on sexual matters before a nurse or physician, a great step toward beneficial action would be taken. In revisits to some of the families in our sample, interviewers found that several women had begun to practice birth control merely because they had talked about it.

[1] Editor's note: An indication of the way in which any such campaign would be exploited politically was made plain during a recent program for mass immunization against tuberculosis by B.C.G. vaccination. The opposition claimed that the party in power was inoculating the poor with tuberculosis in an effort to eliminate them and the problem of poverty at one and the same time. (Correspondence from Dr. Wilson W. Wing.)

As one woman put it, "I'd always been ashamed before. But after talking with you, I was able to talk to my husband about it." The interviewers did no propagandizing. Bringing the subject out into the open had furnished enough impetus to bring about action.

Measures to reduce embarrassment in the clinic would also aid in spreading birth control practice. Utilizing more nurses and female physicians, exercising greater tact, and conducting pelvic examinations only when absolutely necessary, would eliminate a great deal of embarrassment for patients.

Once in the clinic, it is not enough to present the patient with materials and to give instruction on their use. Ill-founded fears concerning birth control must be dispelled, some hints provided as to what to tell the husband, and the importance of continuing control measures stressed. Puerto Rican lower-class women are too modest and too respectful of authority to ask many questions. Their inner questions must be anticipated and dealt with by discussion or lecture methods. Toward the same end efforts could be made to set up discussion groups for mothers, to facilitate the open consideration of problems and tabooed topics.

Finally, it is important that public health personnel themselves have adequate knowledge of the culture of the particular group with which they are dealing. Members of a higher-class group often demonstrate considerable ignorance about lower-class groups in their own society. Discussions with social workers and social scientists working with such groups can teach these people a great deal about their own culture. Moreover, workers should realize the great importance of working simultaneously toward the reduction of fertility and mortality in areas of population pressure. To many public health personnel, the prematernal clinic is just one of many clinics and one whose importance their own training and dispositions may lead them to minimize. Again, staff discussions with medical men and social scientists working in this field can help to stir up interest.

Population Balance and Public Health

The foregoing description of the birth control program in Puerto Rico and its difficulties can be seen as part of a much larger problem that is of growing concern to public health workers. The particular problem faced by the Puerto Ricans, that of serious overpopulation, is just one kind of imbalance that can arise when traditional methods of controlling fertility are disturbed by rapid culture change. It can be seen as part of the general problem of fertility and population balance. To many public health workers, it is becoming increasingly apparent that the successful program in an underdeveloped region is one that aims both at a reduction in deaths and a reduction in births. Only in this way can we avoid keeping more people alive so that they may live badly.[1] But how can this be done?

In every society, culture operates both as a check and as a stimulant to fertility, as Kingsley Davis has shown.[2] A society may restrict its fertility in four ways: it may limit sexual relations, conception, birth, and postpartum existence. Conception may be limited by preventing association of any kind between the sexes, by preventing sexual contact only, or by limiting frequency of intercourse within marriage. Among the Puerto Rican lower classes, for example, taboos on intercourse during the postpartum period and sickness may act to reduce fertility.

Methods of limiting conception by mechanical and other means are old and varied. Similarly widespread are ways of limiting offspring once conception has occurred. In some societies, such as contemporary Japan, abortion is extensively practiced. Some societies condone postpartum infanticide of certain offspring. Limiting the number of conceptions and births is undertaken with the conscious purpose of reducing fertility and thus may be called "manifest" functions, while limits on intercourse may produce the same results without deliberate intent and thus comprise a "latent" function.

In societies where the mortality rate is high, cultural forces must operate to encourage high fertility if the population level is to be maintained. Early marriages and large families are supported by cultural values and social institutions. Such societies are usually agrarian, and children serve as an economic asset.

[1] See Davis, Kingsley, "Puerto Rico: A Crowded Island," *Annals of the American Academy of Political and Social Science*, vol. 285, January, 1953, p. 119.

[2] Davis, Kingsley, *Human Society*. Macmillan Co., New York, 1949, pp. 557–561.

But utilitarian motives for high fertility are generally reinforced by cultural beliefs and values; having many children can be regarded as a sign of virility, a means to good health, or a way of obtaining the good graces of one's ancestors or gods. Christianity, founded in a period of high mortality, exhorts its adherents to "increase and multiply," thus adding more souls to the number of God's worshippers.

Cultural practices that encourage high fertility may be adaptive in societies with a high mortality rate, but if technological and health advances reduce mortality to any considerable degree, these same practices can become "dysfunctional" if they persist in the face of accelerated culture change. This condition is responsible, in part, for the serious nature of the Puerto Rican situation. The United States is an example of a society where cultural values and practices relative to fertility have adjusted themselves to changed conditions; as this country changed from a rural agrarian to an urban industrial economy, the value of large families lessened. As the large family became less utilitarian, values in regard to high fertility changed. In United States middle classes, the father is usually the sole breadwinner; childhood is spent in recreation and education rather than in contributing to family support; increased emphasis on the "glamor girl" and clubwoman aspects of the wife's role tends to take precedence over the mother and homemaker aspects.

Along with the change in cultural values that support low fertility in the United States, the development and mass production of safe, efficient, cheap, and fairly easy-to-use contraceptives have made low fertility available to those who desire it. The result of these concomitant changes has been to produce a fairly stable population equilibrium in the United States. However, this equilibrium did not develop at once. For many years the development of values and practices promoting low fertility lagged behind the rapidly decreasing mortality rate. It took years for cultural values and institutions to catch up with the changed social and economic conditions.

However, in other societies, such as Puerto Rico, fertility practices and ideals have not adjusted themselves to the rapid drop in mortality made possible by modern medicine. In due time and by gradual processes, it is possible that some satisfactory adjustment might occur. The question, however, is this: can we afford to wait for the slow and gradual development of these "natural" processes? By introducing public health measures into societies that are geared for high mortality, we have already upset the operation of "natural" forces; we have substantially reduced the mortality rate, and thus created the condition of dangerously accelerated population increase. Should we demand that public health devote its attention to controlling the rate of births as well as reducing deaths as part of its overall program? The case of Puerto Rico represents one attempt to find answers to these difficult problems.

SUMMARY

This paper has described the difficulties encountered by a program of birth control in Puerto Rico; it has analyzed the social and psychological sources of these difficulties; and it has presented implications both for the particular situation and on a broader level. The study has tried to convey three major points First, we have attempted to show how, in an underdeveloped area with both high fertility and mortality, public health can aggravate its own problems as well as the broader problems of the society by concentrating all its attention on reduction of mortality alone. The situation in Puerto Rico has shown that incisive reduction in mortality without an equivalent drop in fertility can upset the economy and undermine health in a fairly short period. In less advantageously situated societies the problem may become catastrophic, especially since recent medical advances have made possible an even faster drop in mortality than in Puerto Rico.

Second, we have shown that human fertility, in contrast with fecundity, is intimately bound up with cultural patterns. In a society where high mortality has prevailed, cultural forces operate to ensure high fertility; but when mortality is rapidly reduced by modern medical techniques, the culture patterns do not change fast enough to establish a new balance between births and deaths.

Third, we have tried to point out that only by a thorough understanding of the culture of the particular society can a program of fertility control be successful. Puerto Rico, with one of the most extensive birth control programs in the world, has been unable markedly to affect fertility largely because cultural factors have not been taken sufficiently into account. The mere existence of excellent facilities does not provide necessary motivation for small families, guarantee the spread of accurate information about modern means of contraception, or combat erroneous beliefs or prejudicial attitudes toward these methods. As necessary to a birth control program as materials and advice is a combination of high motivation by public health personnel and the use of measures that take cultural factors into account.

All of this does not add up to an easy task, nor does anyone have all the answers on how to proceed. But the difficulty of a problem is no excuse to evade it, especially when such evasion can wreak social havoc. Public health holds great power over human life. To say that with power should go responsibility may be trite, but it is also true.

SELECTED REFERENCES

Annals of the American Academy of Political and Social Science, vol. 285, January, 1953. The entire issue is devoted to Puerto Rico and contains several articles on population, fertility, and birth control.

Cook, Robert C., *Human Fertility:* The Modern Dilemma. William Sloane Associates, New York, 1951. A panoramic view of the problem of expanding population.

Davis, Kingsley, *Human Society.* Macmillan Co., New York, 1949. A scholarly and highly readable introduction to sociology, with a good general chapter on population and fertility.

Hatt, Paul K., *Backgrounds of Human Fertility in Puerto Rico.* University Press, Princeton, 1952. The most comprehensive treatment of Puerto Rican fertility available.

Stycos, J. Mayone, "Family and Fertility in Puerto Rico," *American Sociological Review*, vol. 17, October, 1952, pp. 572–580. This paper explains that high fertility results not from planning on the part of the parents, but as a natural by-product of an interpersonal situation in which the woman's effective role is minimal.

"Cultural Checks on Birth Control Use in Puerto Rico," *The Interrelations of Demographic, Economic, and Social Problems in Selected Underdeveloped Areas.* Proceedings of a Round Table at the 1953 Annual Conference of the Milbank Memorial Fund, 1954, pp. 55–65.

Case 8

ABORTION AND DEPOPULATION
ON A PACIFIC ISLAND
by David M. Schneider

The contrasts between the islands of Puerto Rico and Yap are conspicuous and instructive. Apart from differences in scale, they diverge sharply in ways of life, relations between the sexes, and the direction of population imbalance. From our standpoint, Yap society is minute and its culture exotic. For both of these reasons, we find it easier to see how the several aspects of Yap culture relate to each other and to the environment than to discern the connections between the different aspects of our own large-scale society. But seeing the physiognomy of a far-off culture is like holding up a mirror; we begin to notice that our culture, too, has distinctive lineaments.

Dr. Schneider was one of four anthropologists who spent nine months during 1947–1948 on Yap to study the problem of depopulation. The research was sponsored by Harvard University and the National Research Council. Although the research team was unable to obtain a physician to investigate the possible effects of venereal infection in lowering the fertility rate, medical evidence from neighboring islands supports the assumption that gonorrhea is a factor. The case study focuses on the practice of abortion and its relation to the Yap system of allocating responsibility and prestige. It is clear that the islanders' preoccupation with intricate love affairs has a significant bearing not only on the practice of abortion but also on the possible prevalence of venereal infection.—EDITOR

THE PROBLEM

The Practice of Self-Induced Abortion

Before the coming of the first European explorers to the Pacific Island of Yap, its 39 square miles supported an estimated population of more than 50,000 people. By 1945, when American troops landed on Yap, the island's population had fallen to about 2,500. This spectacular decline in population has had far-reaching consequences for the people of Yap and their mode of life.

The people of Yap had developed a social system predicated on a relatively large population. While the population continued to decline, the form of their organized groupings changed but slowly. Today people bemoan the fact that there is a constant scarcity of individuals to hold the offices and perform the necessary jobs. Political organizations calling for a staff of 15 officials have only four or five men available to fill these posts. Present-day Yap society, with its several thousand people, is still geared to a population 20 times that large, and it is with deep regret that people contemplate the spectacle of unfilled positions and depleted organizations. As they express the situation, something should be done "to have more babies."

In the face of this dramatic population shrinkage and the keenly felt need to refill the thinned ranks of their society, Yap women engage in a practice that produces results exactly opposite to those desired. Evidence indicates that self-induced abortion is widely practiced by Yap women precisely during the years of maximum fecundity. This lowers the fertility rate in a situation where a higher rate is urgently desired. Moreover, the methods of inducing abortion are such as to expose women to the risk of infection. Abortion is widely condemned on moral grounds. A Yap woman will tell of other women who have induced abortion but never admit having done so herself. The admission would create serious trouble with her husband or, if she were single, it would impair her chances of making a good marriage.

In view of the unfavorable consequences of abortion, as well as the moral strictures against it, why do women persist in this practice? Could the very methods devised by the people of Yap to stabilize the population at the optimal level have produced results that defeat their own ends? The enigma of abortion has roots deep in the history of Yap and its people. It is not an isolated practice that can be understood by itself, but is bound up with the totality of Yap culture, its values, moral standards, social organization, and the aspirations of its people.

THE SITUATION

Fertility and Cultural Values

As part of a four-man team of social scientists studying the problem of depopulation on Yap in 1947 and 1948, I became interested in cultural factors relating to the low birth rate. In the course of ethnographic research, I was particularly struck by the fact that 34 per cent of Yap women between the ages of twenty-six and fifty who were interviewed claimed that they had never given birth to a child. In seeking to account, at least in part, for this high incidence of infertility, I began to accumulate information pointing to the prevalence of self-induced abortion. It was next to impossible to get direct evidence. Morally disallowed, this practice was performed in secret. Women readily told about *other* women who had induced abortion. Their knowledge of the precise details of technique, however, left little doubt that this information was based on more than indirect experience. The facts that emerged on the illicit but widespread practice of self-induced abortion are these.

Self-Induced Abortion on Yap

Abortion techniques fall into three classes. One consists in a series of magical manipulations with little apparent efficacy. These were universally recited to me as "ways to abort, but they don't always work." Doubtless they are tried from time to time, however. The other two techniques are empirically more effective. One of these is drinking boiled concentrated sea water. Women described the effect as a general feeling of illness accompanied by vomiting and severe cramps.

The other technique consists in introducing a thin rolled plug of hibiscus leaves (which expand when moist) into the mouth of the cervix and then injuring and scratching the mouth of the cervix with a bit of stick, stone, iron, fingernail, or other sharp object until blood is drawn. Women informants generally agreed that injuring the area about the mouth of the cervix was necessary in addition to inserting the plug; the plug without injury or injury without the plug was subject to failure. The boiled sea water technique was held to be less reliable than the plug-and-injury method, and therefore the less common of the two techniques. One technique common on the Pacific islands of Melanesia and Polynesia, that of massage, was never mentioned by Yap informants and is apparently unknown on Yap.

Induced abortion fits neatly into the Yap way of life, for a woman who knows how to induce abortion can usually do so without the fact ever being discovered. Yap women customarily repair to a special area during their menstrual periods. There they sit within a small but comfortable hut on their voluminous skirts of dry banana leaves and other grasses. When the peak of the flow is over, the woman is free to move around within the menstrual area, and she busies herself with making her new skirt, cleaning up the area, and such basketry work or other appropriate occupation as may come to hand. At the conclusion of her menstrual period, she places her soiled skirt in a place reserved for that purpose in the menstrual area; these old skirts are burned when the pile is great enough to warrant it. She is then free to return to the village and resume her daily life.

It is customary for a woman to keep pregnancy a secret for the first three months at least, for both she and her child are considered to be most vulnerable to sorcery at that time. So whether or not she is actually menstruating, she will repair to the menstrual area about the time she would normally have expected her period to begin. So far as the rest of the world can tell, she is not pregnant and is menstruating regularly. A young woman who becomes pregnant is thus in an excellent position to keep her condition secret and to induce abortion without discovery if she so wishes and knows how.

Contraception, in certain of its forms, is known on Yap but hardly ever used. Coitus interruptus was reported by some male informants to have been learned in relatively recent times from Japanese occupation personnel. It is something some women try once or twice but abandon quickly; men will not tolerate it, and a woman finds that it defeats her own ends in that it drives lovers away. Condoms were made familiar by the Japanese; they were known to be effective in preventing pregnancy, but Yap men were not motivated to use them for this purpose, preferring to make excellent slingshots out of them instead. Other forms of contraception are unknown.

Abortion induced by the plug-and-injury method is likely to produce infection, which in turn may possibly lead to some lasting impairment of a woman's reproductive capacity. On the other hand, it seems clear that more serious consequences of the plug-and-injury method are unlikely, though they may well occur in individual cases. Yap women live in their microbiological environment all their lives without the protection of antiseptics or the habits of cleanliness and hygiene common among us. Consequently, the resistance to infection on the part of those who survive is generally quite high. This does not mean that they never become infected. It only means that were an American woman to try to abort by the plug-and-injury method she would very likely incur a serious if not fatal infection, where the typical Yap woman probably incurs only a mild, localized infection. Medical experts have made actual observations of this sort.

As already mentioned, deliberate abortion is considered "wrong" and immoral on Yap. A husband who discovers that his wife has resorted to abortion may beat her or divorce her, or do both. A woman who becomes known among men as one who practices abortion jeopardizes her chances of a stable marriage. Men are interested in having children, and a woman who destroys her unborn child is viewed as a woman who "throws her child away."

Because Yap abortion techniques are in fact effective, the practice has a critical bearing on the fertility rate. However, the low rate cannot be attributed entirely to the practice of abortion. In all likelihood, there are additional important causes. Although the evidence remains inconclusive, there are good indications that gonorrhea or some other low-grade infection is present and contributes to the low fertility on Yap.

But the practice of abortion by itself is a problem of sufficient gravity to cause concern on the part of American officials charged with the responsibility of administration and on the part of natives themselves. The problem of devising effective means for dealing with abortion requires a searching look at the whole complex of circumstances that surround it. Only by understanding this problem can one hope to plan suitable countermeasures.

The Island of Yap

Yap is a large, eroded mountain top of 38.7 square miles surrounded by a reef and rising to about 500 feet at its highest point. It lies 451 miles southwest of Guam; it is approximately 10° north of the equator and 138° east of Greenwich. Yap is a western member of the Caroline Islands, which in turn are part of a widespread group of small islands and island clusters known as Micronesia. In 1947 Yap had a population of 2,600 living in more than a hundred villages.

Although Yap was discovered by westerners in the sixteenth century, its contact with European and American peoples was sporadic until the last three decades of the nineteenth century, and even so the direct effects of foreign contact on Yap culture have been minimal. Nominal and ineffective administration of Yap by the Spanish lasted until 1899, when the whole Caroline Islands, from Ponape in the east to Palau in the west, were sold to Germany. In 1914 the Japanese took over the former German South Seas Colony in Micronesia and continued effective administration of Yap until 1945, when the American Navy gained control of the islands. Soon after, they became the Trust Territory of the Pacific Islands ultimately under United Nations control but administered first by the Navy Department and later by the United States Department of the Interior.

American administration of Yap since the fall of 1945 saw the introduction of health and sanitation measures, the erection of a hospital and dispensary for the natives, isolation of all known lepers, and the dramatic eradication of yaws. This last task alone, completed before my visit in 1947, went far toward enlisting native support for medical and hygienic suggestions emanating from the American administration.

Yap is known as one of the most conservative islands in Micronesia. After more than fifty years of occupation by a succession of foreign powers—Spain, Germany, Japan, and now the United States—the Yap way of life has altered very gradually, if at all. Missionary efforts are a good example. In the late 1800's, Spanish soldiers and missionaries alternately tried to establish stations on Yap. At first, they were treated with direct hostility, and some missionaries and soldiers were killed. Later Spanish forces were augmented and became sufficient to maintain their position, and fear of retaliation prevented violence from the Yaps. Toward the end of the period of German administration in the first decade of the twentieth century, there were some 60 Capuchin missionaries on Yap, and their published report lamented the fact that for all their work and for all their numbers, but 15 natives could be counted as converts. At the time of my visit in 1947 many natives felt it a gesture of friendliness toward the Americans to claim to be Christians, since in their view all Americans were Christians. In fact, however, the number of regular church-going Christians who had more than a vague notion of what Christianity was, did not far exceed the number cited by the German missionaries.

Depopulation and Its Background

One change of major importance that has taken place over the past hundred or more years is the severe depopulation of the island. Precisely when this depopulation started is unknown. The best guess is that it probably began sometime before 1850, although how long before is unknown. For the people of Yap, a whole series of alterations and adjustments have followed in the wake of the decrease in numbers. The reduction in available personnel simply prohibits certain activities and restricts others to a scale which distorts their meaning and function. Yet these activities of an older day are still thought to be the proper and good ways, while the restricted ways of today are seen as unavoidable compromises to be rectified at the earliest opportunity. It is in this latter sense that the Yap way of life has changed but little; the ideal patterns, so to speak, appear to be unchanged, while their necessarily inadequate realization is universally deplored.

The traditional table of organization for the government of a village lists so many political offices ranging from village chief down to the janitor of the old men's clubhouse that nowadays one man alone may hold four or five out of the 12 or 15 political offices in a given village, while in other villages the complaint is that "everybody is a chief." Such focusing of political function in the hands of one man and such diffusion of offices throughout the whole population distort the concept of evenly balanced political powers implicit in traditional Yap political organization. Furthermore, this situation defeats the traditional intent of restricting the governing function to a selected segment of the society. The Yaps are well aware of this and insist that the time-honored ideal pattern remains "right" but that the present undesirable arrangement is unavoidable because of the shortage of people.

Although the complete history of Yap depopulation is impossible to recover, certain inferences can be made with reasonable confidence. The depopulation trend started during a period of acute overpopulation. According to a careful estimate based on a study of abandoned house sites, the population at one time was in the neighborhood of 51,000 with a density of approximately 1,300 persons per square mile, a figure 20 times that of the present, but no greater than the present density of some other Micronesian islands, according to official sources:

Island	Density per Square Mile
Nama	2,093
Losap	1,892
Eauripik	1,477
Yap (estimated)	(1,300)
Pingelap	914
Kapingamarangi	892

At no time during the depopulation of this island did genuine social disorganization take place. Yap is highly conservative with respect to change of any kind. It is even possible that conservatism increased precisely as depopulation progressed, since barrenness, death, and disease are essentially believed by the natives to be supernatural punishments for breaches of custom and taboo. The frequent occurrence of such departures might well have made the Yaps feel that compulsive observance of customary modes of action was essential to avoid these evil consequences. Associating misfortune with improper behavior is not uncommon elsewhere in the world. The combination of conservatism and absence of severe social disorganization helps to explain why Yap culture, as a blueprint for how life should be lived, remains today in many ways the same culture as obtained during the period of overpopulation. In brief, Yap culture is one that is geared not only to a large population, but in important respects to overpopulation.

If the practice of abortion began during a period of overpopulation, it was at that time a successful adaptation to a pressing problem. These circumstances could account for the origin of the practice of abortion on Yap, and a simple explanation for its current prevalence in spite of a drastic change in population would be that it is a "survival," a custom that has lost its utility but persists of its own inertia. Such an explanation would fail to take account of the interrelated nature of the components that comprise a society's culture. The values and institutions that arose in past response to overpopulation became linked to form a fairly coherent cultural totality with powers of persistence greater than those of the constituent parts.

The Yap Way of Life: Youth and Love Affairs

Insight into the motives that impel abortion can be gained by examining the childhood and youth of Yap men and women. A man's life goes through a protracted period of childhood, lasting well into the late teens, without many responsibilities, without duties of any serious kind, and with a predominant interest in play. As a youth, he has begun to take love seriously, to learn the elaborate code and ritual of love affairs, and has perhaps had one lover and is going on to a second. He has learned that Yap girls are hard to get and harder to keep; they demand much and they are not constant. If he can talk the girl into coming to live with him, he has a firmer hold over her, though her affection is still likely to wander.

Even a married man with a wife and child, however, has few responsibilities. He will have built a house for himself on his father's land (but well apart from his parents' dwelling) when he was between fifteen and twenty. At that time plots for his yams and pits for his taro and trees for his coconuts will have been set aside from those of his mother and father, for he may not share with them food grown on the same land, cooked over the same fire, or in the same pot. He may share food only with men or women of his age-group. A man's wife cultivates and cooks his vegetable food, and the man should provide her with coconuts and fish, and betel nut for chewing; and these he provides as the need arises or as the spirit moves him. Beyond these duties he has but one other, to provide his father-in-law with fish or other gifts from time to time. Otherwise the care of the child, house, and garden falls almost entirely on his wife. She should help her mother-in-law in the house and in the garden and with any small children her mother-in-law may have.

A man's serious responsibilities and obligations do not begin until he is in his late forties or early fifties when, as head of his kin group, he takes part.in the councils and the serious political affairs of his village.

A woman's life need be no different from a man's with regard to responsibilities and work. As a young girl she celebrates her first menses with a year-long residence in a specially designated area outside her village, usually near the inland grassy region. There her friends come to visit and play with her, and she begins her love affairs in earnest. According to the cultural rules, no man can have exclusive claim on her affections during this year, even if she is married, and she spreads her favors widely. After this year she returns to the village, living in a house her father builds for her not far from her parents' dwelling, unless she is married. Except for the fact that she has put on the black neck cord of a mature woman, she continues to lead the life she led as a girl. Her primary interests are in play, in love affairs, and in sociability.

If a woman comes to live with her lover, she is regarded as married, but except for the fact that she is expected to be faithful to him, her life is not radically altered. True, she should do his cooking eventually, but for months after arriving at her husband's house, his mother will still cook for him, and she will share his food. Properly the right to cook her husband's food should be ceremonially transferred from the man's mother to his wife, but since young women do not particularly like the chore, they postpone this ceremony. Often it is just as well, for the couple frequently decide, after a week or a month or a year, that they would rather terminate the marriage. Young people do not get married in the sense of solemnly undertaking the responsibilities of home and family; for them, marriage is in effect a special arrangement to make a love affair easier. When married, they no longer have to meet secretly at night.

The procrastination of the very few ceremonies which are supposed to attend a marriage reflects the instability of this period. There are only two ceremonies, and as often as not one or both are never performed. Besides the ceremonial transfer of cooking privileges, there is supposed to be a small gathering of the bride and groom's immediate families and an exchange of food between them. In this last ceremony the groom's father always makes a little speech which dwells on the hope that the couple will get along together and not fight, will stay together and have children.

There is nothing to prevent the separation (which is divorce) of a couple if they so desire, provided no children have been born. The girl simply goes back to her father's house, taking with her what property she brought—her skirt, her basket, and the knives and jewelry she carries in it. There is no ceremony marking this separation.

On the other hand, considerable social pressure is put on a woman to remain in the marriage if she has borne a child and if the child is alive, for on divorce a child remains with his father unless the child is still nursing, when he will go with his mother until weaned and then return to his father. The mother's parents, her husband's parents, and public opinion bring pressure to bear to keep her with her child. The whole burden of the appeal is laid squarely on her relationship with her child. She is not asked to stay with her husband. She is not appealed to on the ground that she owes her husband's kin group anything, either through her work or her fertility. She is only asked to stay with her child who needs her. It is considered the gravest misdeed for a mother to separate herself from her child and, indeed, the very few children whom I saw whose mothers had been divorced after the child's birth, suffered markedly from the sense of abandonment engendered in Yap in such a situation. A woman who does this is said to have "thrown her child away" and her reputation is badly damaged.

When there are no children divorce is simple, practically without repercussion and consequences; divorce after children are born is a very serious matter and occurs relatively rarely. Out of a group of 28 married women who had each borne one live child, nine had never been divorced at all, 15 had been divorced before the birth of their first child, while only four had been divorced after the birth of their first child.

Thus, when a woman bears a child, her position changes radically. She is primarily responsible for the care and feeding of the child, and she must be with him almost all the time. She will take him with her to the gardens and she will take him along when she goes visiting, but she must be with him. Although her husband shares most of the pregnancy taboos with her and helps with the actual delivery, his responsibility toward the child duplicates his responsibility toward his wife—providing coconuts, fish, and betel. He is not constantly tied to the child the way she is, and a husband's extramarital affairs are not sharply curtailed as are a woman's when she has a child. A woman with a child cannot go "playing about," with her husband or anyone else, at night or by day. A woman becomes tied to a man when she bears a child, and young women on Yap do not like to be tied to one man.

Women up to the age of thirty do not want children because they would no longer be free to fall in and out of love, to attract lovers, to have and break off affairs at will, to practice the elaborate games of love and sociability that appeal to young Yap men and women. They do not want to be tied to a child and to a husband when they are in the best position to gain and enjoy the rewards of being unattached. It is one thing to want to avoid having a child, and something else again to actually do so. Wishing alone will not suffice. On Yap the standard and available means of avoiding children is to induce abortion when pregnancy occurs.

The Yap Way of Life: Adulthood and Prestige

When a woman is about thirty, her attitude changes. She begins to want children. Women say that they want children then because they are lonely and need someone to talk to. This is another way of saying that they find it hard to attract and keep lovers. At this time a woman will have a child if she can. If she cannot, she will resort to a host of magical aids, medicines, prayers, and whatever else promises to bring the child she now desires. If all of her efforts fail, she will try to adopt a child. Adoption is a common practice on Yap, but the supply of children for adoption is, of course, insufficient to meet the demand.

Although women over thirty give as their main reason for wanting babies that they are "lonely" and are tired of running around, it is significant that at this age a woman leaves the age category of "youth" by Yap standards and enters the status of "adulthood." This social transition has important consequences for the people of Yap. Different kinds of rewards are available to people in different age-groups. Older men and women are less dependent on the gratifications that arise from love affairs and sexual conquest and can turn instead to new activities that now become appropriate and available. The reasons for this shift are connected with the basic values of Yap culture.

The dominant value of Yap culture is prestige. People are ranked and assigned differential prestige in almost every conceivable way. Family groups are ranked within a village, and the villages themselves are ranked into a nine-class system divided into an upper and a lower group. This is crosscut by a formal "war organization" now oriented primarily to political ends. Districts are ranked within three major alliances, and these three alliances continually jockey in the political arena for temporary dominance. Organization within the family itself is conceived as a rank system with father taking precedence over mother, mother over children, and older children over younger. Each plot of land within the village has its inherent, almost inalienable rank, and the highest ranking piece of land validates its owner's position as village chief, while lower political statuses inhere in lower ranking plots of land.

Older people, men and women, have more prestige than younger, and the responsibilities which go with age are seen as privileges appropriate to the older people's prestige. It is the old men, the heads of family groups, who sit around in conference, planning large and ostentatious exchanges of valuable shells or exhibitions of dancing by the men or women of the village. Old men and heads of families achieve the available political statuses of chief, subchief, magician, messenger, and so forth. Owing to depopulation, chieftainships today are often inherited by young men and boys, and when this happens a trusted relative of advanced age is often called in to act as regent for them. In the past when population was at its peak, it was only the oldest who could hold such offices, who were admitted to the old men's clubhouse, who could sit with the council of family heads. The young men were the warriors and fishermen, with time on their hands and without important responsibilities.

Closely related to the fact that age, prestige, and responsibility go together is the conception that a man is still a "young man" until he is about forty or fifty years old. Technically a "young man" becomes a "man" when he succeeds to the head of his kin group. Since succession to the position of "leader of the kin group" goes from a man to his next oldest brother, through all brothers in order of descending age, and then to the oldest male among the sons of all the brothers, it was unlikely in the past that a man would succeed to that position until he was nearly fifty. Depopulation has now accelerated this progression, but it has not changed the rules of the system.

Although this elaborate system of ranking is stable, as far as its rules and regulations are concerned, it has a degree of flexibility in that the rank of any particular unit (family, village, district, alliance, plot of land) is not necessarily fixed permanently. Families, villages, districts, and alliances all vie with each other according to prescribed and orderly rules for legitimate improvement in their position; magic, sorcery, and pure chicanery are often used to hasten this necessarily slow process. But whatever the position held by any social unit, the aim is to increase its prestige and better its position.

Prestige on Yap is not correlated with such powers or privileges as make daily life precarious for some and easy for others, as in the United States. For all practical purposes food is now and was in the past equally accessible to all, regardless of rank. High prestige groups do not have the right to exploit the labor of low prestige groups except in ways which are primarily symbolic. Thus, certain families within the upper groups have the right to demand that their roofs be repaired by persons from lower groups. This amounts to a token expression of ranked relationship rather than a continuous work obligation of great magnitude. So far as can be discovered now, depopulation affected all social classes on Yap equally, for all social classes had equal access to the necessities of life and no social class was disadvantaged by being overworked or otherwise penalized in any but symbolic ways.

Why Abortion Persists

I have shown that Yap women induce abortion because they do not want to be tied down with children during a time when they feel they would be better occupied in love affairs and in sociability. In terms of our own standards we might feel that such an attitude was morally "wrong," but they would insist that it was morally "right" and such indeed is the Yap cultural premise in terms of which they act. Young people *should* spend their time in love affairs and in nonresponsible pleasures. But Yap women also feel that they should have children and care for them. The problem is one of timing; after their period of love affairs is over, women want to have children and care for them, but they do not want the children earlier to interfere with the game of love. Yet it happens that children often come before they are wanted.

Yap standards of behavior for young men and women differ from our own standards. This is a matter of cultural relativity, but more than relativity is at issue. What is also involved is the fit between one part of culture and the rest of the cultural totality. Let us suppose that young Americans in their twenties emulated Yap and consistently preferred to engage in love affairs than to assume adult responsibilities. Quite apart from morality, such a shift would set in motion a series of other changes disrupting what we regard as our way of life. Conversely, if young men and women on Yap suddenly decided to settle down in their twenties and rear families, a host of other changes would ensue and the Yap way of life would similarly be disrupted.

I have said that the dominant values of Yap culture center around gaining and keeping prestige. Fundamental to any prestige system is the fact that a kind of scarce commodity (prestige) is differentially distributed; some have a lot and some have a little, but all cannot share equally. For such a system to work, there must be rules and regulations governing who has prestige and who has not, how it can be gained and how it can be lost. These rules must be obeyed if they are to prevent the chaos which would follow a disorderly scramble after the coveted values. One important consequence of such rules is that people must wait, often for long periods of time, before they can obtain the ultimate rewards, and in the nature of such a system some people will be destined never to achieve them. Waiting, along with the possibility of never gaining valued ends, is difficult for human beings. Accordingly, the prestige system of every society has built into it devices that will make waiting bearable and will make the fact that all cannot attain the highest goals a tolerable if not a happy situation. One such device is embodied in proximate rewards, rewards which can be achieved during the waiting period as substitutes for the ultimate goals.

It is likely that characteristic features of Yap culture—nonresponsible early adulthood, love affairs during youth, and induced abortion—originated during a period of ample population. At that time these practices were undoubtedly effective in keeping down the birth rate. When young men and women spent their time avoiding the responsibilities of adulthood, they did not press closely on the high prestige statuses of the old people. When young women were strongly motivated to postpone reproduction until their later years by inducing abortion, they shortened the time span within which they could reproduce and thus limited the overall number of births on the island.

Today, however, underpopulation rather than overpopulation is the dominant problem, and shortening the reproductive span of a woman's life by inducing abortion during her younger years serves instead to aggravate the imbalance. Why, then, does abortion persist? Because they cannot become chiefs or heads of kin groups, women can never achieve the same rewards from the prestige system that the men do. For them, the pattern of repeated love affairs provides pleasure and reward; resort to abortion makes it easier to maintain this pattern of behavior. For men, who must still mark time before assuming positions of prestige and responsibility, protracted love-making offers interim rewards. These practices persist, not merely as useless holdovers from a past era of overpopulation, but as vehicles that continue to serve useful purposes and give psychological gratifications.

IMPLICATIONS

Should anything be done about abortion on Yap? Answers to this question must be predicated on the realization that the abortion problem cannot be considered in isolation but is tied to other aspects of Yap culture. If anything is done, it must be done in a responsible way or not at all. Responsibility implies many considerations. One of these requires asking whether the Yap people feel a need to have something done. The answer is both yes and no. On the one hand, the people of Yap—particularly the men—clearly feel the need to do something about the low population. If they were convinced that eliminating abortion would increase their numbers, they would incline to support such a policy. On the other hand, the felt need of the women depends on their age. After thirty they want children, but eliminating abortion and providing no substitute method would work counter to the felt needs of women under thirty.

Another aspect of the responsibility problem concerns our own moral evaluation of the Yap situation. Among all their felt needs, and there are surely many, which will we try to meet? A program to eliminate induced abortion would have to ponder the problem of introducing another form of birth control to take its place. This inevitably enmeshes us in our own moral values. However we choose to resolve this sensitive issue, we will necessarily become involved in a related one, namely, the responsibility for anticipating the indirect consequences of an action program. Assuming that we were able to increase population by eliminating abortion, could this increase be controlled and kept within practical limits? Yap is a small island in a wide sea, and its resources are limited. At least once before it has suffered from overpopulation, so that food was scarce and people were hungry. Can we responsibly take action that will tend to reverse the population trend without considering the danger of once again bringing about overpopulation? Any program of population control must aim toward a balance adjusted to available or possible food resources.

Overpopulation could be a major undesirable consequence of a well-intentioned but unwise policy. On the other hand, there are other less obvious consequences more difficult to evaluate. Let us assume that we find a means to eliminate induced abortion in such a way as to preclude overpopulation. Mechanical and chemical devices are not and cannot be manufactured on Yap. They would have to be imported and someone would have to pay for them.

So far, the Yaps have scarcely become involved in a money economy. They like tobacco and good steel knives. Today they gather a bit of copra and sail it along the coast to the settlement at Yaptown where they exchange it for money to buy tobacco and knives. But they gather the copra only when they want to, not when the price is right. Germans, Japanese, and Americans have all found the Yaps undependable as a labor force. They far prefer asking for tobacco than to work for the money to buy it with; they assume that any decent human being who has tobacco will share it with those who have none.

If they are to have birth control devices, either they will have to pay for them or the goods will have to be supplied free of charge. The cost of this item alone would not be sufficient to force them into full-time wage labor, but this could become one of a series of conditions that might produce such results. Is this to be seen as a favorable consequence or an inevitable consequence, or as something for a program planner to worry over in advance?

Another facet of the responsibility problem is to foresee to what extent a new item will remain available and a new practice remain possible. If birth control materials could be brought to Yap and successfully introduced, what provision could be made for maintaining the supply over a long-time span? It would be irresponsible to say in effect, "Here is a five-year supply of materials. After the fifth year you will have to figure out some way of getting them yourselves." It is hard to picture how a responsible program could in fact guarantee a continuing supply of materials. Yap has been governed in turn by the Spanish, Germans, Japanese, and Americans. Administrations and policies within administrations have changed time and again. The international situation is not such that we can say that things are now settled. With more certainty, we can say that even within the brief period of American administration there have been some major changes of policy at the upper levels and an interminable series of "shake-ups" at the local level. Would it be wise to initiate a program with far-reaching consequences in view of the likelihood that administrative changes might force its cancellation after people have come to count on its continuance?

Problems of Policy

A sound program to halt abortion would initiate only those changes acceptable to the Yap, would anticipate the major consequences of such a program, and would entail responsible planning, execution, follow-up, and control over ensuing changes. The introduction of some appropriate form of contraception would meet most of these policy requirements and at the same time prove practical.

The outstanding problem is that of the women who do not want children at one period of their lives. To challenge this motivation directly would be futile. It would also be unethical, in the writer's view. A form of contraception that does not cause infection would be an ideal substitute for the current and possibly harmful technique of abortion. During that period of a woman's life when she did not want to bear children, she could safely avoid pregnancy. This plan would substitute one device for another without alteration in motivation or in pattern of general behavior.

The danger of eventual overpopulation would be minimized since contraception is a form of population control. Moreover, the rise in population level would probably be gradual, since only the later years of a woman's fertility span would be involved. Readjustment to increasing population would be easier if the rise were gradual rather than precipitous.

It might be supposed that putting contraceptive devices in the hands of women would increase their power and thus disturb the pattern of interpersonal relations between husbands and wives. I think that this would not be the case. In the first place, the present abortion technique is already in the hands of the women. In the second place, Yap is no fanciful patriarchate in which the men have so subdued the women that a social revolution would follow female emancipation. Yap women do not enjoy precise equality but their status is close to that of men, and women have distinct minds of their own which they do not hesitate to use. A man can abuse his wife only once; she would leave, and her kinsmen would begin vigorous inquiries.

Substituting contraception for abortion would cause very little social change, but two practical problems would arise: the cost of the program and responsibility for maintaining the supply of materials. Continued contact with western European culture almost inevitably will introduce more and more of our standards including a money economy; but it need not be the task of a health action program to initiate these changes. Assuming their inevitability, these far-reaching changes should be the responsibility of the island's civil administration, as part of a carefully planned program including medical service; they should not be tied directly to the tail of a particular health project. The cost of a long-range culture-change program must either be borne by agencies outside Yap or financed with a view to receiving repayment sometime after introducing a money economy on the island.

Problems of Implementation

To implement a birth control plan such as suggested, the sequence of action, the timing, the phrasing, the channels of communication, would all require point by point collaboration between anthropological and medical personnel. Experience has shown that this is more easily projected than accomplished. Two major aims of the project would be to establish the relevant medical and cultural facts on Yap and to generate an atmosphere of trust and rapport. To these ends the program should begin with a period of joint preparatory study by selected members of the anthropological and medical teams. Study and establishment of rapport go hand in hand, provided the study is conducted tactfully and with due attention to the concerns of those studied. Three to four months of preparatory work should permit the action program to begin with favorable prospects of success.

Anthropological research already conducted on Yap points to a number of areas of potential difficulty. Difficulties would probably be encountered; first, in explaining the presence of the persons involved; second, in clearly communicating the objectives in terms understandable to the Yaps; third, in exploring the areas of resistance; and fourth, in minimizing these resistances.

One probable area of resistance will concern medical examination. Yap women are loath to submit to genital examination, and their husbands are even more opposed to letting them be examined. The Yaps have very vivid and bitter memories of medical field work carried out by the Japanese. They were forcibly stripped in mixed groups, subjected to public examination, and several Japanese men sometimes held consultations over the exposed women. Obviously, the job need not be done in this way. In 1947 a conscientious and tactful American medical officer was able to persuade quite a few women to have their children delivered in the Navy-supervised native hospital, although resistance to this suggestion was considerable when he first undertook the task. His success suggests that genital examination could be accomplished. Clear explanation of the necessity for the examination would reduce resistance. The explanation should be made in terms that Yaps can understand, giving assurance of privacy and stressing the desired end of having more babies. Contrary to expectations, employment of female personnel as examining assistants would probably arouse resistance, since Yap women implicitly view any other woman of whatever age as a potential rival for men's attentions. Yap women feel that the worst thing that can happen to them is to expose their genitals, the source of their competitive power, to another woman.

It should not be too difficult to convince the women that contraception would be more desirable than abortion. Once they are past the very early years of their adolescence, Yap women treat sexual relations in a straightforward manner, if the discussion is private and with a man. Women distrust other women, considering them unreliable competitors. While they view sexual relations as pleasurable and desirable in their own right, they also regard them as means to further ends. On Yap a woman's genitals are likened to a man's land; they are her real asset in terms of which she maintains her position in the all-embracing Yap hierarchy of rank and prestige. A woman relies on her genitals to get what she wants: lovers, attention, and the power over men that protects her against being put in a subservient position. At first, she tries to get lovers, and does so by judiciously withholding and granting sexual favors; later, these same sexual powers should provide the children that secure her position as an important and irreplaceable member of a family. Treating sex as a means to an end, not alone as a form of direct gratification, enables women to exercise a high degree of control. The rational appeal to young women to substitute contraception for abortion in their own self-interest would not fall on deaf ears.

A program for the introduction of contraception would probably encounter opposition from the Yap men, from the resident Catholic missionary, and from religious groups outside Yap who exert influence on the administration. Yap men would have to be dealt with directly, for they are all concerned as fathers, brothers, husbands, and potential husbands of the women. I do not believe that Yap men recognize the high incidence of induced abortion. By Yap standards, a man who discovers that his wife has induced abortion would be justifiably violent. Knowing this, any Yap woman who aborts will not tell her husband if she can avoid it. Men have very strong feelings about discussions of sexual matters between their wives and other men. In their view extramarital intimacy, even of a nonsexual nature, constitutes adultery and is punished as such. Further, it is men's conviction that they cannot really exert control directly over the women but can only keep other men away from their wives. A man who suspects his wife of infidelity vents his anger on her, to be sure, but he feels that the only effective remedy is to stop the other man. It would thus be necessary to dissociate consultation between young woman and physician from the sphere of adultery, taking pains to convince the men that the relationship was a purely medical matter.

However, the men are acutely aware of the depopulation problem. In certain respects it has raised more havoc with their concerns than with those of women. It is the male political organization, oriented toward prestige values, which has become extremely difficult to maintain. "Everybody is chief now," they say ruefully. Men are always willing to discuss ways and means of having more babies. Presented to them in this context, a program for contraception would receive a careful hearing. They believe that pregnancy is due to the beneficence of ancestral ghosts and the cooperation of a certain spirit. Older people firmly believe that coitus has nothing whatever to do with conception, except that coitus at the wrong time or place or with the wrong person will offend the ghosts and spirit, and these in turn will deny pregnancy to an offending woman or to the wife of an offending husband. The younger people, having come under Japanese influence, are not so sure about this. Young people believe that the ghosts and spirit have much to do with conception, but that coitus is probably important too. Both older and younger men alike are realists and will try a new proposal if it seems to show any promise at all.

For example, the German and Japanese administrations both treated yaws without success, as did the native magicians, except that the magicians occasionally claimed cures. As the Yaps saw the situation, no one but the spirits could cure yaws. Notwithstanding these beliefs, they tried the antibiotic treatment offered by American Navy physicians and were happily surprised when it worked. They still believe that no one but spirits can cure yaws; but they argue that where the Germans and Japanese and their own magicians had all failed to influence the spirits, American medicine knew the secret. This secret was so powerful that American doctors could gain the cooperation of the spirits without going through the series of ritual steps ordinarily required—payment of shell "money," offering of prayer, and observance of taboos.

Whichever way the Yaps may decide to rationalize the role of contraception in raising the birth rate, they could probably be convinced that it is worth trying, that the doctors' "directions" are a potentially effective ritual. I can see no harm in permitting men or women to regard the mechanics of any contraceptive technique as a ritual; it will be treated far more respectfully and carefully if the "ritual" instructions are clear and simple. On the other hand, I foresee only confusion and resistance if the whole matter is treated in a purely rational or "scientific" way. It will not endear the doctor to his patients if he insists or implies that their beliefs are unfounded and that only his own science is right; they will have a hard time understanding his science and will be offended by his disdain for their beliefs.

The problem of conveying the skills and techniques of contraception and of inculcating the habits necessary for the effective use of contraceptive materials is perhaps the biggest single problem of any such program. Much would depend on the particular contraceptive technique chosen. To be most successful on Yap, the technique should have certain characteristics. First, the technique must be in the hands of the women, not the men. Second, it should be as simple as possible. Dangers of misuse should be minimized even at the expense of a degree of failure to prevent conception. Like most nonwestern European peoples, Yaps do not have the sense of time and routine which we have developed so highly. Third, the materials should be cheap, easy to replace and, as indicated earlier, they should remain available. Fourth, the instructions must be clearly communicated and simple to follow, and there should be routine ways to check that they are understood.

SUMMARY

Induced abortion is a problem on Yap. It is a factor in keeping down the fertility rate and in prolonging the underpopulated state of the island. The practice of abortion cannot be understood apart from its cultural context. Until about the age of thirty, women who become pregnant are motivated to induce abortion, relying on a method that involves at least temporary injury to themselves. But after thirty, women have an intense desire for children. Older men, too, bemoan the low production of babies.

Young women resort to abortion because they have no other reliable means to prevent the birth of unwanted children. They do not want them because children would complicate the most highly valued pursuit available to young men and women on Yap, namely, elaborate and intricate love affairs involving a succession of lovers. The high value placed on love affairs is consistent with the fact that the Yaps consider adult responsibilities as appropriate only to people in their more mature years.

Up to the age of about thirty, Yap men and women are assumed to be "youths" rather than adults, and on Yap the proper behavior for youths is engaging in love affairs. The protracted period of youth is related to the fact that Yap is a stratified society in which positions of high rank are few in number and reserved for the older generation. The rewards of life prized above all others on Yap, the achievement of prestige and high status, are all found in late adulthood and old age. Freed from many of the responsibilities that are thrust upon men and women shortly after physiological maturity in many other parts of the world, young men and women on Yap can afford to pre-occupy themselves with love-making. This preoccupation makes the long wait for high status tolerable and rewarding.

With the knowledge now on hand, it is difficult to estimate how much of the partial sterility on the part of women who are over thirty and who desperately want children is due to complications arising from abortions induced before the age of thirty when children are not wanted, and how much is attributable to the venereal infection of both sexes. But whether, in the interest of repopulation, one is primarily concerned with the control of abortion or with the control of venereal disease, he must recognize the significance of the love-making pattern and its relationship to the entire way of life on Yap. He must be aware that the needs and motivations of a Yap individual vary according to age. He must also realize that the introduction of any one change such as mechanical contraception, if not properly planned, can do as much to disturb the equilibrium as to correct it.

SELECTED REFERENCES

Furness, William H., *The Island of Stone Money*. J. B. Lippincott Co., Philadelphia, 1910. An old but excellent picture of life on Yap.

Gladwin, Thomas, and S. B. Sarasan, *Truk:* Man in Paradise. Viking Fund Publications in Anthropology, No. 10, New York, 1953. An account of culture and personality on another Micronesian island.

Hunt, Edward E., Jr., Nathaniel Kidder, and David M. Schneider, "The Depopulation of Yap," *Human Biology*, vol. 26, February, 1954, pp. 21–51. A fuller report on the probable causes of Yap depopulation.

Schneider, David M., "Yap Kinship Terminology and Kin Groups," *American Anthropologist*, vol. 55, April-June, 1953, pp. 215–236. A technical article on Yap kinship patterns and their meaning for general kinship theory.

Spoehr, Alexander, *Majuro:* A Village in the Marshall Islands. Chicago Natural History Museum, 1949. A very competent and readable report on a community in another part of Micronesia.

PART IV

EFFECTS OF SOCIAL SEGMENTATION

Case 9

WESTERN MEDICINE IN A VILLAGE OF NORTHERN INDIA

by McKim Marriott

This case study, like the one by Dr. Carstairs, Case 4, presents the contrast between western and rural Indian medicine in terms of the doctor-patient relationship. But the two authors use different frames of reference to characterize the Indian point of view. Dr. Carstairs' approach is psychocultural; he relates the patient's expectations to the general cultural climate of the Indian community. In depicting the worldview of the people of the area, he makes only passing reference to organizational features which divide them into different status groups.

Dr. Marriott uses social structure as his primary frame of reference. The social world of the villager consists of three concentric realms. Representatives of each realm command varying degrees of trust; and different degrees of trust and honor are appropriate in dealings among members of groups of the three realms. Despite good medicines and good intentions, the practitioner of western medicine is regarded with suspicion because his conduct usually identifies him as belonging to the remote outside world, or to a low position in village society. To gain greater acceptance, he must penetrate to a suitable position in the zone between the realm of the outsider and the inner realm of kinship. How this might be done is suggested by Dr. Marriott's illuminating comparison of different types of indigenous curers and their methods of establishing relations with their clients.

*In Dr. Marriott's mode of exposition, psychocultural factors are secondary to structural features. Although his approach is different, he is not in disagreement with Dr. Carstairs. Rather, both writers inspect essentially the same phenomena from separate observation points. Like stereoscopic vision, the two views together place the sociocultural context of medical behavior in better perspective.—*EDITOR

THE PROBLEM

The Marginal Position of Western Medicine

"Western medicines are best," I was told by an old carpenter in the remote village of Kishan Garhi, "but doctors never cure anybody." The old carpenter had worked in a large town for many years and knew what doctors were like, but to people who

239

have never lived outside Kishan Garhi, the carpenter's dilemma is equally real. In this village of 850 persons, more than 20 have sought treatment from western doctors,[1] but only two of these— a man saved from hydrophobia by a course of injections and a youth whose crushed and gangrenous arm had been amputated— believed that the doctors' treatments had effected their cure.

The villages of western Uttar Pradesh (United Provinces) are considered to be among the most healthful of India, and Kishan Garhi, a mainly Hindu community in the Aligarh District, is representative of the more conservative agricultural villages of that region. Kishan Garhi lies several miles from any road or town and in 1952 was still far away from any of India's energetic new Community Development Projects. Its 165 families live in houses of mud, crammed wall upon wall around the base of a landlord's fortress. The farmers of Kishan Garhi grow ample amounts of wheat and barley by dint of hard manual labor in the encircling fields. They subsist ordinarily on bread, crude sugar, and a little buttermilk, supplemented rarely by seasonal vegetables and fruits. They quench their thirst on water drunk from open, muddy wells. Villagers pride themselves on their simple life, the purity of their food, and on what they believe to be their exceptional toughness and good health.

But a trained observer might perceive much room for improvement in the general health of Kishan Garhi. The great majority of villagers suffer chronically from dysentery and from trachoma. Dysentery is readily communicated to the mouth either directly by hands soiled with fecal matter, or indirectly by perpetual clouds of flies from the feces which lie exposed in the village lanes. The first of a life-long series of eye infections is passed on to each new infant before his eyes are fully open. The vision of many adults is seriously impaired. In addition, nearly one in five villagers suffers from malaria. Epidemics of cholera and smallpox have taken a large toll of lives, while typhoid, gonorrhea, and tuberculosis still flourish endemically. Deficiencies in the standard village diet are evidenced in the high frequency of boils, skin and

---

[1] The term "western" is used for convenience and should be understood as meaning western in type or tradition. Thus, the designation "western" would apply not only to a European or American medical practitioner, but also to an Indian practitioner trained in the western type of medical institution.

eye ailments, lack of appetite, general fatigue, and in the slow healing of simple injuries, even under medication.

In seeking treatment for these and other diseases, the residents of Kishan Garhi have at their disposal both traditional methods of treatment and the services of western medical practitioners. Western facilities have been provided by government, by Christian missions, and by a few private practitioners, and have existed in all large towns and cities of the Ganges Valley for more than fifty years. Yet they have hardly touched most of the villages. In the lives of most villagers, clinics serve as momentary stopping places on the sick man's pilgrimage from one indigenous practitioner to another, and hospitals serve all too frequently as last resorts of the dying. Many elaborate scientific facilities in the area are unused today, or are used in fits and fragments which rarely effect cure, and tend rather to vitiate faith in the techniques themselves. Even assuming that an increase in clinics and dispensaries of the present type would have some value—an assumption that seems contrary to fact—the cost of such an increase would be far more than any government or charitable organization could support.

The facilities of western medicine are largely ignored by the inhabitants of Kishan Garhi, but indigenous folk-medicine— magical, sacred, and secular—flourishes in every village of northern India. In terms of numbers of patients, amount of expenditure, and frequency of use, patronage of indigenous medicine surpasses that of western medicine one hundredfold. Although the customs and tenets of indigenous medicine are generally at variance with those of western medicine, some indigenous practitioners working in cities appropriate certain palliatives or paraphernalia from western medicine and live well on their trade. Villages will cheerfully pay a rural wizard for the utterance of a spell and will give high reward to an urban practitioner who promises extravagant results from the hypodermic injection of what is actually a bit of plain water. However, the same villagers seem unwilling to take pills from a western-type dispensary unless the pills are given free. Western medicine sits outside the door of the village, dependent upon governmental subsidy and foreign alms for its slim existence.

THE SITUATION

Organization of the Village and Medical Practice

For a period of fourteen months during 1950–1952 the writer lived in Kishan Garhi, making an anthropological study of village social organization.[1] Experiences with the villagers during the course of this study made me vividly aware that there was both a need and an active demand for more effective means of dealing with disease. Hindu peasants brought written reports on their own blood counts, urine analyses, chest x-ray plates, and numerous unfilled prescriptions for foreign medicines; they begged me to help them to decide what they should do next. Many villagers were surprised and disappointed when they discovered that I would not perform surgical operations, that my first-aid medical kit contained none of those prized western machines—the stethoscope, the ophthalmoscope, and especially the hypodermic needle. These and many more devices of scientific medicine are known and desired.

An Exploratory Effort

After six months in Kishan Garhi, I was able to enlist the cooperation of a young English physician who was then in the area. To see at first hand what happens when western medicine is brought directly to the village, we set up a small clinic to run for one week. We publicized our project in advance. We then tried to present western medicine in its most favorable light: patients were dealt with carefully as individuals of equal worth; accurate diagnostic techniques were made available; medicines were offered at cost rates far below those prevailing on the open market; examination, diagnosis, and dressings were given free. The people of the village were encouraged to see how the doctor worked. They were helped to understand the doctor's diagnoses both through immediate explanations and through illustrated talks given later by the writer. Beyond his clinical hours, the

[1] Field study was supported by an Area Research Training Fellowship granted by the Social Science Research Council. The writer is directly indebted to Dr. John B. Wyon for proposing the medical exploration and for carrying it out with great zeal. For comments and suggestions on this paper, thanks are due to Mrs. Gitel P. Steed, to Mr. Albert Mayer, and to many other helpful readers.

doctor participated in many informal gatherings throughout the village. Villagers expressed their liking for his personal manner and their praise for the excellence of his skill.

Yet the results of this brief exploration in Kishan Garhi differed little from the response to western medicine which has been so familiar in other clinics in rural India. Persons soon flocked into the clinic to receive simple palliatives for such complaints as headache, toothache, and inflamed eyes. But out of 150 sick persons examined, barely a dozen were willing to pay in advance for even sample doses of the effective medicines which the doctor had prescribed to cure the causes of their ailments. The doctor was obliged to spend nearly half of his clinical hours in coaxing the patients to pay the tiny amounts charged for medicines in order that the clinic might support itself. Most of the patients pleaded false poverty and begged to be given medicines free. On the other hand, some poor patients put sizable currency notes into the doctor's hand, demanding that he give them only the finest medicines along with a money-back guarantee of certain cure.

At many points, too, the doctor was impeded in his work because of having to disengage the patients, for purposes of individual examination, from the many anxious family members who accompanied them. Frustrating situations frequently arose in which people begged for medicine which then went unused. One Brahman girl, for example, was suffering the chills and fevers of acute malaria during the doctor's visit. The girl's father and her father's brothers came repeatedly to beg that the doctor give her quinine. The doctor sold a full course of quinine pills to the men but discovered three days later that none of the quinine had been permitted to reach the girl. An old widowed aunt who ruled the women of that family had voiced objections, and the whole matter of western treatment was dropped.

A follow-up study of the clinic's patients was even more discouraging. After the doctor's departure, nearly all of those few persons who had begun his treatments soon fell back upon their indigenous practices and practitioners. The only wage-earning son of one poor laborer, a neighbor of the writer, was diagnosed by the doctor as tubercular. Calcium lactate and shark liver oil were prescribed, and a supply was arranged for the boy at nominal cost. A few days after the doctor's departure, the laborer went deeply into debt in order to buy for the boy a preparation of honey and gold which had been made and guaranteed by an indigenous specialist. Among the others, only two villagers ever sought to obtain any of the more extensive treatments which the doctor had advised them to seek from urban hospitals; those two did so only after receiving repeated reassurances and specific help from the writer.

We had brought western medicine to the village and the village was full of sick people, but western medicine did not reach the sick. Why did villagers not accept the doctor's instructions? Why did they seem not to trust him? Why wouldn't villagers shoulder even slight financial responsibility for their own cures? Why did they ultimately prefer treatment by less effective means? Here again was the old carpenter's paradox: "Western medicines are best, but doctors never cure anybody."

Villagers' apathetic responses to the exploratory clinic sharpened the challenge, but in themselves suggest only negative ways out of the dilemma. The exploration had at least narrowed the issues and eliminated some of the presumed difficulties. Difficulties evidently did not lie merely in the physical distance of western facilities from the village, nor in any personal aloofness on the part of the doctor. They did not lie simply in peasant fears of something unknown, nor in objections to scientific techniques, nor in careless diagnosis, nor in high costs—faults which are commonly cited to explain the failure of western medicine to take hold in rural regions of India. While the brevity of the exploratory clinic at Kishan Garhi cannot be discounted as influencing the outcome, it seems clear that other and more powerful factors were at work. Even allowing for the impossibility of demonstrating many cures in so short a time, the most significant difficulties encountered by this clinic were identical with those which continue to trouble many long-established centers of western medicine in India. These difficulties require explanation.

Answers to the dilemma seemed to lie not in gross technical matters, but rather in the system of interpersonal relations. Trust, responsibility, charity, power, respect—these are the issues on which failure turned. These are not technical issues but issues which concern the cultural definition of medical roles. The solution of the dilemma and the keys to greater success seemed to consist in developing an acceptable social place in the village for western medicine.

To discover the reasons behind the difficulties met by the exploratory clinic at Kishan Garhi—and behind the failure of western medicine to take hold in rural India generally—we must understand the nature of the existing social and medical institutions of the village and how these institutions influence the manner in which the villager perceives the western medical practitioner.

The Social World of the Indian Village

Kinship. Village society in India, like most non-European societies of the world today, is very largely a familial society. The groups within which people can always trust each other and cooperate are limited to groups such as the household, the lineage of common descent, and, in northern India, the network of families in different villages that are related by marriage. Fellow members of such familial groupings must help each other by extensive gifts, by loans often without interest, and by first preference in all economic dealings. They must give absolute mutual support in case of trouble. Members of the different lineages that have existed together for centuries in the village of Kishan Garhi tend to regard each other as quasi-kinsmen and may address each other politely as "father's brother," "brother's son," and the like. But such extended relationships are never really so certain, never so free from the fear of treachery as are genuine family relationships.

Beyond the circle of his own true family, the individual must assume the world to be indifferent to his welfare, for it is made up of other closed kin groups, each constituted like his own, and each furthering the interests of none but its own members. A villager does not ordinarily dare to venture out of his village for any important purpose unless he knows where he will find a bed and who will give him bread, unless he knows that he will be able to achieve his purpose through his own relatives or through people of his own village with whom he has some strong, dependent tie.

Some special characteristics of the northern Hindu village are that its kinship groups, with all the loyalties they command, are so small and so numerous, and that they so frequently lack any single leader. Families themselves are sharply divided for almost all activities into separate male and female worlds, each having its separate structure of power. Inside the village of Kishan Garhi, a man can count an average of fewer than 20 persons, both male and female, within the widest limits of his lineage group. A village of average size will contain at least ten—Kishan Garhi contains 46 such ultimate familial groupings. Each lineage group is totally unconnected by marriage or descent with any other lineage in the village, and each is wholly distinct in responsibility. Each gives almost limitless rewards to its members and makes almost limitless demands upon them.

Such extreme subdivision of the people of a single village into a large number of discrete kinship groups puts great obstructions in the way of wider cooperation. Individuals cannot easily form new relationships. If villagers who are not kinsmen try to band together out of friendship or even out of vital interest in some common task, they often risk suspicion of being disloyal to their own familial group. "The village is full of dishonest people, full of thieves," villagers frequently warned me. When a new financial agreement requiring cooperation and trust is proposed, even if its weight is trivial, many safeguards are likely to be felt necessary: witnesses may be called to listen to repetitions of the terms; a single coin may be given, binding giver and receiver in a sacred contract to fulfill all the terms of their agreement. Outside the family, all things must be made doubly sure.

Caste. A second special characteristic of Hindu village society provides a partial answer to the problems raised by the first. This is the use of ranking, or hierarchy, as a major element in relationships among persons and kinship groups. In Kishan Garhi the multiplicity of 46 closed and autonomous lineages is appreciably reduced by a ranked ordering into 24 castes. Each kinship group in Kishan Garhi is merged into one of the local caste groups, and each local caste group is part of a larger regional caste.

Each local caste group in the village holds an approximate caste rank, and holds a stable place in one of the four still larger ranked blocs of castes—Brahman, high, low, and untouchable. The local ranking of the castes and blocs of castes correlates in a general way with differences of wealth and power but more precisely with certain observances between the castes. Ways in which people can eat together, sit together, or address one another serve continually to reaffirm the order of caste ranking which is generally recognized in Kishan Garhi. Thus, a member of the highest Brahman or priestly caste must be greeted by a person of lower caste rank with the sentence, "We should touch your feet, honorable learned man!" A Brahman when so addressed must reply with a blessing, "Live happily!" A Brahman must always be seated at the head of any cot when other castes are present, and only members of the high castes may share the cot with him. A Brahman can eat only those foods that have been prepared in certain ways by members of certain other high or "clean" castes. Each caste below the Brahman also has its special position in the system of ritual and etiquette. Each has its honorific title, the main landlord caste being called by a title that is identical with one name of God, while the lowest sweeper of latrines has the title "headman" or "sergeant."

Most families are obliged to give honorific service to certain families of higher castes and are privileged to demand honorific service from certain families of lower castes. The nature of these honorific services is fixed in tradition for each caste. Some castes have the traditional duty of following certain menial occupations, some of practicing particular crafts. Other castes traditionally grow food; others engage in trade; others conduct religious rituals; and still others wield power and govern. From each of its servant families of lower caste, the patron household may demand some essential, unique service; from each of its patron families of higher caste, the servant may claim a dole of bread upon the performance of the service, a fixed quantity of grain twice during the year and many other kinds of assistance whenever necessity arises. "The point of the whole system," villagers told me, "is to make sure that there will always be someone whom you can depend upon." Without the caste system of honorific rituals and services which arranges everyone in higher and lower ranks, many villagers fear that their society would have no order at all.

Individuals are born into families that occupy particular caste and service positions. Differences in individual achievement of wealth, power, and ability may be acknowledged, but such achievements remain irrelevant to caste; the ritualized caste position into which an individual is born continues always to affect most of his relationships with his fellow villagers. Regardless of a villager's personal qualities, regardless of his learning to practice some new or educated profession, he will continue to receive the formal treatment required by etiquette for all members of his caste. The poorest man of the village, if he is a Brahman by caste, still will be asked to sit at the head of the cot; the wealthiest man of the village, if he is a lowly leatherworker by caste, still sits on the floor or stands respectfully at a distance; and the cleverest man of the village, if he is a sweeper by caste, still lingers below in the street.

Such extreme stability of caste and kinship leaves individuals fairly free to think and to believe as they please. Thus, within one family there may be devotees of as many different gods as there are members; one member of the family may know nothing and care nothing about the gods worshiped by another member. But the requirements of active loyalty to family welfare and observance of intercaste etiquette place severe limits on an individual's social scope. An individual is not free to form friendships or to develop any personal alliances which conflict with the interests of his own caste and kinship group. Beyond the larger family and its caste, the only approved and reliable relationships are the formal cross-caste ties between high patrons and low servants.

Outside the Village. When villagers must deal with strangers, they have their choice of including the stranger either in a family or in an intercaste type of relationship. If strangers are thrown together anonymously as in a bus or in an urban shop and if their common activities are casual ones, then they may classify each other by relative age as pseudokinsmen. Ultimately they may trace more specific kinlike connections through villages with which they share real family relationships.

But when villagers must deal in important ways with outsiders who are more powerful than themselves—with lawyers, officials, urban creditors, and the like—then they generally attempt to extend upward a castelike form of relationship. Whenever possible, intermediaries are used who have some genuine, stable tie both with the villager and with the powerful outsider. When intermediaries cannot be found, then direct flattery and courtesy may be used to simulate obligations between persons of high and low caste where such obligations have not actually existed before. When intermediary negotiations, flattery, and hospitality are rejected or prove insufficient—a situation that often arises in relations with outside government officials—then payment of money remains almost the only way in which the villager can ensure his own interests.

But outside the family and village, monetary gifts cannot create immutable sacred obligations as they do inside. Bribes have only temporary effects which fluctuate with the amount given and with the expectation of more. The poor villager is rarely in a position to give enough money to guarantee more than momentary favor from an official or poor goods from an urban shopkeeper. He gives petty amounts, despises the taker, and suspects the worst of what he gets in return.

The people of Kishan Garhi thus recognize three great social realms—that of kinship and family, which is an area controlled by limitless demands and mutual trust; that of the village and caste, which is an area in part controlled by particular obligations and formal respect; and that of the outside world, of government and the market place, which is an area controllable only by money and power—things which the villager scarcely possesses.

For the people of Kishan Garhi, western medicine has existed up to now only in the third or outer realm beyond family and beyond caste and village. It has remained, therefore, in the realm of contrived dependency and fundamental distrust. Until the day when the relations of the inner and outer social realms may be differently defined and perceived, western medicine seems doomed to languish. If western medicine is to be established not merely in, but as a part of, the middle or inner realms of village society, it must be made to fit the organizational forms of that society. To illuminate in more specific terms these problems of social adaptation, it is instructive to examine the indigenous medical services of the village. Their problems are not dissimilar to those confronting western medicine, and they have solved these problems of social adaptation with noted success.

Indigenous Medical Practice

Indigenous village medical services are overwhelmingly preferred to western medicine. Their strength is due in large part to their successful adaptation to the fundamentals of village social organization. The social roles of indigenous practitioners embody certain elements which no practitioner in rural India can afford to ignore. Some of these elements present incompatible contrasts, while others present rather close parallels with the position and behavior of the physician in western society. Whether these role elements are similar or dissimilar, villagers have specific expectations based on their life-long experiences with relationships between therapist and patient. These expectations affect their comprehension of western medicine and their initial reaction to it.

Indigenous medical specialists in an Indian village such as Kishan Garhi are extremely varied. They include priests, exorcists, magicians, and secular physicians as well as numberless minor technicians such as bone-setters, charm-sellers, cuppers, cultists, surgeons, and thorn-pullers. Like all other persons in traditional Indian society, specialists must occupy relatively higher or lower positions in the village hierarchy of caste and power. Despite great diversity of content among the medical theories and practices of the many specialists, the principle of hierarchical ranking imparts a certain similarity to the whole array of specialized roles.

The Family and Medicine. Specialized medical services are always rendered within the context of the family, and each family tends to occupy a definite position in the village hierarchy. Village families do not isolate an ailing member, as is often the case in the western world, but rather envelop him. Few villagers would think of seeking medical treatment of any consequence without taking family members along with them. Reciprocally, the writer has seen indigenous medical specialists demand that family members be present. The duties of the attending family members are to protect and gain attention for the weakened person, to help the specialist in his work (since ritual rules of intercaste pollution would sometimes hinder a specialist's treatment), to remember directions for home treatment, and to stand security as a group for the costs of the treatment. The larger family in the village thus does what in western society would be done respectively by receptionist, lawyer, nurse, orderly, secretary, and bondsman. It is difficult to see how the western type of medical practitioners in Indian villages could manage to do without such essential family contributions. To use them, of course, is to abandon certain occidental conceptions of privacy and individual responsibility in favor of group responsibility.

Lines of power within village families also affect the utilization of medical treatment. Whatever the treatment may be that is suggested by a specialist, it will be mediated and enforced, or perhaps modified or rejected, according to who is most influential in that particular family. The exploratory clinic in Kishan Garhi encountered this problem directly when courses of treatment were thoroughly "sold" to some members of a family but were later rejected by others who had controlling voices in the family. Since families in villages of northern India frequently lack lines of authority that are obvious to nonmembers, and since the social worlds of men and women are sharply divided, authoritative communication by the medical specialist must aim to include all important family members of both sexes, if it is to be effective. As will be seen, the techniques of diagnosis and treatment used by certain religious exorcists in Kishan Garhi do in fact encourage many members of the family to participate in the cure under the direct guidance of the exorcist.

Resulting in part from this diffusion of power within most village groups is the fact that individuals of the same village—even of the same family—often hold highly varied medical beliefs and follow widely divergent practices. To the same sort of cut or boil, one man will apply a hot mango leaf; his neighbor will apply a paste of wheat flour; his father will apply a poultice of cow dung, while his wife continues to believe firmly in the efficacy of plain butter. If the wife is under the thumb of her husband's mother, then that matriarch's proposal for a magical sweeping and blowing may be added to the other treatments. In case of conflicting ideas, all advisers' suggestions for treatment may be applied in succession, or even all at once. Butter, dung, flour, and leaf may be simply laid on in successive layers—a typical solution to the problem of insistent but varied individual beliefs. Standardized medical treatments scarcely exist, while the internal divisions present in village and family structure are of no help in developing such treatments. Since some kinds of western medicine need to be applied alone and exclusively, the problem of finding an authoritative role for such treatment becomes all the more acute. Until such a role is found, western medicine must reconcile itself to existing in dilution along with its many competitors.

Magical Medicine. In Kishan Garhi and other villages, magical medicine comprises a body of mechanical techniques that can be directed against invading spirits. Its techniques include the wearing of protective strings and amulets and the expulsion of invading spirits by rituals of exorcism. Most young children wear two or three charms purchased from magicians—silver moon pendants, small red beads, capsules containing written spells, tiny bags containing iron, grain, and so on—tied around their necks or wrists. Adults also may wear charms designed for specific ailments which they fear may strike them, or from which they already suffer. When acute infections require that a spirit be exorcised, the magician blows on the infected part through a tube and sweeps it with a broom made of certain leaves, whispering at the same time his secret verbal formula until the spirit departs. In contrast to the mere writing of a prescription by the western doctor, the charm or the performance given by the village magician has an objective existence. Its effect is inherent, and villagers say that they can feel immediate improvement. The magical exorcist is therefore paid a few coins at once for his service, according to his standard low rates.

Blowing, sweeping, and the wearing of charms are appreciated by many villagers because such techniques are painless, quick, and safe. Magical exorcism has the special advantage that if the infection has been caused by a spiritual invasion, the spirit can simply be invited to depart without creating any further trouble. The same spirit is likely to become angered if direct medication is applied to his abode in the body. Only if medication can be understood as cleaning a wound rather than as killing the infection, can it remain theoretically compatible with magical exorcism. Thus, one priest of Kishan Garhi vigorously "cleaned" his son's dog-bite wound with potassium permanganate which I had given him; on alternate days, without conflict, he had it swept and blown by a magician.

But smallpox, a disease that is thought to result from an invasion by the goddess Mata, must be treated circumspectly through magical and religious techniques alone. If vaccination or medication of the skin were applied to any child of the village at a time when Mata was also present in his body, the touchy goddess would be angered and would surely kill or maim those victims whom she had already seized. Government vaccinators ordinarily succeed in inoculating a high proportion of new infants on their visits to Kishan Garhi. However, once during my stay the vaccinator arrived there on his regular circuit when two or three children were sick with chickenpox. The parents of the unvaccinated new babies mistook chickenpox for smallpox, were greatly alarmed, and paid the vaccinator to go away without inoculating anyone.

Despite such obvious differences and conflicts between magical belief and western medical theory, the social role of the medical magician in Kishan Garhi has a good deal in common with the social role of the druggist in western society. The techniques purveyed by both kinds of specialists are, in their respective societies, popular, mechanical, and impersonal. Magic treatments in this Hindu village society, like patent medicines in western society, can be dispensed by persons of almost any social rank and can be applied with little deference to hierarchical differences. Both can be bought and sold much as are other commodities on the market.

But these very similarities lead us to take note of a great contrast between the western world and rural India in attitudes toward technical activities. In the Indian village merely technical and petty commercial activities are of distinctly low rank; in no case do they impart any elevation to those who practice them. In western society elaborate technical competence in the performance of his professional role actually becomes one chief basis of the doctor's high professional prestige and authority. If the prestige of western medicine in a village such as Kishan Garhi had to depend on its techniques alone, its prestige would be no greater than that of barbering or shopkeeping—no greater, indeed, than that of magic itself, which is a relatively low craft commanding little respect. Such low prestige would be incompatible with the authority and confidence required for the more complex and serious kinds of medical therapy. Western medicine clearly cannot establish its full worth in an Indian village through technical performance alone.

Religious Exorcism. Certain religious exorcists in Kishan Garhi stand a notch above the technicians of magical medicine. Their wizardry comprises a rather more difficult art, an art that is inspired and actuated through religious devotion and that is often symbolized by the artist's slightly wild appearance or peculiar manner of dress. As professionals who trade on their intangible talents and on their ability to impress their clients, these specialists have something in common not only with modern faith healers in the West, but also with many western medical doctors of an older time.

Would-be practitioners of religious exorcism must first become "devotees" of a suitable god or goddess whom they will later be able to control by singing special hymns. Devotees may be recruited from many different castes above untouchable rank, although exorcists of higher caste tend to be most successful in developing a large clientele. Learning of the particular arts of exorcism usually descends within particular castes and lineages. In Kishan Garhi certain families of the priestly, weaving, and leatherworking castes carry on the traditions of exorcism, and each controls distinct gods and goddesses. An initiated exorcist is called "wise man." As a sideline, he often practices certain complex magical crafts, such as divining the names of thieves and locating stolen property.

A villager may call on a religious exorcist when he suffers from certain bodily ailments or psychic aberrations, or from any unusually suspicious series of external calamities affecting himself or his animals. The patient visits, or summons to his home, from one to a whole team of performers, who often reside at a great distance. The patient's entire family may be required to assist in the cure over a long period of time, preparing altars, sacrifices, or feasts, and giving clues to the exorcist that may help him identify the troublesome ghost or godling. The exorcists invoke their deity to drive other infesting spirits away. During the treatment the patient demonstrates his condition and its spiritual cause by one of several forms of emotional agitation or trance. The effectiveness of cure is believed to depend on the disposition of the spirits, the devotion of the performer, and the intensity of the performance. Its result is quickly known.

Payment to these religious exorcists works by an explicit principle quite different from that by which magicians are paid in the village and from that by which legitimate physicians are ordinarily paid in western society. The more the exorcist is paid, the better his curing is expected to be. Naturally, a large fee is promised in advance. Gifts of food sometimes are required to precede the treatment and continue at intervals throughout its course. Ultimately, however, depending on the results, a final cash price may be modified by negotiation. By contrast, legitimate medicine practiced according to western customs usually aims to standardize its techniques and to reduce costs as much as possible.

Carrying over the "more-the-better" principle of payment to their contacts with physicians trained in western medicine, villagers of my acquaintance often felt disappointed and distrustful when they learned how cheap and simple such physicians' treatments were. Thus, the doctor at the government dispensary nearest Kishan Garhi was considered unhelpful by the villagers because he usually ordered his pharmacist to dispense the inexpensive remedies subsidized by government funds. A persistent rumor held that the doctor would give better, more costly medicines and more energetic treatment if he were approached and tipped privately after hours. There was no direct evidence to support the rumor; indeed, the doctor was ready at any time to provide such service as injections of penicillin for all patients who needed them and who were able to pay the costs. It appeared that his efficiency and thrift were perceived as unhelpfulness and had served as well to brand the doctor as corrupt.

Western medicine might gain much and lose little if the asking prices of aspirin and bicarbonate of soda, for example, were adjusted upward to create an aura of quality that would engender confidence in the curative value of these useful products. It is true that the enhanced fee is a device that is well known to charlatans both in India and the West, but it also has its legitimate applications.

Sacerdotal Medicine. Domestic priests, who are recruited only from among the highest or Brahman caste, engage in a purely religious medical practice as a part of the profession of priesthood. Priests advise their clients to perform certain religious rituals as means of obtaining good health, prosperity, and children. They prescribe similar rituals as cures for illnesses that are believed to have been caused by religious laxity or immorality. Priestly prescriptions combine or recombine a limited number of fixed ritual elements: making pilgrimages, bathing in the Ganges, pouring water at the roots of sacred trees, praying, conducting sacrifices, offering charitable contributions to priests and beggars. Priests in Kishan Garhi, along with their domestic ritual duties, also give astrological advice, which helps their clients time their activities according to astral omens so as to avoid illness and other misfortunes.

Such priestly medical practice is regarded as ancient and sacred, as notably more dignified than the acquired arts of the religious exorcist. Unlike the western doctor, however, the priest has authority only to advise ritual treatment and to enunciate unintelligible Sanskrit formulas. He possesses no reputation for wisdom in solving a diffuse range of problems, and through his practice he gains no individual authority. Priestly emphasis on fixed formulas conflicts strongly, furthermore, with an inquiring, pragmatic approach to health problems.

The ambiguity of the priest's medical role is brought out clearly by the manner in which he extracts a living from it. In each medical prescription he includes a redundant charitable gift—food, money, or a cow—for himself. For giving astrological advice, as for performing domestic rituals, he demands piece payments. A few of his pious clients may voluntarily send him foodstuffs each month on the day of the full or the dark of the moon, but much of his remuneration is in the form of fixed grain dues, paid after the spring harvest. To collect his dues of unthreshed grain, the priest must hurry to his client's threshing floor whenever he is called and must carry the bundle of grain on his head. For such servile dependence on the farmers' charity the priest is mildly despised. While piece payments or the familiar fixed levy in kind might seem useful devices for financing a village doctor in India, the low prestige that results from such financing would be likely to undermine the authority necessary for the effective practice of modern medicine. And as will be seen below, the highest kinds of village curing require no such debasing devices for their maintenance.

Snake-Bite Curing. The two snake-bite curers of Kishan Garhi are not professional specialists, but they are among the most respected and trusted of all the local medical practitioners. They are respected because of their high ethics, their self-sacrifice, and their devotion to philanthropic duty. Anyone who is considered sincere and fit—usually a person of fairly high caste and wealth— may apprentice himself to a teacher who knows one of the secret spells that neutralize snake poison. To prove his fitness, the apprentice must cook his own food, fast, and sleep on the floor for a year. Then, after the performance of many rites, he may be admitted to knowledge of the sacred spell. He is henceforth bound to give free treatment to anyone who sends for his help. He must drop his plow in the middle of his field, or rise swiftly in the middle of the night to go at once, no matter when, or to what distance, he is called. From the moment he is called he may eat or drink nothing until a cure has been effected. By no means are all of the bites which he treats inflicted by poisonous snakes; and many of his patients do, of course, recover. The curer is not allowed to accept food, water, or anything else by way of pay- ment. His only earthly rewards are the praise and respect and token gifts which are later given him. There are religious rewards, too, and the patient's grateful family assures the curer that he has earned great merit for himself, to be reaped both in this life and in the next.

"Your doctors," a villager told me after watching an arduous snake-bite cure which had taken the whole of the previous night, "can never do anything like that." The Hindu snake-bite curer's great prestige resembles the prestige accorded medicine, ethically the highest profession in western society. But while the western doctor often lays his Hippocratic oath aside, the Hindu snake- bite curer acts out his dedication in every treatment. The Hindu curer's prestige depends, be it noted, not upon his skill as such but upon his spiritual power gained through piety. This piety consists both in his austerities and in his giving service without tangible reward. Psychologically, one might say, it consists in creating a sense of immeasurable gratitude on the part of his clients. Practitioners of western medicine might wish to hold a place in the village that would grant their work the prestige and authority of the snake-bite curer, but they would have literally to fast and sleep on the floor to attain such a place, according to the social logics of the villagers.

Secular Medicine. The indigenous secular physicians of India share some of the snake-bite curer's piety but operate on a more self-supporting basis. They are the most highly trained of all the indigenous specialists. "You needn't worry about medical care here," a man of Kishan Garhi told me early in my stay. "We have many clever country physicians—hakims and vaids—in all the villages hereabout. We villagers go to them, not to doctors." The hakim and vaid share many things with the western doctor— a learned tradition, relative lack of limitation by religious and magical formulas, high respect, and economic solvency. Interestingly enough, the indigenous Hindu physician, like the western doctor, often has the status of an outsider to the villages in which he practices. But, as will be apparent, the indigenous physician's relationships to his clients, which are the key to his success, differ sharply in certain other ways from the relationships typical of most scientific medical practice in the West.

Persons who become hakims and vaids carry on their practice as a kind of *noblesse oblige*. Recruits to country medicine in the villages around Kishan Garhi come from the highest castes and higher economic classes of rural society. By origin they are often the people who reside in the high fortress or in the great brick house above the ordinary clutter of mud huts. For the most part they are landlords, big tenants, or wealthy priests, or merchants. Their medical training sets them still farther apart from ordinary people, since most of them study outside the village for at least a year in order to earn the certificate of a school and the government's license to practice simple medicine. These Hindu physicians study medical texts, those who study in the Unani system being called "hakims" and those who study in the Ayurvedic system being called "vaids." In practice, the two systems differ little. The Ayurvedic and Unani texts are respected; neither is in itself regarded as especially sacred. Still the high original status of the hakim or vaid, coupled with his literacy and urbanization, creates a gulf between him and his patient which requires explicit handling.

The first device that the hakim or vaid uses to bridge the gulf of status between him and his patient is to cultivate a reputation for having a superior and penetrating—almost magical—knowledge of the body. This inspires the patient's confidence. The first thing that such a physician does by way of diagnosis is to grasp the patient's wrist. From the pulse—and from other astute observations which often go unnoticed—he tells everything. He asks no questions, or only indirect ones, for he is expected to *know*. One hakim in a village near Kishan Garhi had the reputation of being able to tell the contents of the stomach by feeling the pulse. He would take the patient's hand and inform him whether he had eaten wheat, barley, or millet bread at his last meal, and whether he had eaten the bread together with sweet milk or with curds. Another vaid was credited with being able to predict anyone's life-span to the day and hour. On one occasion, he felt a very old woman's pulse and said she would die at noon that same day, all treatment being futile. Villagers swear that the woman died on the hour, as if by command. Of course, a western doctor's diagnostic skills and devices would occasionally permit him to play out much the same sort of drama if he chose to do so and similarly to create a reputation of power. Villagers' fascination with the diagnostic and predictive powers of thermometers and stethoscopes has already forced many indigenous physicians to add these to their kits, even though they may understand little about the actual use of such instruments.

A second special device which helps the hakim or vaid create confidence—to make himself a dependable man—is the theory, similar to the theory which surrounds the snake-bite curer, to the effect that he is practicing medicine for piety, for the sake of enhancing his own religious merit. The indigenous physician often seems to charge nothing for his skilled services. Indeed, he is felt to be giving his services as charity. Ragged villagers must therefore approach the lordly, white-clothed physician in a manner of worship. It is usual for the hakim or vaid to hold free clinic each morning at which he advises supplicants as to the diet and regime that may be proper for their ailments and the season. The poor most often seek attention at these early clinics, weaker persons being carried to the physician's house on the back of stronger family members. For the physical labor of walking to a wealthier patient's home, the hakim or vaid charges a substantial fee amounting to a sum two or three times the daily wage of a laborer. One well-known hakim came from two miles away to call on a lone and injured landless laborer of Kishan Garhi; his refusal to accept payment from the lame laborer added a great deal to that hakim's reputation for selfless piety. It is believed safe for a poor patient to deal with a rich physician who is also pious, for then the physician will not exploit the poor man.

The pharmaceutical arrangements of the hakim or vaid are a third device which, perhaps even more than piety and skill, contributes to the financial and social strength of his practice. Since such a physician does not charge directly for his treatment, he must obtain most of his income through the sale of medicines. Himself he travels to distant markets to purchase what are believed to be rare materials. Himself he grinds and mixes the materials. Then when he wraps his powders in small packets and retails them at high prices, he creates an illusion of value and a feeling of confidence in the treatment, here exploiting a logic much like that used by the religious exorcist.

But the hakim goes still farther and guarantees his medicines. If a medicine is very expensive, the hakim may ask for its cost in advance, or may take a small initial payment so as to seal a contract for full later payment by the patient. Such guarantees constitute acceptance of the patient's dependency, and at the same time give the patient a sense of control over the high physician. Any suspicion that the physician is making some economic gain by exploiting the patient's illness is removed from the therapeutic situation by such a contract or guarantee. The physician assumes full responsibility; the patient is reassured; and the two parties are united in a set of mutual obligations, recognizing their respective positions of dominance and subordination.

Such a method of charging only for proven results does require that prices be high and that the physician make a certain capital investment in his patients at the start. In other words, such finances are speculative. To collect his bills after the cure, the hakim or vaid needs to have intimate knowledge of relationships among the families and caste groups in the neighborhood where he practices. A satisfied local patient who may desire treatment for his family members in the future may usually be depended on to pay ultimately. When the patient is unknown or comes from far away, he usually guarantees his good faith by approaching the physician through an intermediary from among the physician's own kinsmen or from among the physician's servants of other castes. The hakim's effective reliance on the particular group connections of his patients contrasts strongly once again with the western doctor's characteristic habit of dealing with his patients as responsible individuals.

Some hakims and vaids pursue their philanthropy almost as far as the snake-bite curer, and treat patients entirely without discussing charges. A villager explained the finances of one such philanthropic hakim as follows: "He never takes money from anyone. If you want to, you can give him something, but he never asks. He is concerned only with curing people. People who are cured just put money into his pocket or go to his house and give the money there. He is like a saint." Thus, the patient, too, can gain the merits of charity by gifts which help to further the physician's pious work. Unsolicited gifts made to the hakim or vaid are thought to assure his good will and careful attention to the patient; they are considered to be more effective than payment of charges. Several young men told me that they longed to have enough money to be able to establish themselves in the virtuous and often remunerative profession of indigenous medicine.

The obvious prosperity of the hakims and vaids near Kishan Garhi and the enthusiasm of their patients testify that the system of spontaneous giving can be a profitable one. There is nothing in the techniques of western medicine that would make a similar set of mutual obligations between a western-trained doctor and his village patients impossible, or financially and therapeutically less effective.

The five types of village medical specializations described above do not by any means exhaust the variety of medical resources that can be found in an average village of the Upper Ganges Valley. Kishan Garhi is served by at least twice that number of medical specialists. The roles of the others are governed by principles only slightly different from those thus far cited. Each specialist has his approximate place in the hierarchy of caste and individual power, and each has his appropriate means for solving the problems of that place. Without detailing other varieties, let us take one more look at the western type of doctor as he is seen through village eyes.

The Western Type of Doctor and Village Society

The doctor, even more than the hakim or vaid, has always been an outsider who stands far above village society. He has had no part in the common understandings of the life in any village, but is rather a participant in Europeanized culture. Whether he is Indian or European, he must speak English, for he must have received his medical training through the medium of English. He would never have learned his profession were he not a member of the wealthiest class of people in the district, were his own family not one of wealthy landlords, moneylenders, or government officials. In village language, the doctor is always a sahib—a "gentleman." Persons of the "gentlemanly" class are often respected as being above the village and, therefore, as being above the petty, corrupting influences of village society. But they are never looked upon as people with whom an ordinary villager dares to establish a relationship of intimacy or mutual trust. The "gentlemanly" class as a whole is believed to exploit villagers by means of its technical superiority and by its possession of special political power. There is little in the usual role assumed by the western doctor which would tend to disassociate him, in the eyes of the villagers, from that class.

In western society any differences of social standing that may exist between the doctor and his patient are generally considered irrelevant to the therapeutic relationship. The doctor strives to discuss the medical problem with a maximum of rationality, inquiring confidentially and arriving at a diagnosis dictated in that particular situation by the doctor's technical knowledge and authority. The relationship may be brief, often coming to an end with the doctor's writing a prescription and the patient's paying the bill, sometimes in advance of cure. Such arrangements are workable and may even be necessary, within the mobile structure of modern western society. They are not necessary parts of medicine as such, nor are they appropriate to the social organization of the Indian village. They are not easily understood by the villager.

In the exploratory clinic, in Kishan Garhi, the western doctor attempted to ignore the general inequality of power and rank which separated him from his village patient, as democratic foreigners often do. Since the villagers regarded the doctor as a person immeasurably higher than themselves and unalterably beyond their control, it is not surprising that many found the doctor's friendly equalitarian bedside manner threatening rather than reassuring.

"No small man would have a mighty friend if the two were not up to some mischief," a wise villager told me. The western doctor's equalitarianism, even when it is accepted as concealing no sinister motive, denies to the villager that subordinate, dependent relationship in which alone he is accustomed to find emotional security when confronted with figures of authority. So long as the doctor denies the relevance of differences of social standing, he forfeits his opportunity to profit from the hakim's best device for creating confidence. When the doctor denies his own general superiority, he compromises his role as a reliable, compassionate person.

Furthermore, the doctor's "confidential" interview cuts out the possibility of negotiation with crucial members of the patient's family, members whose relations with the doctor may determine whether the treatment will be carried on or not, whether it will succeed or fail, and whether the bill will be paid. Next, the doctor's inquiring approach shatters faith in his competence, for the villager rather expects to be told what is wrong with him, as the hakim or vaid tells him by feeling his pulse.

Implicit in the role of the western type of doctor is the assumption that his own known technical competence will itself carry a large part of the burden of establishing therapeutic trust. As noted above, technical competence is the chief basis of authority and trust in the lower forms of village magico-medical treatment, but is not the only basis for establishing interpersonal security in the higher forms of secular and religious therapy. If an outside doctor's great technical competence were in fact demonstrated to the satisfaction of the Indian villager as it is already accepted by the western patient, the villager would have all the more reason to feel uneasy about the possibility of the doctor's exploiting him, since the doctor, as a mere technician, will be bound by none of the usual bonds and sentiments that ordinarily operate to control persons at the top level of village society.

The western doctor, like the doctor at the government dispensary nearest Kishan Garhi, usually deals in few medicines himself. He expresses his diagnosis in a written prescription which the village patient cannot read, and which the patient must have filled by a pharmacist in an urban shop or by a compounder attached to the clinic. In the eyes of the villager, who is used to the elaborate caste-defined division of labor, the doctor's prescription to the pharmacist suggests that the doctor has only limited skill, that he does not himself know how to make medicines, or that he considers such work trivial and beneath him. The village patient may then feel doubly exposed to cheating by the urban pharmacist, another technically superior urban person over whom the villager has no adequate means of social control. Village patients in the exploratory clinic often begged the doctor to treat them himself, however crudely, to give them medicine which he had prepared himself in preference to any other. In my own first-aid work, I found that a villager suffering chronically from toothache would wait weeks for me to bring him "with my own hand" aspirin tablets from a market place which he himself often visited, rather than risk a bargain with an unfamiliar shopkeeper over my written prescription.

Finally destroying the patient's confidence is the western doctor's usual method of presenting a bill simply for his advice or for his treatment in advance of therapeutic results. Here is none of the faith-inspiring dedication of the village snake-bite curer or of the philanthropic hakim. Even looking at the matter technically, villagers argued, if the doctor is sure of his diagnosis and his prescription, then why should he object to payment after the success of the cure has been proved? If, on the other hand, the doctor is not sure, then how can the patient be sure? The doctor's demands to be paid for a mere technical performance are like the petty demands of the magician and the priest. At the same time, the doctor's diagnosis has none of the objective therapeutic value that inheres in the expressive treatment conducted by the magical and religious practitioners. One trusting patient at the exploratory clinic in Kishan Garhi affirmed loudly that the pain in his chest had been quite drawn out when the doctor applied his stethoscope; he was dismayed to learn that stethoscopy was only intended to discover, not to extract, the cause of the pain. Many other patients had to be told when to leave the clinic after receiving medicines, for they had experienced no immediate outward sign of cure. The patient who is required to pay the doctor before he has been cured is left with a sense of financial loss, suspicion of the doctor's moral integrity, and doubt about ever being cured.

In the clinic at Kishan Garhi, the doctor had tried to solve the problems of supply and payment by dispensing medicines himself at the lowest possible wholesale rates. "What kind of gentleman is this doctor?" asked one laborer. "He is not a gentleman, he is a sort of shopkeeper!" was another villager's reply. When there was discussion of the possibility that the writer might set up a regular dispensary on the same basis, a village friend objected. "Surely you are not going to charge those little bits of money!" he said. "That would be beneath your dignity!" When sick people came to me from distant villages, promising me money if they were cured, people of Kishan Garhi frequently bid up their offers, insisting that the amount offered must be commensurate with my status and with what was felt to be the enormous probable value of my own unpriced, simple medicines.

IMPLICATIONS

Difficulties evident in the social and cultural conditions described above have in the past demoralized many workers trained in western medicine. "You see," one skilled surgeon at a half-empty city hospital said to me, "these villagers do not really want to be cured!" More recently, among the more constructive medical workers, the persistent defeat of their efforts has forced them to conclude that western medicine, if it is to be effective, must be brought directly to the villages. Only if western medicine is established within the village, close to medical needs at their source, can it prove its worth on equal terms with indigenous medicine. Only then, these workers argue, can understanding of "scientific" practices and knowledge of "rational" preventive procedures have a chance to spread along with the curative techniques. Only when it is established within the village, will western medicine have a chance of paying its own way.

But beyond this, it is important to note that a distinction can be made between "western" and "scientific" medicine. Westerners conceive of western medicine as a system of curing based on "rational" techniques, and "scientific" concepts of cause and effect. But this characteristic, which forms the basis for the technical practices used by western medical specialists, only partly determines the total range of practices involved in treatment and cure. Treatment is bedded in a social as well as a scientific matrix, and many practices of the western doctor are based on cultural values and on ideas of personal relationships that are peculiar to western society. Without the slightest detriment to the technical effectiveness of western medicine, there seems much scope for divesting it of its western cultural accretions, for fitting the practice of medicine into a role that is appropriate to the social organization of the village and to the therapeutic situation in which Indian villagers live.

Western ideas of personal privacy, of individual responsibility, of the dignity of certain techniques, and of the democratic nature of interpersonal trust are not intrinsic parts of scientific medical practice but are cultural accretions upon it. These ideas are not compatible with the traditional social organization of such an Indian village as Kishan Garhi. Not being supported by the social experience of villagers, such ideas tend to weaken or disrupt any medical approach that attempts to base itself upon them.

In the light of this analysis, it would appear that if western medicine is to find a firm place in the village under present conditions, its role must be defined according to village concepts and practices. The doctor may define his role as that of a philanthropist, a saint. He cannot maintain therapeutic confidence merely as a personal friend who has achieved mastery of advanced techniques. Medical work can be supported by guaranteed charges for medicines, or by the spontaneous charity of the patients. It cannot be supported if it is presented to villagers on the one hand as a low, menial service, or on the other hand as a system designed to exploit them financially.

Study of village social organization in Kishan Garhi as a whole and study of the indigenous medical specialists' roles in particular suggest many ways in which western medicine can be fitted into the scheme of traditional village culture. To bring this about effectively, the methods chosen need only be consistent with each other, with the purposes of therapy, and with the larger organization of village society. Testing of some of these alternative methods in the village may well be made an early subject of scientific medical experimentation.

SUMMARY

This study of medical practice and practitioners in the Indian village of Kishan Garhi has attempted an analysis of the social and cultural problems involved in introducing more effective medical techniques to a conservative Indian village. It describes the overall social organization of the village of Kishan Garhi, then analyzes the village medical institutions in particular, and finally reexamines the role of the western doctor as it appears to villagers in the context of their own social organization and their own medical institutions. Analysis reveals several contrasts and conflicts that have existed in the past between the roles assumed by indigenous and by western medical practitioners, conflicts that have acted as obstacles to the spread of western medicine. Analysis also points to certain resemblances between the roles of indigenous and western medical practitioners and suggests how some of these resemblances might be exploited in establishing scientific bridgeheads. The successful establishment of effective medicine here appears to depend largely on the degree to which scientific medical practice can divest itself of certain western cultural accretions and clothe itself in the social homespun of the Indian village.

SELECTED REFERENCES

Mandelbaum, David G., "Planning and Social Change in India," *Human Organization*, vol. 12, Fall, 1953, pp. 4–12. Surveys a variety of efforts to effect specific changes in peasant life in India. Emphasizes the need for thorough social and cultural knowledge in order to avoid unforeseen obstacles and repercussions. Includes examples from medicine, administration, and agricultural technology.

Marriott, McKim, "Technological Change in Overdeveloped Rural Areas," *Economic Development and Cultural Change*, vol. 1, December, 1952, pp. 261–272. Describes problems of introducing better seed, more manure, and more irrigation water to improve the agriculture of Kishan Garhi village. Stresses the importance of taking into account the contextual interconnections of each new technique to be added and each old technique to be replaced.

Marriott, McKim, editor, *Village India:* Studies in the Little Community. University of Chicago Press, Chicago, 1955. Describes the culture and social life of eight villages in different parts of India. Contains an analysis of the external relationships of Kishan Garhi village, with special attention to political organization, caste, and religion.

Opler, Morris E., and Rudra Datt Singh, "The Division of Labor in an Indian Village" in *A Reader in General Anthropology*, edited by C. S. Coon, pp. 464–496. Henry Holt and Co., New York, 1948. A fuller, formal description of intercaste relations in Senapur, another village in Uttar Pradesh, India, whose social organization is much like that of Kishan Garhi.

Wiser, William H., *The Hindu Jajmani System.* Lucknow Publishing House, Lucknow, 1936. Describes in detail the socioeconomic system which interrelates members of a Hindu village in services, some of them medical services. The village described is not far from Kishan Garhi. (See also Chapter 6 of *Behind Mud Walls* by Charlotte and William H. Wiser, Richard R. Smith, Inc., New York, 1930; also published by Friendship Press, New York, 1946.)

Case 10

AN ALABAMA TOWN SURVEYS ITS HEALTH NEEDS

by Solon T. Kimball

The terms "culture" and "society" have popular as well as technical meanings. In a technical sense all shared human understandings are cultural, but in popular speech only "refined" interests are cultural and only some people are "cultured." Technically speaking, everybody in a community is a member of the society, but in common parlance only the elite are "society"; only some individuals appear on the Society page. Thus, popular usage fixes on that part of the whole it deems important; the rest is not worthy of mention.

In Talladega, Alabama, the same device of making the valued part stand for the whole applies also to the concept of community, according to Dr. Kimball. Like other settlements of the American South, the town of Talladega contains several social segments, differing sharply in their activities, values, and relative power, touching upon each other but remaining separate. Negroes and white workers form distinct groups, and a wide gulf separates these from the dominant segment that controls the town's industry, politics, education, and religion. Although the dominant group forms only one-third of the town, it refers to itself as "the community."

*A self-survey to study the health problems of the total community of Talladega became in fact a creation of the dominant class. As community leaders, members of this class were genuinely interested in improving the health of all the citizens and making the town a better place to live in. But they were even more interested in maintaining the balance of power and the traditional system of intergroup relationships. The health survey made headway where it fitted in with the established order; it fell short where it imperiled this order. Self-surveys are widely advocated as springboards to greater community action. This appealing proposition remains to be substantiated and properly qualified by objective sociological studies of the kind represented in this case study.—*EDITOR

THE PROBLEM

Determining the Health Problems of a Divided Community

In the spring of 1951 citizens of Talladega, a town of 13,000 people in the Piedmont area of east central Alabama, assumed the task of determining their local health needs. They named their project the Health Inventory and planned to carry it out in two phases: an initial investigatory phase and a subsequent implementation phase. Organization of the project was completed by July, 1951, and for about a year a systematic survey of local health conditions was conducted. In the fall of 1952, efforts were begun to carry out some of the findings of the survey.

Those who organized the survey had consulted a team of social scientists from the University of Alabama during the initial planning stages. Members of this team were present in Talladega during the two years the survey was in progress. They acted in the dual capacity of advisers and observers. By watching the people of Talladega going about the job of organizing and executing a communitywide survey, they hoped to derive general principles of community process.

Talladega is a fairly representative town of the southern United States. Like other southern communities, it contains many distinct social divisions, each with its own interests and own way of life. Each of these groups touches on the fringes of the others during the course of the working day, but the groups remain separate and do not mingle. In Talladega there are three main social divisions—middle-class whites, white workers, and Negroes.

It was the aim of the Health Inventory to determine the health needs and conditions of the entire community, not just a part. Its leaders also wanted as broad a base of participation as possible, mobilizing the cooperation of each of the town's social groups to determine the interlocking needs of all.

It was no easy task to attain these aims. The social cleavages dividing Talladega reached deeply into the past. Differences based on background, values, and way of life stood as barriers to cooperation between middle class, workers, and Negroes. Would it be possible to survey the health needs of the entire population or to obtain the participation of people representing the whole community? Would those in responsible positions permit an objective survey of local health needs? Could men whose power and position were tied to the existing order evaluate and alter health conditions in their own domain? Would their influence obstruct or facilitate change? The Talladega story serves to illumine important facets of the community process and of the self-survey method.

THE SITUATION

The Three Social Divisions and the Health Inventory

Organizing the Talladega Community Council

In the early spring of 1951 four representatives of the Talladega Chamber of Commerce traveled to the University of Alabama, a hundred miles away, to find out if the University could help them in a problem of community morale. The stimulus for this visit came from two sources. A Chamber of Commerce committee to raise funds for industrial promotion had met widespread indifference. The committee chairman had discussed the deficiencies in community spirit with the secretary of that organization and others. About the same time a psychologist from the University of Alabama spoke to a local club about community problems. Her remarks aroused the hope in the committee chairman that the University might help to improve the town's civic awareness.

At the University, the Talladega representatives discovered that the Department of Sociology and Anthropology was promised a grant by a health foundation to study social process in a community conducting a self-survey of health. Although the health focus had not been paramount in their thinking, the representatives could see that many of their specific concerns could be included if the problem were suitably redefined. The University of Alabama research group agreed to undertake a project in Talladega on the condition that approval be secured from the County Medical Association, the Board of Public Health, and the community.

The community representatives returned home to set in motion the machinery that would bring the University researchers to their town. Approval was readily secured from the medical and public health agencies. In mid-May, University representatives were invited to Talladega to meet with a larger group of Chamber of Commerce members and about a month later a second meeting was held. In these meetings the basis of a working relationship between University and town was developed. It was agreed that responsibility for all decisions affecting the scope, organization, and policy of the project would rest with the community. Fortunately, this arrangement coincided with the objectives of both groups. The town was wary of outsiders who might come to probe and reform. The researchers, for their part, wished to watch community process unfold with a minimum of outside direction.

During an early meeting between the University staff and local people, the Executive Committee of the Chamber of Commerce approved plans for initiating the survey. They appointed an interim committee and chose as its chairman the man who had carried the major load in creating local interest and making contact with the University.

Two other important decisions were made at the same meeting. The question of including Negroes and labor was raised, and the committee agreed that labor unions should be invited to participate and that Negroes should be encouraged to form a separate group to study their own health problems. The separate organization of Negroes was the procedure regularly followed during Community Chest and Red Cross campaigns. The discussion and decision testified to the general feeling that the survey should be communitywide but in subtle fashion emphasized the special positions of different groups.

The interim committee proceeded at once to establish a formal sponsoring organization for the survey. It arranged a public meeting, inviting each civic, social, and religious group as well as the principal institutions and industries to send two delegates. At this first public meeting, held late in June, delegates voted unanimously to form an organization to be called the Talladega Community Council. Interim officers were elected and instructed to proceed with further organizational plans.

The first concern of the interim officers was the problem of completing the organization and planning a program. Questions such as "What is this all about, anyway?" and "When is something going to be done?" were persistent and widespread. The interim chairman appointed a nominating committee to consider suggestions for permanent officers. He also asked for suggestions about the kinds of problems the Council should consider. The interim committee then decided that the Council would be governed by a Policy and Planning Board consisting of a chairman, three vice-chairmen, one representative each from the medical profession, industry, labor, schools, churches, legal profession, town government, two from the town-at-large, and two housewives.

At a second public meeting a few weeks later, delegates from the separate associations were requested to suggest health problems needing investigation. Some of the proposals stressed correction rather than investigation. Among these were rat extermination, control of insect pests, improvement of sanitary facilities, more effective recruitment for nurses' training, and improved education in nutrition and mental health. Other proposals accented investigation, and these concerned such matters as garbage collection, fluoridation of drinking water, school performance and health, absenteeism and health, Negro housing, stream pollution, and rural health. Those present were divided into six discussion groups, which then discussed these and other topics.

When the meeting was reassembled, each group chairman presented a summary of his group's discussion. There were some significant additions to the original list of problems. These were chiefly concerned with seeking relationships between separate proposals. Emphasis was given the interrelations between physical, mental, and spiritual health. Specific questions were asked about relations between delinquency and recreation, and between poverty and health. Other specific proposals included extension of public health facilities, annual physical examinations for the population, and testing of domestic water supply in rural areas.

No attempt was made to work out details of emphasis and priority, or how to determine the facts and initiate action. That was the responsibility of the newly elected officers. But the range of health problems, called the "Inventory" of the Council, had been decided, and there had been a public mandate defining health problems in broadest terms. Theoretically, at least, every phase of community living had been included within a framework of health.

Elected members of the Policy and Planning Board included two physicians, one of whom was made chairman because of his consistent interest in promoting the survey. The other was a man of considerable influence in the town, in the medical profession, and in the local hospital. Board members included the manager of a textile plant, an official of the American Federation of Labor, two ministers who were the rectors of leading churches, and the editors of each of the two local newspapers. The superintendent of city schools, a lawyer from a prominent legal firm, the mayor, two "old family" women active in civic enterprises, the wife of a physician, and the owner of an old family business were also on the Board. With its organization complete and its objective defined, the Community Council was ready to function. The results of the Council's efforts will be seen in sharper focus against the social and historical background of the community of Talladega.

Talladega's History and Social Groups

Talladega lies in the fertile Coosa River Valley of east central Alabama. It is a county seat with red brick courthouse and square. Lining the square are various business houses that supply retail goods to a town of 13,000 and its surrounding trade territory. Businessmen no longer must depend on the farmer trade as they did half a century ago. Talladega, like much of the South, has been caught up in the great surge of industrialism brought on by the war and postwar industrial growth. The textile mills, for several decades the major source of employment, have been joined by a variety of other industries.

Substantial growth of industry and an increased working population have altered the former pattern of a town geared to the needs of an agrarian hinterland. In 1890, before the advent of the first textile plants, Talladega's population was only 2,000, of whom nearly half were Negroes. During the next ten years the population more than doubled. During the next forty years this figure rose gradually, reaching 10,000 by 1940. Today the population exceeds 13,000, not counting those additional thousands who live outside but work in town.

Growth and industry have brought changes to Talladega. Most workers in the new industries come from small farms in the hillier and less fertile sections of nearby counties. In outlook they resemble the fiercely independent yeoman stock that has peopled great sections of the South and that formerly preferred to migrate westward to new and unoccupied lands rather than settle in towns. With the frontier closed, they have recently turned to cities and towns where they can earn wages. Thus, although these workers are of old American ancestry, they are aliens to industrial work and the cities. In this respect they contrast with town-dwelling Negroes who make up approximately one-third of the present population, and with the business, professional, and skilled segment of the white population.

This last group comprises about half the total white population. It includes all white professional people, businessmen, managers, white-collar workers, and most of those in skilled or specialized trades. This group refers to itself as "community," a term which implicitly and explicitly excludes both Negroes and white workers. This is not seen by "community" members as an invidious distinction; it is rooted in history and the facts of institutional life and social values. Thus, in Talladega, there are three major social divisions: the white "community," the white workers, and Negroes. These major groups make up the social environment within which the Health Inventory was organized.

The Health Inventory and the "Community"

The "Community." The business and institutional life of Talladega is controlled by the "community." From its members come leaders in industry, politics, education, religion, and associational life. Although relatively few in number, those in top positions are not greatly elevated above the rest of the "community." In church, club, and political activity, as well as in business enterprise, they join with others who resemble them in outlook and belief. From their ranks comes the town's leadership. Social distinctions within the "community" are slight compared to the gulf between the "community" as a whole and the Negroes or white workers.

Ties of blood and marriage provide a complicated network of kinship which unites established families with each other and the historical past. Kinship also provides firm links with communities throughout the state. Professional, business, and political endeavors are colored by considerations of family. This intertwining produces relationships of extraordinary stability and influence. Whatever occurs in any part of the "community" is certain to have repercussions in all the others. The world of the "community" provides for its members a firm set of values to guide their response to every event in the flow of life.

The "community" family is female centered. The woman as wife, mother, or daughter generally does not enter into active participation in the workaday world, but it is she who sets the tone of that world and directs the behavior of the men. Although her immediate concern is her family, she exercises wider influence in her own right and through her husband. The male's complementary duties are to provide economic livelihood, protect the family honor, and, in particular, shield his family from intruders. From the family come the basic "community" values: privacy of the home, sanctity of womanhood, fulfillment of obligations (especially those based on one's word), rights of property, defense of one's honor, and resistance to the intruder.

This set of values is not without its contradictions and weaknesses, weaknesses that have become more pronounced under the impact of industrial development. This code best fits an agrarian way of life; inevitable modifications resulting from industrial change are not yet fully apparent. Newcomers—industrial managers and technicians—may not share the values and beliefs of those with whom they live and work. Holding influential positions, their differing attitudes may easily lead to conflict with cherished values of the "community." Moreover, the addition of a sizable group of white workers to the population, and general rise in the educational and economic level of both white and Negro workers pose problems unknown during the agrarian period.

To understand the role played by the "community" in the Health Inventory, one must bear in mind that its leadership is provided from a number of tightly knit families striving to hold firm their traditional values and privileged status in the face of new and disturbing forces. It is not surprising that the Health Inventory became almost exclusively the product of the "community." Despite the expressed desire that the health survey involve the total community, it was in fact the "community" that organized and ran the Health Inventory.

The Committees. One of the first actions of the Policy and Planning Board was to constitute 13 separate committees, each having as its sphere of concern one of the health areas suggested as "problems" during earlier meetings. Inspection of the roster of chairmen shows two things. Each chairman headed a committee whose domain was closely allied to his own occupational interest. Moreover, all active committee heads without exception were people belonging to the "community."

Co-chairmen of the Industrial Health Committee were managers of Talladega's two leading textile plants. Co-chairmen of the Public Health Committee were the chairman and chief health officer of the Board of Public Health. The chairman of the School Health Committee was the superintendent of city schools. A prominent dentist was chairman of the Dental Health Committee. Co-chairmen of the Rural Health Committee were the county extension agent and a veterinarian. An attorney headed the Law and Health Committee. Co-chairmen of the Hospital Care Committee were trustees of the Citizens Hospital. Two mothers were co-chairmen of the Family Life Committee. The chairman of the Committee on Aged and Dependent was the head of the county Welfare Agency. The Sanitation Committee was headed by two members of the Junior Chamber of Commerce. Two nurses were co-chairmen of the Nursing Committee. A member of the city Recreation Board and the high-school principal headed the Recreation Committee. A leader in garden club work headed the Committee on Beautification and Civic Improvement. In their work the committees met with varying degrees of success. With one exception, all committees completed their reports; some effected changes; others produced no tangible results; and a few were blocked by opposing forces.

In the cases of positive outcome, the action taken tended to expand established operating facilities or to further long-term interests of committee heads or to continue programs already initiated under other auspices. The work of the Public Health Committee resulted in salary increases for Board of Health employees and employment of two additional workers. The efforts of the School Health Committee produced health examinations for children in two grades and established permanent health records for all school children. Under its garden club-minded chairman, the Committee on Beautification and Civic Improvement sponsored the organization of garden clubs devoted to civic beautification. The Committee on Sanitation promoted a rat extermination campaign previously planned by the Junior Chamber of Commerce. The Hospital Care Committee, Nursing Committee, and the Family Life Committee presented reports and recommendations all of which served as the basis for changes in existing programs or for new activities.

Several committees either produced no tangible results or else benefited from action undertaken outside committee auspices. The Committees on Law and Health and the Health Services prepared reports but took no action. The Committee on Rural Health never functioned, although the Community Council was able to save the rural phase of its program by giving significant support to a health council organized in a nearby area to combat a severe pollution problem. During the existence of the Recreation Committee, the city Recreation Board expanded its facilities at the request of a youth group.

Three committees were blocked by opposing forces. The details are of considerable interest. The Committee on Dental Health studied the merits and costs of water fluoridation. They recommended favorable action and followed this decision with an educational campaign to win support from various civic bodies. Their activities produced wide public support and the Committee eventually presented its proposal to the city commissioners who voted favorably. Some months later, however, the chairman of the Committee discovered that the administration had failed to take any action. Public opposition had appeared among chiropractors and from a group protesting the increased cost. These arguments were met successfully, and the proposal was again placed before the city commissioners and the Water Board. Both groups acted favorably. The chairman of the Committee then assumed that steps would be taken to purchase the necessary equipment and chemicals. Several months later when he inquired about progress he discovered that action had been blocked by the "inactivity" of the city clerk. When the period of observation ended in the spring of 1953, Talladega still lacked fluoridated water.

The Committee on Aged and Dependent also ran into political troubles. The county gave some tax support to an institution for the aged, but membership was limited to those who could pay some portion of the cost. By this method the truly indigent were not admitted. When the chairman of the Committee, the head of the county welfare agency, was advised by a local politician to avoid this issue, she resigned her chairmanship. The Council then changed the title to Health Services, restated the objectives, and secured a new chairman. The new committee concerned itself with the innocuous task of listing services available to the aged and dependent.

The Committee on Industrial Health, whose co-chairmen were on the managerial staffs of Talladega's two leading textile plants, had set out to measure health facilities in industrial plants and health needs of workers. Committee members represented a variety of industries and were themselves men of prominence. Like the personnel of other committees, they had direct access to the centers of control in industrial concerns. But these attributes proved inadequate to accomplish the objectives of the Committee. Several factors contributed to the failure. Chief among these was the inability of plant managers to agree upon what information would be supplied. Fears were expressed that union representatives might utilize the information to the embarrassment of management. The absence of any previous pattern of cooperation between the industrial leaders found expression in the unwillingness to divulge information which might be used by competitors to their advantage. Fear of union intrusion had some validity. At a public meeting, union organizers had reported that laborers feared reprisals if they made public their grievances. These remarks reached at least a few of the industrial leaders who adopted a policy of caution. The Committee, faced with this array of obstacles, abandoned its immediate goals.

The Talladega Community Council was composed almost entirely of persons occupying high social and professional positions. Although the inclusion of "big names" in an organization can sometimes be a facade behind which the real work is done by others, this was not the case in Talladega. These people had proved their ability to command respect from a considerable proportion of the community. Through the influence and authority derived from their positions they were able to represent their respective groups and to provide a meeting point between their groups' activities and those of the Health Inventory. There are decided advantages to having important people on a civic committee. Acceptance of membership implies sympathy with committee objectives, and presence of the top men gives some assurance that means will be available for furthering the aims of the enterprise. In addition, this arrangement generally makes it easier to obtain pertinent information.

On the other side of the picture, such an organizational plan limits committee participation to those with vested interests in the fields they are investigating. This raises a question as to whether those who hold such vested interests are likely to present information which might lead to unfavorable or controversial response. This kind of organizational plan opens channels to many important areas, but it also imposes limitations. Persons of influence may be able to advance cooperation by opening doors, but at the same time they also have the power to keep doors closed. This method of organization provides an almost certain guarantee that no issue that threatens established relationships, values, or interests will receive much consideration.

Social reformers might well find such a situation discouraging because the cards are stacked in favor of the status quo. Talladega possessed one such reformer, the white president of a college attended primarily by Negroes. He insisted that the survey could succeed only on the basis of an interracial committee. His stand was well known to the town; it had been rejected previously, and it was rejected again. The Health Inventory, as conceived and carried out by the "community," was not a reform movement. The aim of improving local conditions was subordinate to the preliminary goal of determining existing conditions and needs. The survey had actually been so organized as to avoid controversial issues that would have exposed internal divisions within the community.

The Health Inventory and the Workers

The white workers of Talladega are relative newcomers. Like the "community," they are heirs to an agrarian tradition, but one that is vastly different. Their values also stressed family ties and loyalty to neighborhood. But the male is the dominant figure in the worker's family. On the farms, women customarily took their place alongside men when their help was needed. There was no tradition binding them to the home or preventing them from assuming a full share of the economic burden. Thus, women could, without serious conflict, find work in the mills while their men worked elsewhere.

In recent years the worker's standards have been changing, and he has started to utilize his greater income to satisfy new wants. Outward differences in speech, manners, or costume which set him apart a half-century ago have almost disappeared. But his religious and family values remain different. These values change more slowly than his economic status. In any event, the worker participates only indirectly in the civic life of the community. He has no opportunity to do so, but even if he had, he would need to learn new ways of behaving.

During the early stages of the Health Inventory, plans were made to include members of the laboring group. A position was established on the Policy and Planning Board for a representative of organized labor. A union representative was selected for this position, but he never attended any meetings, nor did any representative of the workers participate in any committees of the Health Inventory.

The Committee on Industrial Health could have provided a direct link with industrial workers but, as already indicated, this group was unable to complete its assignment. The original objective, an inventory of all health facilities and needs within the various industrial plants, had been blocked by the fear that plant managers would be unwilling to furnish necessary information. The reasons behind this fear, and behind the schism between the "community" and the workers, can be found in the traditional practices and values of the "community." Industry represented a very sensitive area; conflict between managers and labor was always just under the surface. The labor unions appeared to the "community" as a threat to their basic values of individual independence and rejection of outside interference in local affairs.

The values guiding management were rooted in a tradition based on the operation of farms or family businesses. Such enterprises were intimately connected with the fate and prosperity of the family. Threats to business were also threats to the family and were strongly resisted. Thus, attempted regulation by external sources such as government or unions was resented and opposed. Each man expected to operate his own enterprise without help or interference. There was no pattern of cooperation between specific industrial concerns nor of organized relations between management and workers. Relations between management and workers might be excellent within a given plant, but this cooperation did not extend to relations outside the plant. In the community the two groups were separated by all the factors dividing "community" from workers.

The difficulties faced by the Committee on Industrial Health may now be more readily understood. Its failure reflected stresses within the industrial community. Each plant resisted revealing its particular practices. There were differences in type of industry, size of plant, and local or absentee ownership. These were major factors preventing even a start toward the cooperation necessary to a health survey.

Another major factor was management's relation with organized labor. Some plants were unionized, others were not. The "community" was not unfriendly toward workers as such, but many were unfriendly toward organized labor. Workers in unionized plants were represented by business agents, men who were frequently shifted from place to place and thus remained strangers to the community. These were "intruders" whom the "community" resented and feared. These conditions throw some light on the managers' resistance to any kind of program which might have disturbed their relations with workers.

The difficulties experienced by the Industrial Health Committee in developing a program which involved labor were symptomatic of the separation of "community" and workers. The failure of the union representative elected to the Policy and Planning Board to attend any of its meetings may be considered further evidence. A third circumstance was even more dramatic in its portrayal of the problem of establishing relationships between "community" and workers. The Council chairman, impelled to extend the base of participation and stimulated by complaints that "it was the same old gang running things," decided to generate interest in a residential neighborhood occupied by workers.

The area known locally as the "West End" was composed of several dozen modest single-family dwellings. Only the access street from the main part of town was paved. There were no sidewalks or sewerage, although water mains had recently been extended. Most of the houses were owner occupied, and there were some residents who themselves were landlords and thus secured a few dollars a month rent from transients.

The chairman of the Health Inventory visited a few West End families he knew to find out if any aspect of the Health Inventory activities interested them. He was surprised at the favorable reception he received and by the expressed desire of the people to do something about sanitary conditions in their neighborhood. Local men agreed to call a meeting within a few days when people from the "community" could come to explain what it was all about. The meeting was held at night in a local church. Present were approximately 20 men and two women from the West End, and six "community" people. The meeting was hampered at first by a severe thunderstorm which cut the power, but with the aid of flashlights the local chairman got things under way.

It quickly became apparent that the two groups held different objectives. Most of the local people had come to tell of their needs and to ask what steps they could take to get sewerage and sidewalks, and to correct other conditions. They saw no need to make an inventory of conditions or to hold discussions. Conditions in the West End were already well known to those who lived there. They needed no survey to disclose either problems or solutions. They knew both. What they wanted was help to get action.

But another group of West Enders had come to the meeting because they were opposed to sewerage lines and anything else that meant higher taxes. They were not wealthy men but had accumulated enough capital to build and rent two or three small houses. Any increase in property taxes would pose a threat to their solvency. They also felt that as property owners they should be consulted about new proposals, not drafted into forced agreement. The words between the two local groups were harsh. Each was equally determined, and there appeared to be no ground for compromise. The two groups presented opposing petitions at the next session of the city commission, but no action was taken. The brief excursion of West End into community participation had ended.

Some months later another and more successful attempt to relate the West End to the Community Council was initiated. This time one of the chairmen of the Family Life Committee got in touch with the two West End women who had attended the meeting in the church. The committee chairman then asked the county home demonstration agent to help the West End women to form a club. The club was organized and gradually grew in strength and purpose. After several months club members became interested in developing a neighborhood playground. This project began to interest their husbands. At first they were wary, for they still remembered the bitter experience of their previous encounter with a "community-sponsored" project.

This time Council leadership proceeded much more cautiously. When it became clear that there was local agreement, the Council aided the effort by acting as an intermediary between the West Enders and various community groups, particularly the local government, whose assistance was needed in the enterprise. The greater success of the playground project might suggest that rapport with an excluded group can be established more effectively by working slowly and through informal channels than by the direct approach.

The Health Inventory and the Negroes

The relationship of the "community" and the Negroes in Talladega reflected the influence of the traditional plantation system. Under that arrangement, the Negro was provided a secure position by the established code of the "community." Whites were obligated to care for their "colored" families and could earn the respect of Negroes by decent behavior. Negroes in turn accepted their position of subordination. Values centering around "race" reinforced the separate positions of the two groups.

In recent years this relationship between "community" and Negro has been subject to gradual change. Economic stresses within the agrarian system have made it increasingly difficult for whites to fulfill their paternalistic obligations. Then, too, education, the slow growth of a Negro middle class, and greater economic opportunities for Negroes have done their bit to erode the old arrangement. In Talladega this is made especially evident by the presence of a liberal arts college, primarily for Negroes, with its well-educated Negro instructors and middle-class Negro students. The present relationship between "community" and Negroes reflects this gradual change in the traditionally dependent and subordinate position of the Negroes—a position which has excluded them from the world of the "community"—and the rise of a small but significant Negro middle class.

To "community" members, the college symbolized those who favored social mingling—the "radicals" who opposed the cultural values which kept each system in its customary orbit. "Conservative" Negroes were those engaged in activities controlled by the whites. Their acquisition of property, education, and status could be applauded by the "community" partly because they were in accord with "community" values. Some conservative Negroes were opposed to segregation but were willing to accept it because of necessity.

The white workers, although they were also subordinate to the "community" and excluded from it, did not complain about their status. They may have felt just as much apart as the Negroes, but the social barriers were not seen as insurmountable and were not based on race. On the other hand, those Negroes who had achieved professional and economic status approximately equal to that of "community" members—except for race—readily attributed exclusion to racial discrimination. The vast majority of Negroes, although segregated, did not have to face the recurring problems of status denial to the same extent as those who had achieved approximate educational and economic equality.

It will be remembered that the Executive Committee of the Chamber of Commerce made an early decision to encourage the Negroes to form their own group. Within a few days the temporary chairman appointed by the Executive Committee took steps to stimulate the formation of a Negro group. His first move was to discuss the proposition with the county superintendent of schools. The supervisor of Negro schools on his staff was a respected member of the community, and white officials agreed that she should be appointed chairman of a Negro committee. This agreement, forwarded to her through official channels as a "request," was tantamount to an official order, and she gathered a small group to be instructed by the chairman appointed from the Chamber of Commerce. These activities preceded the public meeting in late June which formally established the Community Council.

The interim chairman of the Council had got in touch with the members of this Negro committee and tried to explain to them the purposes and objectives of a health survey. Feeling that he had failed in this attempt, he turned to the University research team for help. The University group, at the request of the Negro committee, advised that a person trained to work with the Negro community be employed. The permanent chairman of the Council, after consultation with others, agreed to the proposal. A graduate student from the Department of Sociology of the University of Atlanta was employed. After working for several weeks she resigned to take a better position but was replaced by a person with a similar background.

Numerous problems faced the Negro committee. The school supervisor chairman was already overburdened with her official duties and finally requested relief from this new responsibility. The principal of the Negro high school was then appointed cochairman and given the major responsibility. He was given the job in the same way as his predecessor. The superintendent of city schools was first consulted; he then informed his subordinate of the decision.

The respective responsibilities of the Negro committee and the new consultant were never clearly defined. The consultant had been informed that it was not her responsibility to do the work of the committee. Committee members apparently understood otherwise, and they reported that she was not meeting her responsibilities. This problem also arose from time to time in the relations between the Community Council and the University research team.

Contact between the white and Negro committees was uncertain and infrequent. The white chairman was burdened by his load of civic and professional duties and could devote little attention to the Negro group. The University research team did not feel responsible for directing the Negro group, although on several occasions they raised the problem of integrating the two groups. The Policy and Planning Board discussed the issue many times and finally appointed a liaison committee of two to work with a similar committee from the Negro group. The joint committee met several times but had a hard time working together. The Board also suggested that white committee chairmen work with their opposite members in the Negro organization, but this was never done.

These difficulties in organization and communication undoubtedly hindered understanding by the Negroes of the objectives of the Inventory, resulting in a correspondingly reduced commitment to its activities. Nevertheless, there was one phase of Inventory activity in which there was considerable joint effort by whites and Negroes.

One objective of the Health Inventory was a communitywide survey using a questionnaire. Committee chairmen and the Policy and Planning Board began serious planning for this survey in early fall. Each committee suggested questions. By December a several page questionnaire was completed, with the help of the University team. The Negro committee had been encouraged to develop its own questionnaire and had made some progress. When the draft of the questionnaire for the white community was presented to the members of the Negro committee for their information, they decided that it fitted their needs and voted to adopt it.

Information on the questionnaire was to be gathered by volunteer workers interviewing every fifth family in Talladega. The Policy and Planning Board requested various civic groups to supply volunteers. The Negro committee also called for volunteers but its chairman, the Negro high-school principal, placed the major responsibility on its teachers. Some of these teachers felt that undue pressure was used to secure their services in an enterprise not appropriately related to their school duties. With the exception of this difficulty, the interviewing program proceeded smoothly and concurrently among both Negroes and whites.

It is evident that considerable effort was made to secure Negro participation in the Health Inventory; certainly more attention was devoted to the Negroes than to the white workers. The effort was directed toward involving the Negroes in the activities of the Inventory rather than its organization, and this was a reflection of traditional white-Negro arrangements in Talladega.

Enough has been presented on the background of Negroes in the community and of the activities of the Negro committee to enable one to appreciate the problems involved in the relationship between whites and Negroes engaging in a community enterprise. The superior position of the white "community" was traditionally established. Initiation of action was a right and a responsibility of the whites. Neither joint nor coordinated efforts could find precedent in past events. In Talladega the nearest approximation to an activity similar to the self-survey were the fund-raising drives for Community Chest and Red Cross. In both of these a Negro headed the canvassing for his own group, but under the supervision of a white chairman.

The separate but partially integrated activities of the white and Negro committees created resentment on the part of those who opposed segregation. But it also proved awkward to the whites who had difficulty in bringing themselves to work with Negroes in other than a relationship of superiority.

The Role of the University Team

The role of the research team merits some attention. Members of the team defined for themselves the double role of researchers and consultants. In actual practice they performed both these functions and others as well. Through their association with the Health Inventory and participation in other affairs in the town they began to find a place in the world of the "community." The team had been in Talladega several months when one of the townspeople remarked that at first he had reserved judgment of the team, but after he got to know them they seemed to be "sweet and gentle" people. Undoubtedly others made widely different evaluations.

The University team assiduously attempted to avoid becoming involved in public direction or leadership of the survey. They offered no gratuitous suggestions or criticisms. This position was not completely accepted or understood by some townspeople, who felt that the University should have been fully committed to the success of the venture and that the prestige of the University could have been helpful in getting through certain difficult situations.

The neutrality of the team in policy matters, however, did not mean that they isolated themselves from the survey. As consultants they were able to discuss the advisability of various courses of action. The local plan to form a Community Council composed of representatives of selected civic groups was discussed in great detail with the researchers before specific action was taken. Each public meeting was a problem in joint planning. The research team gave technical assistance in constructing the questionnaire and selecting an interviewing sample. They also instructed the interviewers and did much of the tabulation. The researchers performed a few other routine duties they felt were not properly their responsibility, because the work needed to be done and no one else was available.

By and large, however, they avoided involvement in major policy matters. This was in line with their research objective of observing developments with as little interference as possible. Once policy was made, however, the team might raise questions or offer suggestions they felt might lead to smoother operation. For example, they frequently pointed out the need for improved communication with the Negro committee.

IMPLICATIONS

Collective Participation and Separate Values

A major problem of Talladega's health program was that of extending the program throughout the entire community. Events in Talladega indicate that the relative success of the Health Inventory within the "community" was due to the fact that it was skillfully organized to conform with existing patterns. If this had also been the case for the workers and Negroes, results might have been different for them. These segments of the population have all too often been ignored in health and other civic programs because of their relative social isolation and the difficulties of intergroup communication. Methods should be developed to bring these groups into health programs on some other basis than the prevalent mandatory and authoritarian basis.

Because of the way it was organized, the Health Inventory became a creation of the "community," that segment of the town that dominated its organizations and its values. The belief that the Inventory was "a good thing for the town" was in keeping with the "community's" conviction that Talladega was a good place to live and a town where people are friendly toward one another. The "community" accepted the Inventory out of a general desire to see the town progress and the feeling that "although there is nothing really wrong now, there is still room for improvement." The leaders of the Inventory were respected because that respect had been earned. Sentiments of this kind made possible ready acceptance by the "community" of a plan to conduct a self-survey of health needs.

But there were also sentiments that the activity should have been, in reality, communitywide. Attempts to cross the lines of class and caste have already been described. The success of the effort was hampered by the separate values and organizational methods of each of the three main segments of Talladega's population.

The world of the white workers, revealed through events in the West End and the trials of the Industrial Health Committee, both resembled that of the "community" and differed from it. It was a male-dominated society, individualistic and separatist; it believed in direct action, resented bossiness, and was inexperienced in the processes by which the "community" worked out its problems. White workers shared with the "community" the assurance that Talladega was a good place to live but were unsure as to whether they really "belonged."

Despite the existence of marked differences between the worker and Negro groups, they shared certain characteristics by virtue of their common status of subordination to the "community." Other similarities derived from coinciding aspects of their respective subcultures. Neither group perceived the basic objectives of the Inventory as did its organizers. Both groups were dependent upon leadership from above. Neither group possessed a tradition of civic participation and responsibility. And both groups were characterized by conflicting attitudes toward the dominant "community."

Basing Communitywide Action on Existing Organizations

The Talladega Community Council was composed of representatives of existing civic associations. This familiar method of setting up a new organization proved useful but imposed some limitations. On the favorable side, participation was made as extensive as possible within that segment of the community that joined organizations. On the other, those who were not members of clubs or associations were effectively excluded.

Those who build community programs upon a base of membership in associations are often unaware of the limited representation that results. The "joiners" in American society are found mainly in the middle classes. They are the people who serve on committees concerned with community welfare, who join luncheon clubs, fraternal organizations, and professional groups, and who rally to causes that promise to better their lot or that of others. Middle-class Talladegans are like other Americans of the middle class in their propensity for joining associations. They are also the ones sought out for the never-ending requests to support worthy causes. In responding to the call of the Health Inventory they followed a familiar pattern.

Despite the fact that its members are capable and dedicated, such a group does not represent all social segments. In a community that separates races, it obviously excludes Negroes. But in Talladega this arrangement also effectively excluded all the white workers. Civic leadership is found within the middle class. Workers, in Talladega, live outside the pattern of "joining." They are not acquainted with the procedures and rituals of middle-class group life.

How Far Off "Dead Center"?

There is growing acceptance of the idea that change cannot readily occur unless one works within the framework of a community's traditional culture. Although the techniques of social science have been particularly helpful in determining existing patterns of interaction, traditional behavior, and values, this knowledge in itself is not enough. One needs to understand, in addition, the actual processes by which a community, or some segment within it, accepts and incorporates change.

An overwhelming sentiment in favor of good health is no assurance that people will rush to support a program that promises health improvement. Health, like sin, can be controversial. You may be for the former and against the latter, but you also wonder how action by others is going to affect you. The proponents of the Health Inventory did not make the mistake of openly proclaiming that their activities would improve existing conditions. Such assertions would immediately have been interpreted by some as reflections on themselves or as a possible threat to their position. Only those with great authority can afford the illusion that their actions are immune from the consequences of unfavorable response. The leaders of the Inventory were fully aware that crosscurrents and pitfalls might impede their progress. Whether by conscious design or intuitive response, they directed their efforts along lines which coincided with community traditions and values.

The history of the Health Inventory has shown both the advantages and disadvantages of such a policy. With the organization and execution of Talladega's survey resting in the hands of its dominant powers, there was little likelihood that anything would be done to upset the existing system or threaten established interests. Thus, it was possible for the Health Inventory to continue for two years, undertaking health surveys and effecting certain modest changes. There is little doubt that if the organizers of the project had stressed a "reform" policy, or proclaimed their intention to push extensive interaction among the "community," the Negroes, and the workers, the whole project would have had short shrift. Any hint that the project favored racial or class intermingling on a basis other than the established system of dominance and subordination would have threatened basic values close to the core of "community" subculture—the sanctity of the family.

It may thus be understood why change is so difficult in Talladega. Change means the establishment of new relations, new procedure, new ways of thinking about the world. If recommended measures conform to existing patterns, then these may be accomplished without serious difficulty. But if they contradict or destroy established values, they are resisted.

The Health Inventory worked successfully to the extent that it conformed to prevailing values and worked according to existing patterns. The Community Council and its program had strength where it gave expression to the prevailing order. It failed in exactly those spots where there were no traditional procedures or where values kept social groups apart. The Health Inventory moved the town off "dead center," but not so far off as to upset the balance of power and the system of intergroup relations.

SUMMARY

The survey of local health needs organized and carried out by the people of Talladega, Alabama, was successful where it ran with the grain of existing traditions and social conventions, and unsuccessful where it ran against the grain. The community was divided into three major social divisions—"community," white workers, and Negroes—and each of these groups perceived, participated in, and benefited from the health survey in different ways. The dominant group participated more and benefited more than the subordinate groups. Basic differences between these groups, as well as the strength of the barriers that separated them, were revealed by difficulties in intergroup communication.

The case of Talladega points to solutions for some of these difficulties, but leaves many others unresolved. Attempts to overcome basic divisions in the community were inadequate to meet the objectives of a communitywide program. The question may be asked if any attempt, irrespective of the skill available, can successfully bridge social and cultural chasms as deep as those in Talladega. Methods and techniques developed during the Health Inventory program suggest that while the job is extremely difficult, it is not impossible.

SELECTED REFERENCES

Cash, W. J., *The Mind of the South*. Alfred A. Knopf, New York, 1941. A penetrating analysis of historical, economic, political, and social factors as they have contributed to the growth of southern culture. Explains southern agrarianism and the impact of industrialization.

Hunter, Floyd, *Community Power Structure*. University of North Carolina Press, Chapel Hill, 1953. An analysis of the leadership pattern of a southern city. Provides insights into the kinds of problems which those who work for social change must face. Shows how decisions affecting civic welfare are made.

Kimball, Solon T., "Some Methodological Problems of the Community Self-Survey," *Social Forces*, vol. 31, December, 1952, pp. 160–164. An analysis of relationship between social scientist and community in the self-survey process.

Kimball, Solon T., and Marion Pearsall, *The Talladega Story*. University of Alabama Press, University, Ala., 1954. A report of observations on a self-survey of health conditions and needs made by citizens of a southern community over a two-year period. Describes processes of community action in relation to social environment.

Miller, Paul A., *Community Health Action*. Michigan State College Press, East Lansing, 1953. A report of the contrasting pattern of citizen action in five small American communities, to acquire hospital facilities. Illustrates regional variations in social process.

Poston, Richard Waverly, *Small Town Renaissance*. Harper and Bros., New York, 1950. A documentary description of the impact of a social action program in a number of Montana communities. Useful for illustrating how citizens act on local problems.

Sanders, Irwin T., *Making Good Communities Better*. University of Kentucky Press, Lexington, 1950. A working guide for the intelligent citizen who wishes to learn more about his community, to initiate a program of social change, or to improve on the effectiveness of existing organizations.

Case 11

A MENTAL HEALTH PROJECT IN A BOSTON SUBURB

by Kaspar D. Naegele

Directed by Dr. Erich Lindemann and originally supported by the Grant Foundation, the Wellesley experiment in preventive psychiatry has had few signposts to follow. The new agency had to provide useful services in order to gain community acceptance. Yet it was difficult to know what service would be useful before studying the community and discovering its problems. From the outset, therefore, the staff consisted of two classes of workers, social scientists and social practitioners. Dr. Naegele, who was one of the social scientists, includes in his case study a perceptive section on problems faced by the two classes of personnel in their attempt to achieve mutual understanding.

He makes no effort to cover the entire gamut of service and research undertaken by the agency. The case study is essentially confined to the agency's relations with representatives of two other institutions, the church and the school. Like the agency itself, each of these confronts the task of shaping character and guiding behavior. But psychiatrists, teachers, and ministers approach the problem from different standpoints and are governed by different values. In order to work together effectively, these groups must perceive their differences and recognize the varying institutional traditions and arrangements responsible for these differences.

The divergence of value orientation between psychiatrist and minister invites comparison with the divergence between the worldview of the western physician and of the Indian villager described by Dr. Carstairs in Case 4. In rural India, priest and doctor have never been clearly separate; in suburban Wellesley, they are now seeking common ground on which to meet and cooperate.

Of course, school and church are social segments of a different order from those represented by Talladega's "community," workers, and Negroes. The latter divisions, in fact, contain segments of the former kind; ministers, psychiatrists, and school authorities can well belong to the same social class. The differences between the various social institutions in Wellesley and elsewhere are by no means so great as those separating the three major groups in Talladega. Members of these major groups had trouble conducting joint sessions because of the extent of their mutual differences. In Wellesley, members of separate social institutions had no trouble meeting but found it difficult to recognize the existence of real divergences in their conceptions of mental illness and the functions of a mental health agency. Yet the discrepancies did and do exist and, as Dr. Naegele's study demonstrates, can be accommodated only with much patience and resourcefulness. —EDITOR

THE PROBLEM

Recognizing Divergent Expectations

Early in 1949 a project, called the Human Relations Service (HRS), was established in Wellesley, a residential town of 20,000 in Massachusetts. This project was born under the auspices of Harvard University. It had originally been suggested by an active citizen of Wellesley who cooperated with the director of the HRS in establishing an organization, the professional staff of which was drawn mostly from the University. The form and purposes of the project had been planned only in the most general terms. It was to render service and engage in research in the area of "mental health." How this was to be done, to a large degree, was left to that continuous and often haphazard process of trial, error, and change, which carries most of us along much of the time. Yet we all had preconceptions as to what constituted mental health, how it might be created, and what price one should be asked to pay for it. In addition, there were many misconceptions as well as gaps of thought on various issues.

Informed citizens of Wellesley would, for instance, have various notions about "mental health," but would often have given little thought to the relation between mental health and particular practices of social institutions such as church and school. Or again they would have various expectations as to what service we should render and thus force us to explain the value of the kind of service we considered appropriate, given our own conception of mental health. As for research, there was only little appreciation of its nature, its concern with issues not necessarily of immediate and practical relevance, and the difference between doing research and giving advice or service.

The task of our agency, then, consisted in solving several problems. We had to learn how the different worlds of the school, the church, the home (and other worlds as well) produced different perspectives concerning the same issue—the "right kind" of human behavior, an issue with which we, too, were concerned in yet another way. As psychiatrists, social workers, and social scientists, we also differed among ourselves. We had to learn to accommodate our internal divisions and not to read these differences into our relations with the world around us.

These were not merely intellectual issues. They were involved in practical decisions which affected the lives of specific people. Furthermore, the outcome of our trial and error could be assessed in concrete terms. We arrived as volunteers sustained by a foundation, and at the end of five years hoped to become well enough accepted to win financial support from the community itself. We wished not only to be tolerated in Wellesley but to have our services wanted and hence to be paid for.

In 1954 the town did assume the responsibility of supporting the HRS as a service agency. This case study is not concerned with the immediate events that led to this important decision, nor with the subsequent history of the agency. It cannot deal in detail with the entire range of activities undertaken by the HRS, or with the many sectors of the community with which it came in contact. The case concentrates on relationships during early years between the HRS and the clergy, between the HRS and the school, and between the divisions within the agency itself.[1]

The church, the school, and the agency had different views on mental health and what should be done to promote it. To work out a satisfactory division of labor between these institutions it was not enough to write this situation off as mere difference of opinion. We had to understand the basis for the differences in order to know which of these could and should be changed and in order to respect the differences that remained. The three institutions had different, though overlapping, purposes and correspondingly different methods of organization. These differences in turn affected the actions and expectations of those who per-

[1] I wish to acknowledge the support of the Grant Foundation, which financed the Human Relations Service project and of the Anti-Defamation League, which made my initial participation in it possible. Obviously, none of the experiences reported here would have been possible without the cooperation of many people in Wellesley and the general acceptance by that community of our efforts. My special thanks are due Dr. Erich Lindemann for his support and cooperation in allowing me full scope to follow my own ideas. K.D.N.

formed the role of clergyman or teacher or psychiatrist. How did the clergy conceive of their relationship to us and how did we conceive of this same relationship? How was our relation to the school distinct from our relation to the clergy? Which of our own ideas did we have to defend, elaborate, or give up?

THE SITUATION

Varieties of Assessment of the Wellesley Project

The Human Relations Service

The HRS was founded in 1948 and established in a house in Wellesley by 1949 to accomplish an array of purposes. It was to provide without charge limited psychotherapeutic services to any citizen in the community who wished to avail himself of these. It was to consult with teachers, ministers, doctors, social workers, and others whose occupations gave them access to the private struggles of others. It was to facilitate discussions about common concerns among such groups as nurses, mothers of young children, and the like. It was to do research on the volume, etiology, and predictability of various kinds of emotional disturbance. And it was to work toward a change in its administration so that at the end of a five-year period, the service functions of the HRS would be financed by the community itself.

To implement these aims, the HRS gradually developed its own special type of organization. It had a staff with a director, who was to a degree limited in his decisions by an executive committee. This included citizens of Wellesley and was chaired by a local Unitarian minister who had been very influential in helping the HRS become established; he remained one of its most active supporters throughout the period discussed here. The HRS also had an advisory committee, consisting of professors in medicine, public health, and social science at Harvard University. The University, especially through its School of Public Health, acted as guiding mother to an infant field station which needed the reputation of his parental sponsor, though this infant often went his own willful way and at times became suspect precisely because of his academic connections. The advisory committee helped to formulate general policy but bore less responsibility for the implementation or repercussions of such policy than did the executive committee or the staff itself.

The staff consisted of workers in adult and child psychiatry, clinical psychology, psychiatric social work, social anthropology, and sociology. Its size varied, as did the amount of time specific members of the staff gave to the project. Throughout, the psychiatric social worker was employed full time and provided a needed constancy in contrast to the more partial involvement of the others. Being the main "intake" worker, she accumulated the sort of detailed and informal knowledge of acquaintance and hearsay concerning Wellesley, its arrangements and citizens, which even part-time workers in such an institution need to have, but which only a persistent and full-time association with its clientele and staff makes accessible.

Members of the staff differed in the tasks they were to carry out as well as in the experience and training at their disposal. For some of us, indeed, the HRS was more of a training than a practice ground. The double aim of the project—service and research—provided an important basis for the division of labor among the staff. The psychiatrists did therapy, consulted in various contexts, and engaged in a certain amount of public speaking. The clinical psychologists administered tests, conducted or observed discussion groups, and engaged in research on the assessment of specific preschool children or the possibilities of assessing the community's committed or domestically cared for psychotics. A group worker and a person interested in small groups carried out observations of children in kindergartens and early grades.

We wished to supplement the assessment of individual preschool children by reasonably detailed and systematic accounts of pupils and their teachers. In that way, we could think of classrooms as "social systems." Our concern was the variation among these social systems and the consequence of such variation for the emotional status of specific children. How, we wanted to know, is authority expressed and accepted in different classrooms, how is help given, or what is the relative importance of specific achievements, like reading or writing, compared to more intangible matters, such as manners or getting along with others? Children could then be understood as members of such social systems, facing different forms of confinement and liberation; similarly, teachers could be understood as agents and creatures of these same systems.

Two anthropologists worked on the ecological and organizational features of the community and were later joined by a person interested in voluntary associations. Together with one of the anthropologists, I engaged in some research on the problems facing a parent in a community like Wellesley. This was later followed by some explorations into questions of social isolation and friendship, which a social anthropologist and social psychologist examined in the elementary schools and a clinical psychologist, psychiatrist, and I investigated in the senior high school.

These diverse efforts and different combinations of people were all to converge by providing, piecemeal, answers to the inclusive questions: What is the actual and potential "case load of emotional disturbance" in the community? How could one recognize emotional disturbance early and see it in relation to the social arrangements in which people live? What would be an appropriate agency to help deal at an early stage with some of the identified neurotic and destructive patterns, and deal alike with the creators and victims of these patterns?

Our differences in assignment, discipline, gift, and experience, moreover, were to be balanced by an organization of the staff which would combine equality with freedom and allow each a say in the decisions that had to be made. These were to be discussed at weekly or biweekly staff meetings at which we were to be kept informed about future plans, each other's activities, and developments in the community. Guests, it should be added, were to be accommodated at such meetings as well. The fate of such hopes is discussed below.

The work of the staff was to be extended through a series of joint committees for exchanging views on matters pertaining to mental health. These included a clergy committee and a school committee, a committee with doctors and one with the local social work agency. By comparing notes, the HRS was to gain a better understanding of Wellesley and its resources and to be advised on the effectiveness of its program. Through these committees, too, it was possible to spread more realistic notions about the value and meaning of social research as distinct from social service.

It is important to add that it was part of our aims to see in "cases" more than the particular persons who first appeared for advice. Usually these were young mothers who came with one of their children. We assumed that troubles ran in families and that the critical persons in a disturbed equilibrium are not necessarily those who first present themselves. We tried to see as many family members as possible. Yet, on the whole, the HRS gained more access to the worlds of women and children and schools than to the world of men and occupations. But then Wellesley is a "bedroom town."

The Community of Wellesley

Wellesley is a well-to-do suburb of Boston and consists of about 20,000 people. These tend to order their lives according to standards of the middle and upper classes. The husbands, as a rule, commute to the city and are engaged there in professional work or as business executives, salesmen, and the like. There is no local industry, although there are, of course, shops and restaurants. Officially the town is dry. The wives, servant-less, look after their children and balance household routines with diverse activities of their own or for their children. The community contains mostly single houses, surrounded by tidy grass and flowers. Almost everyone owns at least one car. In riding and walking through Wellesley one gets the impression of material comfort. There is much living on one's economic toes, yet the HRS seldom dealt with people who had to wonder where their next meal might come from. "Relief" was not our concern. Neatly dressed, our clients came in cars, protected from outer insecurities, concerned with the inner present, past mistakes, and a better future.

Predominantly Wellesley is Protestant and "Yankee," although it has both a Catholic and a very small Jewish group. For some purposes, it is a convenient and appropriate shortcut to speak of Wellesley as "the community." Yet it clearly embraces several styles of life and different levels of income. Neighborhoods vary by cost and size of house and garden, by degree of privacy or individuality. One or two recent housing developments are worlds unto themselves; one or two main thoroughfares create barriers for children's play. Schools vary in size and condition, some containing children with similar backgrounds and some including children from a wide range of backgrounds. There is mobility within the community as well as into it. Seen as a whole, the community represents a desirable "end station" in a person's upward journey out of the nearby metropolis.

Wellesley is a suburb, but geographically and psychologically, if not economically, it is a fairly autonomous town from which husbands leave by train or car or bus on weekday mornings to be in their offices in half an hour, and to which they return at the end of a day reading the newspaper. In the evening Wellesley is quiet. There are one or two places where one can eat out, but no nightclub. The town has a movie theater and stores but no legitimate stage, except in summer. On its outskirts there is a college, but Wellesley is not a university town. It has churches, a public library, and a Friendly Aid Society, as well as a town government with vigorous citizen participation. But I still do not know in what manner the place itself is important to the sense of identity of those who live there. "Our town" as an affectionate expression is a dispersed community which recedes from busy streets to quiet hillsides and has no geographic and symbolic center around which it is architecturally grouped.

Perhaps the pride of its citizens lies less in the town as such and more in its particular advantages: its public schools, its protection from the big metropolis, and its well-kept appearance. In such a setting a psychiatric agency plays an ambiguous role, at least in the beginning; it is a reminder that external orderliness has its limits; it is also a valued means for extending orderliness from the outside to the "inside."

The Clergy and the HRS

The clergy was one of the first groups with whom we met regularly. This was a logical step, since the local Unitarian minister had been active in establishing the HRS in the community. Besides, he was also the chairman of the executive committee. He became as well the organizer and chairman of the clergy committee, which met monthly on a weekday morning from nine to eleven, over doughnuts and coffee. It met at the quarters of the HRS and not in one of the local churches. The meetings were informal and not too punctual. Previous meetings were orally summarized; no minutes were prepared. The Unitarian minister and the director of the HRS were co-chairmen of the committee. Discussion was quite spontaneous. Attendance varied; sometimes three of the possible total of ten ministers were present, sometimes nine. From the HRS side, at least three staff members usually came.

It is interesting to note that this committee provided the only occasion in Wellesley when all the local clergy did or could meet in one body. It should be noted, too, that Wellesley contains a sizable Roman Catholic population and that as time went on, one of the Roman Catholic priests became reasonably well integrated into a group which, apart from him, was almost exclusively Protestant. There is no organized Jewish congregation, but a Jewish group does meet at one of the churches and a rabbi associated with this group was later asked to join the clergy committee. After one or two of the meetings, incidentally, the Protestant clergy remained to transact clerical business of their own, usually involving arrangements for joint services.

At the outset we hoped that they would consider us one of their resources, as an agency to which they could send parishioners for early treatment or which could advise them about other psychiatric facilities; that they would help us in our task of "case-finding" so that we could assess the extent of emotional disability in the community; that they would discuss with us their way of managing human situations with which our work also brought us into contact. How, for instance, we wanted to know, did they cope with death or divorce or infidelity? To accomplish our aims we had to acquaint the clergy with our intake and referral policy. We also worked out informal ways of keeping them informed about the people they had sent to us, without violating the confidence of our clients.

The clergy saw their relationship to the HRS in characteristically different terms. Their first concern was with our values. What did we stand for and against? When we gave no immediate nor clear answers, they wondered whether perhaps we were indifferent to moral considerations. Perhaps, so ran the doubt, we condoned in the name o.' freedom a range of conduct which from the point of view of the churches was undesirable or even sinful. Indeed, might not psychiatrists wish to implant in their patients their own psychiatric values in place of religious values? Were we collaborators or rivals?

It is the clergymen's calling to declare their commitments; hence in the beginning we were likewise challenged to declare ours. For reasons of our own we did not comply. We succeeded in shifting the discussion to more technical concerns and thus left behind, unresolved, a residue of thorny issues: What is the real cause of juvenile delinquency and what is the right kind of discipline for children? What about sexual experience before marriage and what about divorce? We shrugged our shoulders, said something about "mental health" and "freedom from anxiety," and urged that we discuss instead the concerns with which parishioners approach their ministers. We then made modest attempts to explain psychiatric theories about particular symptoms.

Meanwhile, some parishioners were referred and were helped. This helped to establish our competence and gain respect. Given respect, we could discuss the basis for a division of labor between clinicians and clergymen. Respect yields trust and trust suspends many questions. Our discussions from then on could become concrete. For instance, the clergy wanted information about the values of different kinds of psychiatric treatments. What are the risks of shock treatment? Why cannot psychiatrists intervene in a home where someone obviously in need of help refuses to present himself at a clinic of his own accord? We could then explain about the difference between home visits by a minister and the usual office-boundness of psychiatric treatment. In our discussions we could make clear as well that there were differences of perspective within the psychiatric profession as there were denominational differences within the Christian church.

As time went on, we learned much from the clergymen as well as much about them. We learned about the clergy's views concerning the meaning and efficacy of specific rituals, including prayer and confession. They learned something about psychotherapy. We learned about the difficulties of getting proper leadership and curbing unsuitable volunteers for various church-connected organizations or activities. Through their reports we came to understand more about the daily concerns and conditions of life of the citizens of Wellesley. We discussed their management of marital counseling and had general discussions about research work in Wellesley or elsewhere pertinent to this and other issues.

Still, the clergy did not lose all their suspicions of us. Our willingness to accept many varying religious philosophies as they were expressed by our patients could not be regarded with equanimity by men committed to advancing the doctrines of a particular religious system. In addition, after hearing us discuss human motives and social arrangements in the secular terms of psychiatric theory, the clergymen began to wonder if we were also subjecting them, and not only our clients, to the same kind of observation and interpretation. One might hear a clergyman introduce a tale of some social situation with the comment: "I don't know what this reveals about me, but the following thing occurred the other day. . . ."

In other words, there were always three "we's": the "we" of the clergy, the "we" of the HRS, and the "we" that for various occasions bound these two together. How can one account for our differences and for the emergence of a mutual understanding that made a division of labor possible? In the beginning it was precisely our like concerns that tended to keep us apart. Both groups were concerned with the well-being and problems of people. But we stood for different ways of viewing people's well-being and their quandaries and debilities, and for different ways of affecting them.

Medicine is no longer confined to the body but approaches spheres which were formerly the exclusive province of the church. "Neurotic conflicts" involve questions of alternatives in the "meaning of life" which cannot be decided on purely scientific grounds. Moreover, the experiences of isolation, threat, or despair which express the impasse of an emotionally ill person are facts on which different religious traditions also have distinct views. Uneasiness typically marks the relation of two groups of people who promote like matters in different ways; they have an ambiguous sense of being in competition, each seeking success that brings failure to the other. In retrospect, it would seem that in the case of the relation between HRS and clergy this uneasiness was resolved when two specific steps were taken.

We first had to recognize the difference in the social situation of our respective professions. Typically, the psychiatrist stays in his office or in a hospital. His patients come to him and leave him again more fully informed about themselves than they are about him. He remains anonymous in many respects, even if he does not confine himself to the stereotyped poker face. His obligations are limited to treatment for which he is usually paid.

The minister represents and teaches a specific religious tradition which defines standards of conduct and answers man's ultimate questions. These standards and answers explain and bind. The faithful become committed to them. By that token the clergyman is a model, if not an authority. In some cases, furthermore, he is an intermediary between laymen and God; in others he is a representative. As one of the ministers phrased it, "People pay us to do their praying for them." The statement underlines the fact that the clergy becomes a symbol of standards, such as "charity" for Christians or "learnedness" and "justice" for Jews. The clergy helps to define evasion and may help to expiate it once it has occurred.

The minister, therefore, like the psychiatrist, becomes a confidant, especially if he is sympathetic. Yet unlike the psychiatrist, the minister, priest, and rabbi are public figures; they are not anonymous. The minister participates in the affairs of his parishioners and they in his. His house is open in many respects. The limits to his duties are wide and his life and work are distinctly fused. Yet he also stands apart. In that he resembles the psychiatrist again. He participates in more than one world. The world of his parishioners, however, is organized; it is solidified as a congregation. The patients of a psychiatrist form no such bonds to one another. He faces each of them alone, or selects them himself to form a group.

The minister, moreover, is a member of a church, which may give him a distinct place in a hierarchy transcending local circles.

As a member of the church he is, however, specially privileged, so that his clients are laymen to him, as they are patients to the psychiatrist. The psychiatrist, too, is integrated into a larger body —the circle of colleagues organized in professional association— but this body does not include the patients whom it serves. The minister faces the parishioners as a congregation, in corporate worship or in confession. He participates with them in joint ritual that goes beyond the act of speaking.

It follows from these differences that the clergy would naturally ask about our values—and that we would be at some loss to answer. We could not, as an agency, be committed to a moral order so specific as that of any of the denominations. Admittedly, health and salvation may be similar states. But we assumed that health can accompany different forms of salvation, and that there are methods of managing emotional disturbance which are not an explicit part of any religious tradition.

Second, once we understood our differences we were free to imagine some division of labor clarifying our respective limitations as well as common ground. By this road we became in fact a resource to the clergy. They came to acknowledge that they could not adopt our mode of procedure without altering their own role or at least without creating many conflicts for themselves. They remained active agents in the world, while we constituted a refuge away from it where they could discreetly send their parishioners. We compared our way of assessing human situations with theirs, while they in turn informed us of the range of problems brought to their doorsteps. This increased our knowledge of the community in a manner we could not have accomplished on our own.

In retrospect, it seems that one reason our differences ceased to compete lay in our common marginality: both the clergy and our psychiatrists participate in two worlds at the same time. The HRS participates in the worlds of the healthy and the sick, the clergy in the worlds of the sacred and the secular. These dual participations are not wholly analogous, but they made both of us "outsiders" in certain respects, whatever else we were. Under favorable circumstances, common marginality can bind people by providing a common fate.

The School and the HRS

Just as we had regular meetings of the clergy committee, so we met regularly with the school authorities. At the time there were eight elementary schools and one junior and one senior high school in Wellesley. Each of these schools has its own building and principal. Only the senior high school has an explicit guidance program. This is in the hands of two people, one for boys and one for girls. The elementary schools have a director of elementary education, whose office adjoins the superintendent's in the basement of the senior high school.

In the course of time, the HRS initiated the formation of a school committee. It was encouraged to do so by at least two people with important positions within the school administration. Unfortunately, both of these left the community shortly after plans for joint action had gotten under way. Our task of establishing cooperative enterprises with the schools was thus complicated by having to work with people who were also new and feeling their way. Our presence, although intended to be helpful, must have been an added burden to school administrators who were in one or two instances unfamiliar with the community.

In addition to the assistant principal of the senior high school as chairman, the school committee consisted of the superintendent, the director of elementary education, the school doctor and nurse, and later a representative from the junior high school, as well as the boys' counselor from the senior high school. Neither teachers nor parents were directly represented, although such extension was discussed and tabled several times. On our side participation varied. At the beginning the director of the HRS, one of the staff psychiatrists, and the psychiatric social worker always went. Later our representation tended to include more of the research group. Six or more of us would go to these monthly meetings, which usually followed the meetings of the executive committee the previous Wednesday evening and were held on Thursday mornings before the regular staff meetings of the HRS. This schedule helped to make our relation to the schools a matter of much discussion and attention.

The purposes of the HRS called for a whole series of cooperative arrangements with the schools and school authorities. Specifically, we wanted the schools to help parents with the decision, where warranted, to seek our psychotherapeutic advice. We also wanted the schools to let us do research. We wanted to explore ways of assessing the emotional status of children at early stages of their life, create opportunities for checking our predictions, work out ways of describing a classroom as a distinct social world made up of a teacher and children, in which children must come to terms with the two tasks of learning school subjects and learning the art of getting along with peers and elders. Later we also wanted to do research on problems of friendship and social isolation.

But the schools thought of us in other terms. They expected help in managing difficult problem children and wanted a set of precise instruments for drawing lines between "disturbed" and "normal" children. They hoped, further, that although we were independently financed, we would consider ourselves part of the school system. Yet they hesitated to phrase their aims as needs which we might fill. To acknowledge a willingness to cooperate with a psychiatric agency would be, they assumed, an admission that they needed such services. Such a need might reflect unfavorably on the schools' capacity to handle their problems. The schools, therefore, tended to oscillate between demanding specific measuring devices: "handing over" problem children, yet wanting exact information as to what we were doing with them and to them; denying the need for the HRS service, yet wishing to have its equivalent wholly under the jurisdiction of the school system. We felt that we could not and should not provide the measuring rod; we did not want to become the repository of unsolvable problems; and we jealously guarded our autonomy.

When we first began to work with the schools, we were asked by the school committee to prepare a checklist of criteria for measuring "mental health." Such a list, similar to other specific psychological tests, was to be used by the teachers. It was to enable them to classify each child and to indicate, along with the impressions of the teacher, where therapy was needed. Such therapy could then be given by us, provided the teacher was able to persuade the parents, where necessary, to consult us.

We opposed the request. We did not think that emotional balance or imbalance is of one piece; there are modes and stages of balance, depending on character and social situation. It was, in fact, this conviction which led to the establishment of the HRS in the first place. It would, therefore, have been inconsistent to set about developing a simple measure of emotional functioning. We believed that our interests called for devising ways of assessing the situations of specific people, normal and otherwise, rather than measuring these along some one continuum. We wanted to discuss with teachers how they felt about members of their classroom. We wanted to work out joint and tentative agreements, based on observations and inferences. In other words, we preferred a more inclusive, but less conclusive, approach. They began by demanding a more specific and impersonal instrument.

The differences between the school's view and our view of the therapeutic services we could offer reflect the differences between our purposes, values, and social structure and the school's purposes, values, and social structure through which it carries on its work. In contrast to therapists who treat patients individually, teachers must work with a whole group of pupils—and "behind" these their parents and "above" themselves their various superiors. Principals are also gatekeepers and although school children may like visitors as welcome distractions, these must be limited so as not to interfere with a full program of activities. Teachers, as public servants, act in public. Therapists act in privacy. Teachers, like ministers, have various common values to impart: absorbing knowledge, doing one's best, obeying rules of honesty and cooperation. These values influence psychotherapy only indirectly.

In contrast to the schools, the HRS had a looser and much less routinized organization and on the whole dealt with specific individuals and their worlds and not with the emergent world of people who form a class of pupils in charge of one teacher. We were not concerned, furthermore, with getting people to learn specific skills like writing or reading, or specific bodies of knowledge like ancient history or geography. We wanted to help them be free to learn such skills and areas of knowledge.

Meeting the schools' request for a checklist of mental health criteria was our first difficulty and we resolved it in two ways. We ran a seminar on personality development in children for teachers. This provided an opportunity to present a view of personality which would suggest the severe limitation of simple mechanical devices for gauging a child's mode of adjustment. It also provided an opportunity for discussing problems in general, without going into particular cases. This kept us away from specific instances of troubled relations between a particular teacher and particular pupils.

Second, we established definite policies of referral. If a teacher thought a child needed outside professional help because the pupil had difficulty in learning or getting along within the classroom, he would bring this to the attention of the parents directly or through the principal. It was the parents' decision to come or not to come to us. A school could not refer a child to us directly, although it could facilitate such referral.

Again and again came the complaint: "When we, the school, help a family bring a pupil to you, we never hear any more about the matter. Why do you not tell us what you think of the case and let us know what we can do under the circumstances?" The solution, in other words, led to a new difficulty, as solutions usually do.

To meet the reproach that we were not giving the teachers the benefit of the knowledge acquired from their pupils, we developed a consultation program. Our clinical psychologists, psychiatrist, and psychiatric social worker visited each of the elementary schools at least once a month. By arrangement of the school principals, any teacher could consult one or more of these HRS representatives. They could discuss pupils who were our patients or children we did not know, or they could discuss general problems which concerned the teacher, such as restlessness, seeking attention, and the like.

This arrangement allowed the therapist to see at least some of his patients in the setting where teachers had to cope with them. It also allowed the HRS to make clear to the teacher that psychiatric therapy involves confidential information. Just as the school entrusted us with information it wished to go no further, so parents, in bringing their children to us, acquainted us with matters not to be relayed to the school or anyone else.

The consultation service created a further problem, however. By claiming competence in the treatment of emotional disorder, the HRS implied that the teacher was incompetent in that respect. Yet we declared ourselves interested in increasing the teacher's awareness of children's behavior and the meaning of the teacher's response to it. In the beginning we failed to see clearly that the teacher has his or her special competence in a school setting and that we, as clinicians or consultants, are in many ways incompetent in that setting.

Teachers became aware that in discussing their pupils they were also discussing themselves. It is always possible to wonder whether the "disturbed" child is not rather the "disturbing" child. This would make his disturbance a measure of one's own stability. Besides, so the logic ran, psychiatrists were given to "analyzing everything." Teachers could thus imagine themselves "looked through" or feel themselves looked down upon, for physicians enjoy higher status than teachers. Finally, the encounters between teacher and psychiatrist entailed the problem of specialized vocabularies. All professional groups have these as part of their standards. Such vocabularies could easily act as barriers rather than roads to clarity. What, for instance, was a teacher to make of the assertion that one of her pupils is "seriously compulsive"?

Just as some researchers are likely to perceive people as subjects, so are clinicians prone to change them into patients or cases. The consultation program courted these same risks. Indeed, teachers were our colleagues, for they asked to have a report on our assessment of some specific child. But they were also our clients, for they requested advice as to what to do with him now. This question readily implies further questions: What can I do under the circumstances? Perhaps there is something wrong with me, too, that makes me ask for advice? Teachers thus were our clients as well. In discussions away from the school it is all too easy to speak about them in categories usually used to assess the labyrinthine ways of patients. But the relation between therapist and patient is not one of equality. When we recognized these things, we were able to balance the notion that teachers were colleagues and clients but certainly not patients, with the notion that their work, partly overlapping with ours, was of necessity carried out in a far different setting.

We took other steps in our work with the school. In spring, we participated in preschool clinics, inviting mothers whose children were to enter kindergarten the following fall to come to our quarters for discussions. In this way we hoped to build a cumulative record on each school child which would add meaning to later symptoms or successes. Invitations were issued by members of our staff when the mothers came to the elementary schools for the yearly advance registrations. At this time children also received medical and dental examinations and became acquainted with the kindergarten teacher.

In one year we extended our participation in these clinics by observing children and their mothers in the doctor's office and the dressing rooms. Although we had no systematic way of recording our impressions, having no definite purpose in mind other than to build up records of successive generations of Wellesley citizens, we were impressed by the wealth of things to be seen when a mother brings a partly undressed child into a strange room occupied only by a doctor, a nurse, a pair of scales, and an improvised examining table. The four actors in this drama played quite a variety of roles. At times the mother went through the examination with the child, as it were. At times she left the child to its own devices and to the doctor and engaged the nurse in a separate conversation. At times she remained outside the triangle of doctor, nurse, and child.

We also learned at these clinics that some mothers, not knowing who we were, thought of us as teachers. This assumption made it difficult for them to see why they should give us personal information they felt was none of the school's business. In fact, we had to abandon an attempt to use the school premises for conducting a rather simple survey of facts about the play life of Wellesley children; we had to confine ourselves to gathering a few identifying data during the school clinic and issuing an invitation for more extended conversations about the child at our own quarters.

Extension of our activities during the preschool clinic necessarily prolonged an already long afternoon for mothers and children. This interfered with domestic routines and the needs of young siblings who came along or impatiently waited elsewhere. Time and routine are certainly to be taken seriously in America.

HRS representatives tended to be less constrained by time and routine and unrealistically expected others to exempt themselves in the same way.

As time went on, we succeeded in establishing the consultation program on a mutually satisfactory basis. In addition, a fair amount of research was undertaken with the cooperation of the school. Indeed, after receiving "free" service for five years, the school was willing to begin paying the HRS for its share of service.

Within the HRS

The HRS necessarily began its work with a vague and extensive array of goals, and the staff included specialists who performed a great variety of roles. Such circumstances stimulate internal differences of emphases. These, in fact, were present, in different forms and degrees, throughout the five-year period here under discussion. In the HRS at least two kinds of worlds were united in a single organization. One was the world of psychiatry, social work, and clinical psychology, devoted to service. The other was the world of social psychology, anthropology, and sociology, devoted to research. Clearly enough we had a common ground. We wanted to understand various aspects of mental health.

We differed in the way we sought such understanding and in the degree to which we wanted to apply our knowledge or assumptions. This difference became frozen into the opposition of "service" and "research." Much of this opposition rested on misunderstanding, so that the genuine differences between these two orders of activity and the way in which they could complement, and also limit, one another could not at first be properly assessed.

To the clinician, the researchers seemed compulsive and superficial. They seemed to gather material by asking specific and direct questions, thus cutting loose from its emotional moorings information which thereby became distorted, besides arousing undue anxiety in the informants. The researchers seemed, finally, to look at people from the outside and had little direct acquaintance with the intricate meanderings of human emotions as known to those who are more dynamically oriented.

To the researcher, the clinicians seemed to hold firmly to assumptions and interpretations which lacked decisive confirmation or appeared as only one among several possible alternatives. Nor did they seem to apply to themselves and to their relations with patients the same logic they used for assessing the situation of the patients. It looked as though they did not see therapy as a social situation in which they and their patients played social roles that remained constant regardless of who the patient was or what his symptoms happened to be.

Two further aspects of these images should be noted. On the one hand, the therapists used the word "research" to cover a whole range of things from clinical investigations to research on population growth. Then, exaggerating the preciseness of research, they wrongly contrasted it with the more qualitative and intuitive work of detection and healing. This led to a certain rejection of research and at the same time to very high expectations of it.

The researchers, on the other hand, expected the clinicians to provide them with well-formulated problems for which they could find the solutions by going out and gathering the appropriate information. Half of one's investigative work, however, is over once a problem is defined. The formulation of problems, moreover, assumes a particular way of thinking about phenomena. It is quite misleading to imagine that a clinical frame of reference can be enlarged simply by adding a sociological one, or a sociological frame of reference enlarged by adding a clinical one. The process is rather one of transforming each side. This takes much time, good will, and imagination.

We made progress toward defining common problems for clinical service and for research when we understood the roles of clinician and researcher better. Then it became clear that a clinician has responsibility for making specific decisions that affect others, often rather noticeably. He cannot afford skepticism, just as the researcher can ill afford not to have it. The time perspective of the researcher, on the other hand, is necessarily longer and his attitudes to his informants more impersonal. He sees them as representatives of various social arrangements or as members of various groups, not as cases and instances of clinical syndromes. This way of thinking, however inefficient it might appear at times, yields an economy of concern which keeps a particular clinical problem within manageable bounds.

Disagreements between therapists and researchers—and within both groups, since neither was in turn homogeneous—had, however, another aspect. As has been suggested, the HRS started out with ideals that would make it an equalitarian and permissive organization. It was to be a far cry from the status-conscious arrangements of hospital staff meetings or the orderliness of bureaucratic procedures. Yet we had a director who had employed us and could ask us to leave or stay. We had not come together as equal colleagues; we had been brought together by one or two people. Under these circumstances, it soon developed that our organization was subject to the exigencies of all other human organizations, that we, too, had to have our inner differences and had to have some authority and inequality of right and privilege.

We clung to the ideal of maintaining a relatively informal and personal organization, yet we were not merely a group of friends. We were cooperating not just to be sociable but to do some work by which we were to be judged and which was to remain behind us. Such aims always demand discipline and impersonal regulations. Nor can the outside world be entirely ignored. In it, doctors have higher prestige and greater responsibility than, say, sociologists. Such differences necessarily affected our inner arrangements. These status differences became expressed also in different emphases as to our twin aims of research and service and, more particularly, as to the appropriate ways of implementing them. These differences, moreover, affected our dealings with the outside, so that it was never easy to know to what extent the opposition we received from outside represented a reflection of our internal divisions.

IMPLICATIONS

Cooperation Through Conflict

People are kept apart by being grouped together in various ways—through their work or their pleasure, their faith or their station. This is common knowledge. One anticipates that a hospital will be run differently from a bank, that a teacher will have a somewhat different image of a child than will a psychiatrist. Social institutions differ, and their representatives will therefore look at an identical person in different ways. Thus perceived in various ways, the person will ultimately come to look upon himself in a number of different ways. Moreover, a single institution often performs a number of purposes, and so an institution, too, is usually looked at in more than one way. The HRS, therefore, was in a sense a different agency to every group it dealt with, because of its own and the groups' diversity of aims and outlooks.

The psychiatrists seek to heal, but health, especially "emotional health," can assume many forms. The school teaches specific skills but is concerned as well with "character" and "happiness." Clergymen, as functionaries of religious organizations, represent a moral tradition that creates and solves quandaries. Social scientists, restricting their immediate responsibilities, seek to clarify the order of social arrangements in which they and others participate. These several worlds, however, also overlap. They are ultimately concerned with the same phenomena, and their efforts represent a division of labor. The life of a clergyman, a psychiatrist, and a social scientist involve one another and thus imply shared concerns.

We would have made a grave mistake had we minimized the persistent differences among the divergent expectations of teachers, ministers, and other groups. We would have erred had we assumed that just because people are using the same words they are saying the same thing. It is an essential step toward cooperation to recognize the existence and persistence of conflicting views. Moreover, such conflict can actually be productive. Within the HRS, for example, researchers kept therapists on their toes by asking, "How do you know?" And therapists kept researchers on their toes by asking, "So what?"

Cooperation, whether within an organization or between representatives of different organizations, needs both agreements and differences. Given mutual appreciation, some kinds of disagreement are useful. One is kept alive to one's own assumptions. In this way, as a sociologist, I learned much from the clinicians, who could teach me how to listen to people. I learned much, too, from trying to recast their explanation of this or that case in terms involving regularities of social arrangements so that, for instance, the perennial "unsolved oedipal conflict" could be seen within the context of middle-class family structure. In that way, too, likeness and difference between minister and psychiatrist came into sight and thereby also the meaning and relativity of such concepts as "health" or "illness" or "salvation." All involve assumptions that as such cannot be proved.

Disagreement Versus Misunderstanding

Sometimes, Americans, who place such high value on cooperation and education, are prone to talk as though all disagreements are the outgrowth of misunderstanding and so can be done away with by conferences and by enlightenment. Sometimes this is carried to a point where it seems that someone were saying, "Everything would be all right if everybody knew everything about everybody." This essay argues differently. It suggests that all social arrangements involve gaps and differences between people. These lead to or confirm differences of interest, competence, and value. They can, but need not, lead as well to misunderstanding. The latter arises especially where one fails to see how the same matter can be viewed differently by another who stands in a different relation to it, and how differences in social position affect the kind of knowledge of human affairs that can be associated with these positions. Understanding, on the other hand, does not preclude disagreement. Disagreement over what is to be done and why, or how it is to be done, is deeply rooted in social organization, just as the latter invariably depends on some measure of agreement.

Our social arrangements involve the persistence of a variety of positions or social roles, like those of minister, teacher, therapist, and researcher. People occupying these positions tend to differ in their evaluation of the same matter, in this case a specific mental health agency. These differences, however, need not constitute obstacles for a program of service and research.

The social arrangements through which particular purposes are achieved affect the way in which these purposes are understood, both on the inside and the outside. Relative to the school, the HRS was a loosely organized agency. This was congenial to the clergy committee but led to certain obstacles in our relations with the school representatives. We appeared to them somewhat unreliable; they appeared to us somewhat compulsive, demanding figures, written reports, orderly schedules. When we became aware of the difference in our form of organization and the reasons neither could readily become a model for the other, then we could maintain our differences and yet achieve cooperation.

In some respects ministers, psychiatrists, and teachers have like concerns; they are interested in the welfare of others. At the same time they differ from one another; their obligations and privileges are not identical, and their prestige is unequal. Moreover, the boundaries between their respective tasks are not always clear and may even shift in the course of time. Under these conditions, it is not surprising that the division of labor between specialists is subject to certain strains and abuses. Two dangers stand out: the temptation of role incorporation and the error of overextension.

The first danger is that incumbents of one social role will incorporate functions and practices appropriate to another category of specialists. This is especially likely where two groups enjoy unequal prestige. One group can hope to improve its status by taking over some of the characteristics of the other. Ministers, for instance, might be tempted to incorporate psychiatric functions into their own role. To a degree this is feasible and can be done in the name of pastoral counseling. Beyond a certain point, however, such role incorporation can lead to conflict. Ministers, as distinct from psychiatrists, represent another world and a fairly articulate moral order. They are expected to draw moral lines and to make judgments. Ministers may vary in the manner in which they do this, but within the accepted boundaries of their social role they can never be so permissive with parishioners as psychiatrists can be with patients.

For their part, psychiatrists are likely to see in the permissive therapy situation a model of the good society, and accordingly judge what they find in the real world as pathological or pathogenic. Part of the efficacy of the therapist-patient relationship, however, stems from the very fact that it is a special situation. In failing to see that a special situation by its nature can never be a general one, psychiatrists would be committing the complementary error of overextension.

Cooperation usually involves some revision in the points of view of people who previously worked apart. Such revision proceeds slowly and in stages rather than by sudden enlargements of awareness. Individuals who seek to cooperate will find it easier to make this adjustment if they realize that their initial divergence of views is a product of their different social worlds and their different institutional arrangements.

SUMMARY

This account relates in part and from a sociological point of view what occurred during the first few years after the Human Relations Service, a mental health agency providing both service and research, was established in Wellesley. The report has centered on the divergent expectations concerning the HRS held by the clergy, by the schools, and by different segments of the HRS staff itself.

The HRS began as a free service to the community. It was accepted in different degrees by different parts of the community. Primarily, the service dealt with the world of mothers and young children, on the one hand, and the school and church on the other. To become more firmly established it had to recognize its limitations and work out a division of labor within its own ranks and in its joint efforts with the school and the clergy. This required agreement on common goals, recognition of appropriate differences in procedure, and delimiting controversial areas in which the cooperating parties agreed to disagree. One measure of the success of the project was its financial acceptance by the community which had invited it without initially having to support it.

Some general implications can be drawn from this study. Recognizing the presence of persisting conflicts of values and goals is an essential first step toward establishing cooperation. Divergent views of the same issue are not merely the result of misunderstanding. Differences in approach and emphasis are inherent in a cooperative division of labor. A division of labor is made possible by the mutual relations of different social roles. Some of the latter, notably those of psychiatrist, minister, and teacher, are closely allied. This can lead to mutual misperception; it can also lead to profitable cooperation. Working together requires an understanding of the irreducible differences and an agreement to differ with respect to certain matters. Such a cooperative state of affairs can only come about slowly.

SELECTED REFERENCES

Aberle, David F., "Introducing Preventive Psychiatry into a Community," *Human Organization*, vol. 9, Fall, 1950, pp. 5–9. This article gives a detailed account of the very early history of the Human Relations Service in Wellesley.

Aberle, David F., and Kaspar D. Naegele, "Middle-Class Fathers' Occupational Role and Attitudes Toward Children," *American Journal of Orthopsychiatry*, vol. 22, April, 1952, pp. 366–378. This article, one of the research products of the Human Relations Service, describes the relationships between the social and occupational position of the father, the goals for which he trains his children, and his evaluation of their behavior in terms of these goals.

Lindemann, Erich, and Lydia Dawes, "The Use of Psychoanalytic Constructs in Preventive Psychiatry" in *The Psychoanalytic Study of the Child*, vol. 7. International Universities Press, New York, 1952. The director of the Human Relations Service and its consultant in the field of child psychiatry here provide a preliminary account of the aims and theoretical underpinnings of the service aspects of the agency.

Lynd, R. S., and H. M. Lynd, *Middletown in Transition*. Harcourt, Brace and Co., New York, 1937. Chapter 12 of this classic community study of a midwestern town is a still relevant presentation of the general values by which a majority of people in the United States attempt to live. The more recent concern with "mental health" can be better understood within the framework of these general values.

Parsons, Talcott, *Essays in Sociological Theory*. Rev. ed. The Free Press, Glencoe, Ill., 1954. Chapters 1, 2, and 18 analyze different professional roles, especially those of the doctor. These are contrasted with business roles. Implicit in this analysis are many of the ideas concerning the possibilities and difficulties of cooperation between different occupational roles indicated in the present paper.

Stanton, Alfred H., and Morris S. Schwartz, *The Mental Hospital*. Basic Books, Inc., New York, 1954. Though confined to the walls of a single institution and a women's ward within it, this report of a cooperative enterprise by a psychiatrist and a sociologist contains suggestive proposals for a sociology of mental illness as well as detailed accounts of the roles of doctor, nurse, aide, and patient (Section III) and an analysis of various processes of information, misinformation, and misunderstanding (Section IV).

PART V

VEHICLES OF HEALTH ADMINISTRATION

Case 12

THE CLINICAL TEAM IN A CHILEAN HEALTH CENTER
by Ozzie G. Simmons

One way to learn what a particular organ contributes to the functioning of the whole organic system is to see what happens when that organ is altered or removed. The same method applies in the study of social systems. Parts of the system can be deliberately altered; this is done, for example, in small-group research conducted in a laboratory setting with volunteer subjects. Another way is to take advantage of so-called natural experiments where customary team combinations have been disturbed. What happens in the clinic when the public health nurse is removed from the conventional triad of doctor, nurse, and patient?

As a social scientist studying health beliefs and health programs in Peru and Chile, Dr. Simmons recognized an opportunity to collect evidence on this issue when he came to the San Lucero Health Center serving one of Santiago's ten sanitary districts. There the nurses had been relieved of duties in the prenatal and well-child clinics so that they could spend all their time promoting health education in homes. The useful but unofficial functions they performed in mediating between doctor and patient became fully apparent only when communication between patient and doctor in the clinic virtually broke down in the absence of the nurse.

Dr. Simmons' account touches only a limited aspect of the overall San Lucero program. The part-time and peripheral involvement of the doctors described in the case study is now being modified as a result of legislation providing for a unified national health service, which will enable Chilean public health doctors to spend more time with fewer programs than heretofore and to have comparable salary scales if they continue to participate in more than one program. But these qualifications do not diminish the merits of the study, which provides instructive case material on the social role of the health worker, particularly the nurse, and on the significance of intra-team communication.

Along comparable lines, Dr. Wellin's study contains material on the social role of the grass-roots hygiene worker in Peru, and the India cases by Carstairs and Marriott concern the social role of the physician. Dr. Cassel describes how the health team works together in the home as well as the clinic; the public health doctor in South Africa travels out to the neighborhood and the home, along with the nurse and the native health educator. Problems of intra-team communication are treated in the Guatemalan case by Dr. Adams and in Dr. Stycos' Puerto Rican study where concern is with the husband-wife team rather than the clinical team. Indeed, the parental team and the clinical team have much in common; both exhibit features characteristic of small-group systems. —EDITOR

THE PROBLEM

An Impasse in Health Education

The director of the San Lucero Health Center in Santiago, Chile, faced a dilemma. The Health Center, established a few years earlier, was part of a broad program instituted by the Chilean government, a program designed to bring improved health services to a larger number of people. The core of the program was a group of community health centers, strategically located throughout the country. These centers were to concentrate on preventive medicine, on communitywide service, and on an extensive program of basic health education, aimed at the family group.

The director of the San Lucero Center subscribed fully to the general aims of the national program, but he was especially interested in family-focused health education. He had taken over the directorship of the Center in 1943 when it had a staff of seven—with himself and one medical student the only staff physicians. By hard and assiduous effort he built up the Center until by 1950 it boasted a staff of 102, including 15 doctors, 12 nurses, and three social workers, housed in two buildings containing offices and clinics.

In 1950, however, despite proliferation of services and great strides in the sanitary and epidemiological control of the district, the Health Center director felt that he had arrived at an impasse in the critically important educational program. He and his senior nurses were discouraged by a situation in which they seemed to be repeatedly exposing the same patients to the same educational materials and were reaching few new people.

Troubled, the director cast about for some way to increase the effectiveness of his lagging educational program. He had at his command the services of more than 100 trained personnel. The Center operated daily infant, prenatal, dental, and tuberculosis clinics, an epidemiological service, sanitary inspection, and a program of home visiting by nurses, social workers, and a nutritionist. Each of the Center's 15 doctors spent two hours a day on clinic duty. The nurses engaged both in clinic duty and home visiting, attempting to promote health education in both settings.

Keeping in mind his available facilities, the director pondered a number of alternatives. Should he add a corps of specially trained health educators? Should he try to train the staff doctors to become more effective agents of health education? Should he rearrange the schedule of his nurses so as to increase their home visiting time, giving them increased contact with a larger number of expectant and nursing mothers?

He realized that each of these alternatives would have its limitations or drawbacks, but that it would be impossible to evaluate in advance the full effects of his decision. To appreciate the rationale behind his decision as well as to appraise its effects, we must first examine the background of the director's problem.

THE SITUATION

Utilizing Center Personnel for Better Health Education

The Municipality of San Lucero

The metropolitan area of Santiago, a city of 1,700,000, is divided into a number of *comunas*, or municipal districts, each with its own administration and services. Within the last decade, sanitary districts have been set up for public health administration, and these districts usually coincide with the comunas. Public health activities in these comunas are administered through the health centers.

The San Lucero Health Center is located in the comuna of San Lucero and is one of ten centers serving Santiago. The estimated population of the comuna in April, 1952, was 145,442. The population increase of San Lucero in the past fifteen years has been phenomenal, with 35,293 in 1930, 65,463 in 1940, and an estimated 75,168 in 1943. Situated on the southern edge of the city, much of San Lucero is urban in character, but its outlying sectors merge with surrounding rural communities. In San

Lucero there are 364 factories manufacturing textile, paper, chemical, rubber, leather, glass, ceramic, and metal products, and a wide variety of other commercial enterprises. Most of the residents are employed by these factories and businesses, but some residents such as professional people, businessmen, white-collar workers, peddlers, or day laborers work in other parts of the city.

As this list of occupations indicates, the whole range of socio-economic statuses is found in San Lucero. The comuna's housing reflects this, with "residential" sectors characterized by four-bedroom houses averaging 1.3 persons per bedroom at one extreme, while at the other are the rapidly growing "mushroom" populations strung along the banks of the sewage canals on public domain and housing an average of 5.2 persons per room in one-bedroom shacks. The socioeconomic pyramid has a very broad base and a thin spire. Low-income groups living under hardship conditions make up the vast bulk of the population. Fifty per cent of the comuna's housing is considered substandard and an additional 20 per cent is classed as "uninhabitable." The comuna has 17 public schools and 12 private schools. Physically, public schools are extremely crude, many having very much over-crowded classrooms with dirt floors. Only about half of the school-age children in San Lucero attend school, as in other parts of Santiago.

By mutual agreement, the Health Center has little contact with the upper-income group of the population. Health Center personnel concentrate their efforts on those who have greater need of their services. Most upper-income people resent intervention in what they consider their personal affairs; they prefer private physicians and are annoyed by suggestions that their personal and domestic hygiene or dietary practices are not all they should be. The rest of the population is classified by the Health Center into two groups, those who can be "educated" and those who cannot. The standard of living of the first group enables it to comply with the health worker's teachings, while the second group is considered too poor and too unlettered to do so, even if willing. This group receives only minimum services, such as immunization and essential medical care.

Before the Change: Doctor and Nurse as Health Educators

The director of the San Lucero Health Center had given a good deal of thought to the problem of how the health needs of this sprawling and heterogeneous community could most effectively be served. He had come to the conclusion that a well-planned program of health education was the best means at his command to bring better health to the largest possible number of people. On the Center staff, the most logical people to do this job were the doctors and nurses, and the director had tried to outline their duties so as to maximize their effectiveness as agents of health education. Like any other organized enterprise, his program was administered on the basis of an official "charter" specifying the formal duties of staff members and based on such factors as the technical specialties of individuals and the organization and objectives of the program.

The official philosophy of the Center was based on teamwork. Doctors, nurses, social workers, and other health workers were expected to be sufficiently aware of one another's activities and spheres of competence to help one another and to make intelligent and appropriate referrals. Teamwork, it was felt, was especially important in health education, and there was a general expectation at San Lucero that everyone would cooperate in health education "from the director down to the porters."

According to the "charter" of the Health Center, doctors were to practice both curative and preventive medicine and to carry on health education. Preventive medicine was defined as measures for preventing illness or reducing its probability. This included physical examinations, height and weight control, vaccination and immunization, and indication of hygienic and dietary precautions. Health education, on the other hand, was conceived of as the inculcation both of good personal health habits and a sense of responsibility for the maintenance of good health. In accordance with these objectives, the principal effort of doctors was to be directed equally toward preventive medicine and health education, with curative medicine practiced only to the extent necessary to expedite effort in the other two areas. All doctors attended clinics on a part-time basis and were expected to give two hours of their time, either in the morning or afternoon, for consultations with a standard quota of about 15 patients.

The doctors themselves, however, tended to define their duties quite differently. For the most part, they felt their primary function to be "control"—checking the physical condition of patients, prescribing whatever was necessary, explaining the importance of their instructions, and doing a "little educating" when time permitted. Viewing their proper functions in this way, doctors paid little attention to health education and not much more to preventive medicine.

Officially, nurses had two main duties: supplementing the preventive medicine practiced by the doctors and conducting health education. Until 1950, nurses performed these duties in homes and in the prenatal and well-baby clinics. In the clinic health education was focused on ideas appropriate to the clinic setting and the immediate situation of the patient. For example, in the infant clinic mothers were instructed concerning proper infant diet, while demonstrations in preparing nursing bottles were held in the home. It was felt that education in the clinic was as essential as education in the home. Clinic procedure was arranged so that nurses saw mothers after their consultation with the doctor, repeated the doctor's instructions as indicated on the patient's record, gave mothers a copy of these instructions to take home, and lastly undertook to educate the mother on details relevant to her particular case.

Nurses also administered vaccinations and immunizations in the clinic and issued authorizations for milk, distributed free or at low cost. On the day following clinic visits, the nurse went to the patient's home to see if she was following instructions. A nurse would be on clinic duty on the days when patients from her home-visiting district were scheduled to appear. Thus, the nurse could inform the doctor on the individual situation of patients whose homes she visited. Since the doctors considered health education of minor importance in their own work, the main burden of health education fell to the nurses. The nurses, for their part, accepted the importance accorded to health education by the director, commenting that "our work is mainly accomplished through health education" or "wherever a nurse goes, she has to educate."

Doctors, on the other hand, conceived the role of the nurse as supplementary to their own and felt that her principal duty was to reinforce and clarify their instructions by means of practical demonstrations and to carry out the controls they had indicated. Doctors characterized the nurse as a sort of personal assistant and tended to ignore her health education duties. They believed that the nurse's attention should be directed to the family, the doctor's to the individual.

The nurses, for their part, frequently complained that the doctors did not carry on even the minimum health education necessary to complement their own work. They claimed that their most useful assistance to the doctor lay in providing him with otherwise unavailable data on the living conditions and dietary practices of his patients rather than merely supplementing his instructions.

It should be stressed that the doctors at San Lucero were competent physicians who made a real contribution to therapeutic and preventive medicine. The doctor's limited contribution to the health education effort was not a matter of willful neglect. The limits to the amount of help he could give to this aspect of the Health Center's total program were set less by factors of individual motivation than by the peripheral nature of his relation to the health education campaign.

Reorganizing the Health Education Program

The director was thus faced with a difficult problem arising from the fact that the Center doctors shared neither his enthusiasm for health education nor his conviction that it was an effective means to bring about maximum community health coverage. Not only did the doctors devote little of their own time to health education, but their use of the nurse as a personal assistant limited the amount of time nurses could devote to an activity they endorsed.

Taking into consideration the personnel resources he commanded as well as the lack of agreement among staff members as to their proper duties, what arrangements could the director make to achieve his goal of improving health education? He considered adding specially trained health educators to his staff. But this plan, however desirable it might have been, was not feasible.

His budget provided no funds for this purpose. Moreover, only a few health educators were available and their schedules were arranged by the Ministry of Health so that each of Chile's health centers had the services of a health educator for only a few weeks at a time.

The director also considered the possibility of persuading the doctors to conduct more health education and offering them training to that end. This alternative posed certain serious difficulties. One of these was the peripheral position of the doctors in the Health Center program, which severely limited the degree of administrative and technical control the director could exert over them. Doctors were isolated not only from the director and other health workers, all of whom had some contact with each other, but from their fellow doctors as well, since they worked on staggered schedules and rarely met in their comings and goings. The two doctors who had worked longest at San Lucero had not seen each other for years, except for chance encounters outside the Health Center, nor had they exchanged opinions about their work at San Lucero since the early days when the Center was small.

The reasons for this thoroughgoing insulation of the doctor from the program were not hard to find. Until recently the vast majority of doctors recruited for Health Center programs had a "clinical" rather than a public health background. Unlike many recently trained doctors, the older men did not understand public health objectives nor were they very sympathetic toward them.

Another reason was the part-time employment of doctors. Health center administrators have long realized that this has severely handicapped the development of the clinics as an integral part of their programs. The customary practice for Chilean doctors who work for government or other large-scale enterprises, and most of them do, has been to devote two hours a day to each of two to four different medical programs. Although the amount of time and technical competence required by different organizations are about the same, the pay scales are different. In consequence, doctors tend to give more time and attention to the better paying jobs, despite the fact that they are formally under contract for two hours at each post. Since the doctors were beyond the reach of the director's authority and only mildly committed to the Center's program and ideals, it would have been difficult to effect any appreciable changes in the situation of the clinic doctors.

In view of the impracticability of other alternatives, the director turned to those staff members over whom he did exercise administrative control and who were committed to the goals of the Center's program—the nurses. Along with the senior nurses, he had come to the conclusion that conditions did not allow the nurse to do much educational work in the clinic. The doctors were not putting in their full two hours in the clinic and were rushing their patients through so that the nurse had little time with each patient. Moreover, because he was always in such a hurry, the doctor made little effort to convey his instructions to the patient, depending on the nurse to do this according to indications he entered on the record. In consequence, the nurse had to spend what little time she had with the patient explaining the doctor's orders, thus performing "therapeutic" rather than "preventive" education work. The director believed that this did not justify the services of nurses and that the doctor should make his explanations directly to the patient.

Basing his decision on these immediate considerations as well as others, the director decided, after consulting with his senior staff members, to relieve his nurses of all clinic duty and assign them to home visiting on a full-time basis. To perform the irreducible minimum of clinical duties that required nursing supervision, he obtained one nurse from a nearby hospital to work full time in the clinic.

The director thought of his decision primarily as an administrative shift and regarded the innovation as a "technical modification" in the duties of the nurse. Along with the assignment of nurses to full-time home visiting, efforts were made to streamline the diffuse subject matter discussed in the home visit by focusing on three basic points: personal and environmental hygiene, disease prevention, and nutrition.

Reactions to the New Policy

Shortly after the shift of nurses to full-time home visiting, the single nurse on duty in the clinics found herself beset by all man-

ner of complaints and requests from patients, which she herself
could not begin to satisfy. Many women complained to the nurses
visiting their homes about conditions in the clinic. One of these
nurses reported that patients came to the clinic with less confidence than before. She added that it was more comfortable for
them to be attended by a nurse whom they knew and felt close to,
and that no relationship of this sort was possible with the new
nurse who took over the supervision of the clinics.

Another nurse said that patients expected to be able to discuss
family problems with the nurse but since she was not in the clinic,
this was impossible. It meant that the patients had to wait until
the nurse came to their home.

These reactions showed that the patients had been depending
on the services the nurse in the clinic had provided and keenly
felt her loss. Other reactions by patients seemed to indicate that
the clinic nurses had been acting as an important intermediary
between doctor and patient and that this role was no longer being
filled. One nurse reported that mothers felt "disconnected" because they did not have the same confidence in the doctors as in
the nurses. Sometimes they even went off without having their
prescriptions filled because a nurse was not there to explain why
this was necessary and they themselves did not attach much
importance to the prescription.

Another nurse related that patients were accustomed to seeing
their own sector nurse in the clinic and felt strange when they
did not see her. Nurses were no longer on hand to tell them
where to go for different things, such as medicines, milk, and so
on. And since no one was there to guide them to the various
services, which were spread around, the mothers wandered from
one place to another with their children in their arms.

One nurse said that in visits to the homes after the change
occurred, it was common to find mothers confused about items
of infant diet—for example, when to give fruit juices and when
not. Also, the mothers were often uncertain about administering
prescribed remedies, both with regard to frequency and quantity.

The patients' dissatisfaction, however, did not become chronic;
complaints became less frequent and after a time virtually disappeared. This did not necessarily mean, however, that patients no

longer missed the nurse in the clinic. The single nurse supervising the clinics stated that many patients still came to the nurses' office in the administration building after a visit to the clinic looking for their own sector nurse to help them with their problems.

Two of the doctors had been working at San Lucero before the new policy was put into effect. They differed as to the consequence of the change. One doctor expressed mild regret over losing the nurse's assistance in getting across his instructions but felt that he could handle the situation alone, and that the nurse was more useful in home visiting. But the other doctor said that the nurse was essential for amplifying and reinforcing his instructions and for giving him information about the patient's home situation. He lamented the loss of direct communication between himself and the nurses and considered this the most serious defect in the functioning of the Health Center program. Unable to speak with the nurses directly, he felt the loss of coordination between doctor and nurse on a particular case. He illustrated this lack of coordination by pointing to a patient's record in which he had indicated in August certain measures to be undertaken by the nurse, but which were not carried out until the nurse had visited the patient the following March.

If he made a special request, he said, the nurse would visit a patient soon after the consultation, but he was reluctant to make many such requests since the nurse had her own home visiting schedule to follow, and too many special requests would upset this schedule. A lack of coordination also resulted, he said, when the nurse failed to record fully the measures she had taken in a home visit. He gave as an example the fact that nurses sometimes forgot to indicate that they had administered a vaccination, and when the doctor would recommend one later on the patient would be very much confused.

Most of the nurses substantially approved the decision to relieve them of clinic duty. A few were rather unhappy at first when they found that some of their patients were not receiving so much care in the clinics as formerly, but they had less reason for this concern when a public health nurse was substituted for the hospital nurse assigned to supervise the clinics following the shift. In general, the nurses said they preferred the new arrangement because it gave them more time for home visiting and increased their effectiveness as health educators. Many nurses expected the change to force the doctor to fulfill his educational obligations more faithfully by making it necessary for him to give instructions formerly given by the nurse.

A few nurses, however, expressed dissatisfaction with the new policy. One nurse said that she was not content with the change in the beginning and continued to feel that she should have at least one day a week in the clinic. In this way she could see the people in her sector who attend the Health Center but whom she had no time to visit. She said she would also be able to help those of her people who did not have enough money for milk and medicines, a service she could not perform in the home where these problems did not arise. Another nurse said she would prefer to return to the old system, but only if it were possible to do some educational work in the clinic. If she worked in the clinic in addition to her sector, she said, she would know whether or not the patient actually attended the clinic and in what ways she benefited by attending.

The director himself felt that the changes resulting from his decision were, on the whole, beneficial. Although the Center did not undertake any systematic evaluation of the results of the new policy, the director gained the impression, by personal observation of the overall program, that the change considerably increased the effectiveness of the health education program.

He realized that direct communication between doctor and nurse had been virtually eliminated. Instead, they communicated by means of the patient's record, which was much less effective than direct conversation in revealing the particular environmental and psychological situation of individual patients. The director felt, however, that the loss of direct contact between doctor and nurse was not critical since the doctors had not been much involved in health education anyway. He felt that the nurses' freedom to concentrate their full attention on health education in the home more than compensated for loss of communication effectiveness in the clinic.

No attempt was made to substantiate the director's impression that gains in the overall health education program outweighed the losses in clinic effectiveness. However, the complaints of mothers who visited the clinic and the feeling by some staff members that something had gone wrong can be taken as a good indication that a fairly fundamental change in the system of relationships within the clinic had occurred when the nurses were removed. The following sections will analyze the nature of interpersonal relationships in the clinic before the nurses were shifted and the effects of the shift on these relationships.

The Relationship Between Doctor and Patient

Several causes lay at the root of the difficulties in the relationship between doctor and patient. One reason was that the doctors considered their work in the Health Center clinic to be of no greater importance than their other commitments and were not wholly conscientious in their dealings with patients. Another was that ready communication between doctors and patients was hindered by the fact that they belonged to different social classes and held different convictions by virtue of belonging to those classes. Moreover, doctors and patients subscribed to two different systems of medicine, and each group was unfamiliar with the other's system. The nurses were impelled to assume many unofficial duties in order to compensate for these deficiencies in the doctor-patient relationship.

The doctor's participation in the San Lucero program was but one of his professional activities, and the other professional interests generally took precedence over his clinical practice at San Lucero. In the clinics, contact between doctor and patient was brief and formal, and the doctor's procedure standardized and routine. Questioning was usually perfunctory and superficial. Relatively detailed verbal instructions were fired rapidly at the patient. On the rare occasions when the doctor asked if the patient understood the instructions, he invariably received a perfunctory affirmative reply. Only when the patient obviously and grossly misconstrued his directions would the doctor repeat them and even then he did not write them.

Doctors rarely concerned themselves with anything beyond conventional curative considerations. Their almost exclusive concern with immediate therapy usually diverted their attention from the "nonclinical" factors involved in a particular case. The doctors were always in a hurry to finish their clinic work and rarely remained for the full two hours even when they had to attend their maximum quota of 15 patients. The following incident illustrates a consequence of the narrow focus on purely clinical aspects of a case.

The mother of a seriously underweight infant brought the child to the clinic weekly in accordance with the doctor's instructions. During one visit the doctor noted that the child was not gaining weight despite the fact that he had authorized a given quantity of milk to be provided by the Center. He asked the mother if she had been giving all this milk to the infant and when she did not reply berated her for not remembering his instructions. There was no use in telling this woman anything, he said, because she could not remember and did not seem to care whether the child became healthy or not. At this point the mother burst into tears and the doctor, disconcerted, asked her why. Hesitantly, the woman explained that her husband was unemployed and that she had used part of the milk ration for an older child because she had no food for him. The doctor, now apologetic, arranged to have a larger milk ration provided.

Other attitudes on the part of the doctors contributed to their insensitivity to difficulties in their relations with patients. In fact, the doctors did not feel that there were any problems in their relationship to patients. They assumed that their professional status and technical competence assured the respect of patients, as well as an automatic compliance with orders. Nurses, sanitary inspectors, and others confirmed the doctor's judgment that many people regarded him as the final arbiter in medical matters. Unlike the doctors, however, the nurses and other health workers did not assume that this necessarily brought about willing compliance with the doctor's instructions or unlimited confidence in him. Indeed, the nurses unanimously maintained that clinic patients had been much more frank with them than with the doctors. A few nurses went so far as to say that the doctor never inspired confidence, and all nurses agreed that patients were timid and apprehensive in his presence. They seldom volunteered any information about their personal affairs or dared question him.

Patients did evince respect for the doctor, but this respect was based not only on the doctor's technical competence, as he believed, but also on his social position in the Chilean class system. Most Chilean doctors are of upper-class background, whereas those served by the health centers ordinarily belong to the lower classes. Patients defer to the authority of the doctor as an upper-class person as much as to his authority as a medical expert. Government health workers claim that most Chilean doctors working in public health put social status considerations before professional responsibilities in their relationships with patients. Doctors encourage a tendency to "deify" them and prefer to command and impress their indigent patients than to deal with them strictly as patients. Thus, the doctor's superior class position increases the amount of deference that would normally be accorded him by virtue of his professional status and makes free communication even more difficult. He is regarded with respect but seldom with confidence. Nurses, on the other hand, generally come from the Chilean lower or middle classes and are accorded less prestige but more confidence.

Another attitude related to class position blocks communication between doctor and patient. Many doctors believe the capacity of people to understand and thus to cooperate is directly related to their formal education and economic status. One doctor said that although the people were willing to accept his advice and recommendations, their intellectual level was very low, and they had great difficulty understanding new ideas. Another doctor indicated that he measured the mental capacity of his patients by the number of years of schooling they had and equated illiteracy with mental deficiency.

While there is little doubt that poorly educated people have difficulty in understanding certain kinds of instruction, it is also true that the doctors' facile assumption of inherent incapacity caused them to expend little effort in trying to make themselves understood. Rather than resulting from ignorance or mental defectiveness, the patient's failure to understand could well have resulted from the doctor's use of technical medical terminology.

Indeed, the nurse's principal task in "explaining" the doctor's instructions, when she served in the clinic, was to convert the doctor's terminology into language understandable to the patients.

An additional reason for the mother's failure to understand the doctor and to accept his precepts was her belief in folk medicine, the theories of which are often in direct competition with those of modern medicine. In Chile, as in other Latin American countries, belief in folk medicine pervades even the most highly urbanized communities and plays a substantial part in determining attitudes toward modern medicine. Most doctors are only dimly aware of these folk beliefs which frequently limit understanding and acceptance of modern medicine. The followers of folk medicine tend to look with disfavor on modern doctors.

These unfavorable attitudes are directed at doctors in general and not in particular at Health Center doctors, some of whom occasionally are praised by patients. Discussing doctors in general, patients frequently say that they know nothing about internal ailments and can only treat the "outside"; that they know only how to give injections and thereby kill people; that doctors will never admit that they cannot cure certain illnesses; that they know nothing except surgery, giving injections, and prescribing drugstore remedies. Some say surgery is the main reason for seeking a doctor's services, but many maintain that doctors just slash away the flesh indiscriminately. One patient told of a young man whose arm became greatly swollen as a result of a spider bite and said that a doctor cut all the flesh off his arm, leaving nothing but skin and bone.

Health Center patients told many stories about the failures of doctors. One woman said that a Health Center doctor had erroneously diagnosed her daughter's affliction as mange and for a long time treated her accordingly, but it turned out to be a venereal disease. A woman suffering from tuberculosis was treated by the "best" doctors to no avail and was finally cured by a folk curer. A few patients felt that doctors are ignorant because they did not act in accordance with folk beliefs. One woman complained angrily that a doctor had advised her to bathe and wash her hair even though she was menstruating, a combination which can result in serious illness, according to folk belief. Another said a doctor had prescribed a remedy for her child's diarrhea, but this only partly cured him since it was also necessary to "bring up" the object that was causing the diarrhea. She said the doctor's knowledge did not extend that far, and she finally had to use a home remedy to complete the cure.

Despite generally unfavorable attitudes toward doctors, patients were not above buttressing folk beliefs by the doctor's sanction, showing that they both rejected the doctor and at the same time acknowledged him as an authority on medical matters. A patient would extol the virtues of a particular folk remedy and add that the doctor also recommended it, or claim that an herb remedy was so good that the doctors themselves prescribed it.

The Relationship Between Nurse and Patient

The nurse was the Health Center representative the patient came to know best. On the mother's first contact with the Center under the old policy, it was the nurse who explained to her the nature of the program, what the Center expected of her, and what she might expect from the Center. After an initial home visit by the epidemiologist, the nurse was also responsible for communicable disease control and whatever preventive medicine was practiced outside the clinics. The general outlook the nurse brought to her work, derived largely from her formal public health training, motivated her to assume the job of intermediary in the clinic and provided a "humanistic" conception of the patient that contrasted with the doctor's conception. In spite of some occasional lapses, most nurses made a genuine attempt to learn about those problems of the patient and family that might affect their teachings and to adapt their recommendations to the family's means and resources.

The role of the nurse made it possible for her to be closer to a patient than any other staff member. Only she had direct access to the patient's home environment. On home visits she obtained extensive information on incomes, occupations, schooling, domestic economies, and dietary practices, and made an inventory of sanitary facilities, sleeping space, and so on. In the home nurses could gain the patient's confidence and observe at first

hand the more subtle aspects of her situation. The head nurse at
San Lucero said:

> Since the nurse knows the patient in her home condition, the pa-
> tient cannot hide anything from her. There the patient is disposed to
> tell the nurse about herself because she knows the nurse will discover
> these things anyway, and she knows the nurse will not be contemptu-
> ous of her in any way when she does know these things.

The frequency and duration of the nurse's contacts with the
patient also promoted closeness. The nurse directed her attention
to all members of the family. She made periodic visits to expectant mothers, nursing infants, and preschool children, and made
contacts with children through school health programs operated
by the Health Center. Home visits could last as long as an hour.
The patient enjoyed continuity of contact with the same nurse
through her prenatal and postnatal periods, whereas she had to
change from obstetrician to pediatrician after her baby was born.

The relative absence of social barriers between nurse and patient has already been cited. Patients were generally relaxed and
poised in the presence of the nurse and asked questions freely.
Nurse and mother were of the same sex and spoke the same
idiom. The many married nurses with children of their own were
able to use a "mother-to-mother" approach.

In view of the barriers that existed between the doctor and
patient, and the closeness of nurse and patient, it is not surprising
that the nurses in the clinics assumed duties and responsibilities
that their official job outline did not call for. Trained to view the
patient as a "whole" person and to value mutual understanding,
they developed "unofficial" functions to compensate for the doctors' deficiencies in these areas. The duties they assumed can be
characterized as "intermediary" functions, designed to bridge the
gap left open by the doctors. The nurse acted as a protective
buffer between doctor and patient, and as interpreter of doctor to
patient and patient to doctor.

As a buffer between doctor and patient, the nurse could protect the mother from possible erroneous judgments and offer her
the emotional support that trained insight made possible. As interpreter of doctor to patient, nurses translated the doctor's

terminology into comprehensible language, restating his recommendations in keeping with the patient's level rather than simply "explaining and amplifying" them. One nurse said:

> If a child came to the well-child clinic and the doctor found him ill, he would prescribe and no more. The patient would come out knowing nothing about what was wrong. Then the nurse would explain in detail the nature of the illness, how to prevent it, and the reasons behind the treatment. She also pointed out the consequences of the illness if it were not treated. If the mother left the clinic after seeing just the doctor, she would have learned nothing about any of this.

Nurses also tried to bring about some sort of rapport between doctor and patient. According to one of the nurses, for example:

> The patient never dared question the doctor and had a great deal of fear of him. To the nurse the patient recounted all her difficulties. Nurses tried to teach patients to lose their fear of the doctors. When patients, through fear, could not remember what the doctor said, the nurses tried to make them change so that they could listen to him without being afraid.

Lastly, the nurse was the interpreter of the patient to the doctor. Most nurses did not make moral evaluations of the people or of particular groups in the community, asserting instead that there are "all kinds." One nurse commented that when nurses were asked for employment recommendations for their patients they did not feel qualified to say anything about character; they confined their remarks to those pertaining to cleanliness and state of health. This conception of the patients helped to counterbalance the doctor's practice of measuring mental capacity in terms of income and degree of formal schooling.

It is probable that the nurse made her greatest contribution by using her knowledge of the patient's situation as a check on impractical recommendations by the doctor. For example, a nurse would tell a doctor who had recommended individual beds for children that the entire family was living in one room where the only bed was reserved for the parents and the newest child, while the rest slept on the floor.

Effects of the Change

This background picture of the official roles of doctors and nurses and how they worked out in practice makes possible a more informed evaluation of the effects of removing the nurses from the clinics. There is little doubt that health education in the clinic has suffered, along with other aspects of clinic operation. Removal of the nurses has impoverished the doctor's contribution to the Health Center program, imposed limitations on the nurse's contribution, and reduced the benefits patients could derive from their relationships with these two professional groups. Since the nurse had served as the communication link between doctor and patient, communication between doctor and patient has been impaired.

The doctor no longer has access to information, formerly provided by the nurse, about those aspects of the patient's particular situation that bear on the immediate clinical problem. Nor can the nurse be an intermediary between doctor and patient, acting as protector, buffer, and interpreter. Thus, the limited contribution the doctor had been making has been reduced even further.

The doctor-nurse relationship has also suffered. The nurse no longer has any knowledge of the doctor's work and has lost the opportunity for the special insights into the patient's situation to be gained from mutual participation in the clinic. Under the present system, communication between doctor and nurse takes place indirectly through the patient's record, in which both enter their observations on the case. The record is quite inadequate for conveying to the doctor the nurse's full knowledge of a patient.

It is the clinic patient who has suffered most from the change. She no longer receives the benefit of coordinated effort in her behalf by doctor and nurse. The continuity between the health program in the home and in the clinic has been severed. More important, her experience in the clinic is now a mechanical affair. At best, it takes cognizance only of her immediate illness problem. All the "nonmedical" problems relevant to long-term good health are lost in the clinic setting.

Did the director's decision advance the Center's overall program? This question cannot be definitively answered until more is known about possible educational gains in the community stemming from full-time duty in the homes by nurses. No such check has yet been attempted. This study has focused on the effects within the clinic resulting from the change and not upon the effects within the neighborhood. Whether the losses incurred in the clinic setting were balanced by increases in community health education, as the director maintained, must remain an open question.

Although no certain assessment of the overall effects of change is possible, removing the nurses from duty in the clinic has provided an excellent opportunity to gain insight into the inner workings of the clinic team. Removing from an established system of relationships one of its traditional elements approximated an experimental situation that threw into clearer relief typical characteristics of the role of the public health nurse. It also made more visible the discrepancy between official duties and actual practice.

IMPLICATIONS

The consequences of removing the nurses from the San Lucero Health Center clinics draw attention to a number of characteristics common to most public health programs and indeed to most organized enterprises. The case of the San Lucero Health Center points up two important implications. The first is that there is always a difference between expected "official" behavior and what people actually do and that actual behavior is strongly influenced by existing cultural notions. The second lesson is that relationships within an organization form a system; removing one of its elements disturbs the whole arrangement and impairs communication within the system.

Cultural Determinants of Interaction

All public health programs involve a system of social interaction. People relate themselves to one another in such a system partly in terms of what their official duties demand and partly according to the culturally defined attitudes and predispositions they bring to their job. Officials frequently make decisions on the assumption that relationships within their organizations are based only on the official version of staff duties. Such decisions can produce unexpected consequences, since the actual system of relationships is greatly influenced by attitudes, ideas, and beliefs acquired by its participants outside the immediate organization.

In San Lucero, for example, the relationship of doctor, nurse, and patient was influenced not only by the official expectation of how people in these roles should behave toward each other, but also by their respective social classes, which already determined in large part the nature of their mutual interaction. Similarly, the training of doctors and nurses produced very different attitudes toward health education and its value, and it was these preexisting attitudes rather than the Center's official specifications alone that strongly influenced their actual behavior.

The Organization as a System and Its Communication Channels

Relationships within any organization can be thought of as forming a system whose parts are interconnected. Such a system can function effectively only when there are effective channels of communication between its parts. Two aspects of the San Lucero case highlight the importance of communication. First, it was the ineffective communication between doctor and patients in the clinic that originally impelled the nurses to assume the unofficial but necessary role of intermediary. Second, the removal of the nurses from the clinic cut off this communication link and severely impaired the system of relationships within the clinic.

In addition to the relationships within the doctor-patient-nurse triad, the nurses as a group were systematically related to other units of the program, such as sanitation and epidemiology. Thus, the removal of the nurse group had repercussions for the total organization of the San Lucero program.

Dislocations within the total program were offset to some extent by the strategic and influential position of the director. Communication between the various technical groups was habitually channeled through him. Thus, although the removal of the nurses placed them outside the immediate system of the Center, nurses could still relate to the rest of the organization through the director. However, the communication gap between doctor and nurse was not materially helped by this link, since the director himself had little direct contact with the doctors.

Exclusive attention to the official versions of organizational positions and a tendency to view each component of the program as an entity in itself can lead to the pitfalls of mistaking the ideal for the real and sacrificing the real for the ideal. The San Lucero program encountered both these pitfalls.

SUMMARY

The San Lucero Health Center emphasized health education as the most effective means for realization of program objectives. Originally it was assumed that the nurse could work most effectively at this task by undertaking educational work both in the home and in the clinic. When the health education program arrived at an impasse despite the substantial strides that had been made in other programs of the Health Center, the director decided to remove the nurse entirely from the clinic to promote health education on a full-time basis in the home, free of the limitations imposed by clinic conditions. The director thought that such a move would also compel the part-time doctor to comply more faithfully with the public health role defined for him by the San Lucero Center.

It developed that the removal of the nurse from the clinic led to a serious impairment of communication between doctor and nurse. The doctor was insulated from the nurse's special knowledge of the patient, while the nurse had little access to the doctor's clinical activity. The doctor became even less effective in getting across to the patient any health education message, and the nurse lost those insights into the patient's situation derived from her participation in the clinic. Effects of the change on the education program in the homes were not determined.

In conclusion, it should be pointed out that attention has been focused on an aspect of the San Lucero program where things did not go especially well. When viewed as a whole and in terms of its total development, the San Lucero Health Center is one of the most progressive and effective in Chile and has made substantial contributions to the health and welfare of the community it serves.

SELECTED REFERENCES

Caplan, Gerald, "The Mental Hygiene Role of the Nurse in Maternal and Child Care," *Nursing Outlook*, vol. 2, January, 1954, pp. 14–19. A discussion of the potential role of the mental hygiene consultant nurse by a psychiatrist dedicated to the development of community programs in preventive psychiatry. The characterization of the nurse's position vis-a-vis the patient offers some parallels with this case study.

Homans, George C., *The Human Group*. Routledge and Kegan Paul, London, 1951. A systematic and readable treatment of interpersonal relations in small groups. Of particular relevance is Chapter 10, which deals with the elements of social behavior and their mutual dependence as parts of a social system.

McBride, George M., *Chile: Land and Society*. American Geographical Society, New York, 1936. An authoritative account of the human geography of Chile by an expert whose treatment of agrarian social institutions, particularly the interrelations between social class and the land tenure system, is sensitive and perceptive.

Simmons, Ozzie G., *The Health Center of San Miquel:* An Analysis of a Public Health Program in Chile. Institute of Inter-American Affairs, Santiago, 1953, mimeolithed. Available on request from the Institute in Santiago, this report deals primarily with the development of a district health center program in relation to the community. The roles and mutual relations of supervisors, doctors, nurses, social workers, and sanitary inspectors are analyzed in some detail.

"Popular and Modern Medicine in Mestizo Communities of Coastal Peru and Chile," *Journal of American Folklore*, vol. 68, January–March, 1955, pp. 57–71. A description of the key etiological concepts, illness syndromes, and curative practices of folk medicine, and an analysis of their implications for the reception accorded modern medicine.

Subercaseaux, Benjamin, *Chile:* A Geographic Extravaganza. Macmillan Co., New York, 1943. (Also available in Spanish: *Chile:* O, Una Loca Geografía. 5th ed. Ediciones Ercilla, Santiago, 1943.) Customs and points of interest in Santiago and the provinces as seen through the eyes of a Chilean who writes in a popular, guidebook vein.

Case 13

A COMMUNITY IMPROVEMENT PROJECT IN BRAZIL

by Kalervo Oberg and José Arthur Rios

Health improvement programs cannot proceed beyond a certain point without the collaboration of other agencies. The necessity of combining health work with programs of agricultural improvement and economic development is clearly demonstrated in the South African case study by Dr. Cassel, Case 1. Conversely, programs of agricultural and educational improvement are equally dependent on progress in public health. Sick farmers cannot carry out an extensive agricultural program, as Dr. Oberg and Mr. Rios remark, nor can children suffering from intestinal parasites become good students. Government-sponsored combined programs create special administrative problems, however, since the activities of diverse services and various governmental levels need to be carefully coordinated.

In the present study the authors describe the administrative funnel through which agricultural, educational, and health services were directed into a demonstration community located in the Rio Doce area of Brazil. The people were apparently willing to accept new techniques and ideas, particularly in regard to health. In retrospect, one shortcoming of the project lay in the establishment of a community council, an arrangement which proved to be disruptive; a new and so far successful attempt to carry out a village improvement project in another Brazilian community proceeds without a council. In a community unfamiliar with voluntary and nonpolitical administrative devices, the council served as a platform for political disagreement rather than a means of enlisting cooperation. This does not mean that the community council is a defective mechanism. It means that the council, like other products of a particular ideological environment, cannot readily be transplanted to locations with different social and political climates.
—EDITOR

THE PROBLEM

A Carefully Planned Project Encounters Difficulties

In January, 1951, specialists and technicians in health, education, and agriculture began to arrive in the small Brazilian village of Chonin de Cima, located in the Rio Doce Valley and within the state of Minas Gerais. They were about to inaugurate an

349

experiment in focusing the usually independent efforts of separate service agencies on the problem of a single rural area. The technicians were well trained and experienced in their respective fields and were well informed on the latest methods and material devices. Furthermore, they were reasonably familiar with the physical and social features of the region.

Supporting them on higher administrative levels was a body of experienced technical consultants who had planned and organized efficiently. Generous financial contributions had been made available to the project. A baseline social survey was to acquaint all concerned with the details of the community and its problems. Outside experts in the fields of agriculture, health, education, and community organization were to make periodic visits to the project in order to make certain that nothing would go amiss. In a gala opening the project received the blessing of important state and federal officials.

The most promising features of the project were its democratic basis and use of combined services. The people of the community were to participate in the solution of their problems, the agencies providing the means, both technical and advisory, in tackling these problems on a broad front. No overly ambitious goals were contemplated. The project was to run for three years with possible extensions if things worked out satisfactorily. There was enthusiasm and good will on the part of the planners, technicians, local officials, and the people.

The health, agricultural, and educational programs continued actively for two years. Then at a money-raising party sponsored by project officials a violent dispute between local leaders and the coordinator over matters of dress and admission forced an abrupt termination of the entire project. What was behind this sudden and unexpected breakdown? Could an apparently trivial incident and the whims of a few individuals have the power to upset what appeared to be an intelligently planned and well-accepted program? Was it really this incident that scuttled the program, or had some major dimension been overlooked in the planning? The case of Chonin not only throws light on these questions, but shows how knowledge gained from troubles there can be and has been put to good use in similar projects elsewhere in Brazil.

THE SITUATION

An Operational Plan Conflicts with Local Realities

Planning and Establishing the Project

The idea for a combined project grew out of the experiences of men active in the joint Brazilian-United States agencies that have operated in Brazil for some years. Observing that disease, illiteracy, and poverty were generally found together in many rural communities, they reasoned that greater and more rapid progress could be made if the separate agencies dealing with these problems joined forces to concentrate their efforts on a restricted area. The philosophy underlying the project stressed joint effort. Each agency, it was felt, could work more effectively in combination with the others than when working alone. Through teamwork, joint effort, and simultaneous advances on all three fronts, the rural dweller could be helped to enjoy higher living standards and a more meaningful life. A primary purpose of the Chonin project was to develop the means by which these ideals could be put into practice. In this sense Chonin was considered both an experimental and a demonstration project. If the techniques developed here proved workable, it was planned to extend them to other areas.

The process of developing these techniques involved a number of problems. A practical and economically feasible formula had to be worked out whereby federal, state, and local agencies could work together effectively, utilizing public funds to improve both the human and economic resources of a specific rural area. These agencies had to be convinced of the importance of a cooperative and coordinated approach in such fields as agriculture, education, health, and transportation, and of the value of securing community participation for "helping the people to help themselves." It also became necessary to demonstrate the practicality of the nuclear system which combined an area center with radiating subcenters for providing services in a rural zone.

Those who initiated the Chonin experiment planned to get personnel and the financial support for the project from five sources: the Brazilian-United States rural public health service;

the Brazilian-United States agricultural services; the Brazilian national rural education service; the state health, agriculture, education, and public works departments of Minas Gerais; and the local municipio government.

Administrative Machinery. Once the necessary support and financial backing had been obtained, the project's planners proceeded to set up administrative machinery. Three administrative groups were instituted: a Joint Committee, an Executive Committee, and a Community Council. The Joint Committee was composed of the directors of the participating agencies who met once a year in the state capital. It was responsible for overall policy, program, budget, and personnel.

The Executive Committee was composed of appointed or special representatives from each participating agency who were to meet once a month in the state capital to guide the operations of the project. This Committee was authorized to act for the Joint Committee in lesser policy matters and to decide specific operating details. The Joint Committee appointed the chairman of the Executive Committee; the chairman also acted as liaison officer between the various participating agencies and between the Joint Committee and the field workers.

The top official at the local level was a coordinator appointed by the Joint Committee and given responsibility for the entire local project. He presided at regular staff meetings of field personnel. These meetings were called for the purpose of planning project activities, coordinating its undertakings, and developing cooperation. The coordinator was given limited technical and financial authority. He was in charge of receiving and spending funds authorized by the Joint Committee, but he was not to decide technical or professional matters outside his own field. He was not authorized to employ separate personnel nor to commit any of the agencies financially without approval by the Joint Committee, nor was he to take action involving personnel or project contrary to the administrative policies of the participating agencies.

On the local level a third administrative group called the Community Council was set up, with a local resident as chairman. The group was to be the link between the project administration and the people of Chonin and was designed to secure the active participation of the community itself. This Council was to include from eight to ten leading members of the community selected so as to represent farmers, shopkeepers, craftsmen, and housewives and was intended to be nonpolitical in character. The coordinator with the aid of the local chairman was to arrange weekly meetings to be attended both by the Community Council and by representatives of the participating agencies. At these meetings he would explain to the Council the nature of the project's activities and solicit their wishes, advice, and aid in planning for the future.

The meetings would also give the agency representatives an opportunity to talk about their respective activities, answer questions, and generally to get their message across to the people. The coordinator was assigned the job of showing films and distributing educational material. He was also responsible for renting and maintaining the local project headquarters and for making monthly overall reports to the Executive Committee, describing progress and suggesting future action. Finally, the coordinator was responsible for organizing the villagers to carry out those enterprises requiring joint community action.

Program Policy. The base of the project's various activities was to be a strategically located headquarters building in Chonin de Cima that would house the personnel of all agencies and serve as the center of the nuclear system. Smaller community centers were to be established at two other villages in the District of Chonin. Personnel of the base were to visit the smaller units on a regular schedule known to the residents of the entire area. These secondary centers were to serve as focal points for reaching the rural residents with the three principal services of health, education, and agriculture.

Health personnel in the main clinic were to provide medical examinations and treatment, nursing services, and health education. In addition, they were to stage demonstrations and furnish information on sanitation activities such as the building of privies and well construction in all the three villages. Health work was to have top priority, particularly in the opening phases of the project. Sick farmers could not carry out an intensive agricultural program; children suffering from intestinal parasites made poor students. The community had first to be cleared of infectious diseases.

Both general and vocational programs in adult education were planned. The vocational program was to be devoted mainly to agriculture. The general education program would draw on subject matter furnished by the State Secretariat of Education. Both the agricultural and health services would continue their established policy of working through the schools. In agriculture the Center in Chonin de Cima was to be the source of information on financial credit, technical assistance in agronomy, and home economics. Classes in homemaking were to be held for adults in cooperation with the expert in adult education and the nurse or health educator.

The several participating agencies furnished specialists to implement the programs of agriculture, health, and education, directing them to work in close association with the local coordinator. The agricultural service appointed one full-time agronomist and one full-time home economist; the health service provided one part-time doctor, one part-time nurse, one full-time sanitary assistant, and one part-time health educator; and the educational service provided a teaching supervisor on a part-time basis.

The Smithsonian Institution of Washington furnished a social anthropologist to make a survey of social and cultural conditions. This information was to be used in the planning and organization of the program. The anthropologist was assisted by two graduate students from the School of Sociology and Political Science of São Paulo. During the course of the action program, in June and July of 1951, the research team made a study of the village of Chonin de Cima, and from January to April, 1952, studied the surrounding rural zone. This survey concentrated on factual information that would be of greatest use for the various activities of the project.

Chonin de Cima and Its Surroundings

Like other Brazilian states, Minas Gerais is divided into a number of countylike administrative units called municipios.

Each municipio has its own governmental organization, the *prefeitura*, consisting of a top official (prefect), an elected council, and several appointed officials. The prefeitura is housed in the town or city that serves as the municipio seat; it governs all the cities, towns, villages, and the countryside that make up the municipio. The municipio and the municipio seat bear identical names. Chonin de Cima is part of the municipio of Governador Valadares. The local government (prefeitura) of the municipio is located in the city of Governador Valadares, which had a population of 25,000 in 1950. Members of the municipio council, which meets in the city of Governador Valadares, represent the various districts that make up the municipio.

Each district, like the municipio, has a seat (usually a village) which has the same name as the district. Each district has one or more justices of the peace to try minor disputes. Chonin is a district within the municipio of Governador Valadares and comes under the jurisdiction of the prefeitura at Governador Valadares, having no separate government of its own. The District of Chonin contains three villages and surrounding farms. The villages are Chonin de Cima (Upper Chonin), Chonin de Baixo (Lower Chonin), and Vila Matias. The plan of the Chonin project was to serve the whole District of Chonin, although personnel and physical facilities were located in the district seat of Chonin de Cima.

The community of Chonin de Cima involves more than the village itself. Like others in Brazil, this rural community is organized around a village center with its church, stores, craftsmen's shops, school, and registry office. The people living on the surrounding farms use the facilities of this center. They never have any doubt as to which community they belong to. Each community has its own history and is identified by its church and patron saint. The people of Chonin de Cima also call their village Chonin dos Cunhas, referring to the Cunhas family which first settled there, some of whose descendants are still in the community. They differentiate themselves from Chonin de Baixo by calling it Chonin dos Baianos, or Chonin of the people who came from the state of Bahia. There are many other terms used for differentiation but the basic distinction is that of a different patron saint. The social survey conducted by the research team concerned the natural community of Chonin de Cima, its organization, and the conditions existing within it.

The community of Chonin de Cima is fairly representative of rural communities in the large agricultural and mining state of Minas Gerais. Still in full use are many old style devices—the muzzle loading gun, the outdoor beehive oven, and the *monjolo*, a unique type of water-operated mortar and pestle. Farmers raise cattle and cultivate corn, beans, and rice. They prepare their land by the slash-and-burn method, using the hoe, bill hook, and axe. Most land users occupy unsurveyed parcels of land to which they have no legal title.

In 1952 the population of Chonin de Cima and its environs was 1,986. Of this number, 635 people in 125 families lived in the village proper, while 1,351 in 237 families occupied the outlying area. The population is a mixture of white, Negro, and some Indian. On the basis of external characteristics, about 20 per cent of the population are white, 25 per cent black, and the rest mixed. These color distinctions, although not associated with any pronounced race feeling, correspond roughly to social ranking. The whites are at the top, with the largest families, best-paying occupations, and the largest and best houses. They are the landowners and have the lowest illiteracy rate. The Negroes, as a group, are socially at the bottom. The mulattoes are in between.

As in most rural Brazilian communities, the important social groups are the immediate family, the larger group of kinsmen and godparents, the church, religious associations, political parties, and social classes. Leadership is personal and paternalistic, resting largely in the hands of family heads, priests or other religious leaders, large landowners, and political leaders.

Although national political parties are represented on the local level, local political units are largely splinter groups under the control of local leaders. Differences between political opponents do not diminish to any considerable extent after election day but continue on a permanent basis. Solidarity between the leader and his followers is maintained by a system of patronage. The relationship between officials in power and the people is paternalistic. What the people get in the way of roads, schools, parks, and other public works is regarded both by the officials and the people as a gift. These gifts often bear the name of the official and thus perpetuate his memory. The attitude of the people toward the administration and its head depends on how much he gives. A good political leader gives much, a bad one is niggardly.

Health conditions in Chonin de Cima resemble those in many other rural Brazilian villages. Prior to the experimental project, roughly 95 per cent of the houses were without privies. People used the shrubbery at the back of the house for disposing of human waste. Approximately 90 per cent of the families used water from the nearby stream, a carrier of schistosomiasis and other water-borne diseases. Customary diet lacked protective foods rich in vitamin and mineral content. These conditions, in large measure, were responsible for the high prevalence of dysentery, anemia, tuberculosis, and malaria. Yet the people did not recognize these conditions as causes of illness.

The people of Chonin de Cima attribute some diseases to physical causes, such as intestinal worms, insects that penetrate the skin, and certain food combinations. Other diseases are thought to be caused by fright, anger, or jealousy. The people believe that breaking taboos or religious regulations, such as working on one's saint's day, may produce illness. Some individuals have an "evil eye" which can unintentionally cause illness. Sorcery is frequently cited as a cause of illness. Some diseases, such as tuberculosis, are thought to be due to the will of God. A wide variety of herbal remedies constitutes the most common means of healing. Many of these are widely known and each family is able to prepare its own remedies. Some special herbal remedies, however, are bottled by local curers, experts in the art of healing. Since witchcraft and sorcery are important causes of illness, magical counter-cures must be performed by magicians.

The illiteracy rate for the community of Chonin de Cima was roughly 75 per cent in 1952. A single school building was located in the village. Although the building was new and well constructed, it lacked sufficient seating accommodations, pure water, privies, and teaching materials. Moreover, learning was hampered by the low educational level of the teachers themselves, the fact that they considered their positions political appointments, and the general lack of appreciation of education by parents.

Poor roads, poverty, migratory habits of many families, and living far from the school all contributed to low attendance.

Two Years of Combined Service

The first step in the implementation of the project was the acquisition of a satisfactory building to serve as the headquarters of the nuclear system in the village of Chonin de Cima. The project was fortunate in being able to rent a large house belonging to the local church organization. Under the direction of the project agronomist, who acted as local coordinator for the first six months of the program, this building was repaired and offices for the various agencies' representatives were established.

A demonstration kitchen, sewing room, and a model bedroom were established for the use of the home supervisor. A small building was outfitted as a carpenter shop. A water tank built at the back of the house was connected to a well that was equipped with a pump. The basement of the building was fitted out as a clinic, including a kerosene refrigerator for the storage of medicines. Sufficient beds, dishes, and furniture were provided for the members of the staff who had not yet found accommodations in the village. The headquarters building itself and the headquarters staff became known, both in English and Portuguese, as the "nucleo."

These preparations began in January, 1951, and by April the clinic was ready for use. Once initial preparations were complete, the three main programs—agriculture, education, and health—were ready to get under way.

The Agricultural Program. The agricultural service based its plan for improving and modernizing farming methods on a system of supervised credit. Under this system, a farmer is given a loan to buy equipment, seeds, and insecticides and to hire necessary labor. Once the loan is approved, the agricultural service provides the technical assistance of an agronomist to see that equipment, seeds, and labor are used to best advantage.

The first agronomist sent to Chonin de Cima was also appointed acting coordinator. He resigned from both positions when the regular coordinator was appointed in July, 1951. At this time also a second agronomist was selected for the project; he remained until December, 1951. In the spring of 1951, despite the fact that the agronomist was busy with the nucleo headquarters building and other administrative details, he began to work on the agricultural program. He very shortly discovered that only 20 per cent of the properties in the Chonin District had clear legal title, that 60 per cent were in various stages of survey and claim, and that 20 per cent were occupied under squatters' rights alone.

This discovery dealt a severe blow to the whole agricultural program. The actual loan upon which the supervised credit plan depends is made not by the government but by a Brazilian bank, and the bank imposes certain conditions as prerequisites to granting a loan. One of these is that a piece of land, either occupied or rented by a farmer, must be surveyed and have a legal title. This meant that at least 80 per cent of the farmers in the Chonin District were in no position to apply for a loan under supervised credit. Of the remaining 20 per cent, the agronomist found out that many of the properties that could request a loan were too small to warrant improvements or that the soil was so depleted as to make improvements difficult. In addition, some landowners declared that they were not interested in supervised loans. This meant that the loan program, which was to have been the foundation of the agricultural program, had to be given up completely.

An attempt was then made to continue the agricultural program without loans. Late in 1951 the State Secretariat of Agriculture sent to Chonin de Cima a lightweight tractor to be used on a number of farms in the community under the supervision of the agronomist. But the tractor could not reach the areas to be plowed because of the swamps and unbridged streams surrounding the fields. After plowing the land of one farmer near the village, the tractor was withdrawn. It thus became clear that no immediate large scale improvement in agriculture could be carried out, and in December, 1951, the second agronomist was withdrawn. The mistake of predicating the agricultural program on conditions that did not in fact exist thus virtually cost the project its program of agricultural improvement.

During the remainder of the project agricultural activity continued on a limited scale. To replace the agronomist, the state furnished a resident agricultural technician to the project in the beginning of 1952. He maintained demonstration vegetable gardens in the village and made available hybrid corn seed, modern tools, barbed-wire fencing, insecticides, and improved types of poultry to those farmers who wanted them. In addition, the home economist held classes in cooking, sewing, and domestic carpentry for all housewives and young girls who wished to attend. She also visited homes in the village, giving advice on the care of children and home management. Her work was well received and produced lasting benefits for local domestic life.

The Educational Program. The educational program had two basic aims, improving the physical facilities of the school and improving teaching methods and curriculum. The first aim was successfully accomplished. The school building, formerly one large room, was partitioned into four classrooms, making possible separate teaching in each class. The rooms were equipped with desks, maps, books, and other teaching materials. The schoolyard was provided with a fence, a cement walk, and a flower garden. A well with a pump was constructed and four privies were built.

Considerable effort was made to improve teaching methods. The State Secretariat of Education provided for the hiring of a fourth teacher to augment the teaching staff and conducted two teachers' training courses in Chonin de Cima during the holiday seasons. These courses were designed to acquaint the teachers with current ideas in teaching methods and curriculum construction. To oversee school conditions and improve teaching efficiency, a school board and a parent-teacher association were organized.

These efforts to improve education by helping the teachers ran into difficulty, however. Teachers in Chonin de Cima are hired by the local authorities and remain under their direct administrative supervision. Both the teachers and their employers construed the attempt to improve teaching standards as a reflection on themselves and saw the new organizations as a means of undercutting their authority. When the newly created school board and parent-teacher association insisted that the teachers follow some of the "new" educational ideas, the teachers complained to the local officials that outsiders were interfering with their work. Further attempts by the new organizations to win the cooperation of the teachers only produced increased resentment. As a net result educational standards, teaching methods, and low school attendance remained substantially unchanged.

The Health Program. The health service planned improvements in three main areas: medical assistance, environmental sanitation, and health education. Fortunately for the project, there already was an established Health Center in nearby Governador Valadares, seat of the municipio. Health personnel maintained headquarters at this Center and set up a subpost in Chonin de Cima. During the two years of the project, health activity moved ahead on all three fronts.

The medical assistance program was carried on by a doctor and a nurse who came to Chonin de Cima once a week from the Center at Governador Valadares. They received and treated patients at the clinic from 8 a.m. to 5 p.m., and during the remainder of the week a resident sanitary assistant was on duty. He gave injections and treated minor injuries. The residents of Chonin District were quick to avail themselves of clinic facilities. The chief difficulties encountered by the medical assistance program related to transportation. In December of the project's first year, two bridges on the main road between Governador Valadares and Chonin de Cima were washed out, and for some time the doctor and nurse were unable to reach the clinic. Even when the bridges were in, they frequently had to spend hours getting through mudholes in the road. Despite these difficulties, however, clinic attendance remained high. More than 2,000 patients from Chonin District and other areas, who had never before received modern medical care, visited the clinic. During the two-year period, 6,519 clinic visits were recorded.

The principal project of the environmental sanitation program was the construction of pit privies. This was planned as a co-operative program. The houseowner was responsible for digging a pit and constructing the privy building, while the health service provided a concrete basement slab to be placed over the pit. The sanitary assistant helped the householder choose the location for the pit and construct the privy building. The privy construction program proceeded rapidly at first, but during the second year difficulties began to arise. The wealthier families were able to pay for the excavation and construction and responded readily. However, the poorer families claimed that they did not have the money to build a privy. These families were of two kinds: those in which the father had died, left the family, or was too ill to work; and those in which the father was a migrant agricultural laborer. They lived in rented houses, and neither tenants nor owners were interested in building privies.

To meet this problem, the health service assumed full responsibility for digging the pit, supplying the slab, and building the enclosure for those willing to make small monthly payments until the privy was paid for. This still left a number of absentee-owned, rented houses for which privies could not be provided. In the course of the two years, 90 pit privies were installed in the village. This left 35 out of 125 families without privies.

In addition to his work with the privy construction program, the resident sanitary assistant inspected backyards, instructed the people in proper methods of garbage disposal, advised them about water-well construction, and warned them against using water from the stream unless it was first boiled.

Health education was carried on in two ways. Doctors, nurses, sanitary engineers, and other public health personnel were encouraged to spread the basic ideas of health education in the course of their regular work. In addition, a special health education campaign was conducted with public film showings, talks, home visits by nurses' aides, posters, and pamphlets. During the course of the project in Chonin, 688 health pamphlets were distributed, 172 posters displayed, 54 public talks given, and 35 films shown.

It can be seen that the medical assistance, environmental sanitation, and health education programs were well organized and carried out. Much of their success was apparently due to the fact that the health program had much to offer in the way of free services and demanded less active cooperation than the agricultural program. In the latter part of the second year, the health program expanded its activities to include the nearby villages of Chonin de Baixo and Vila Matias.

An Explosion at the Spring Fiesta

In October, 1952, almost two years after project personnel first arrived in Chonin de Cima, the program was progressing fairly well. The health program, on the whole, was running successfully. Although an important part of the agricultural program had fallen through and the educational program had run into difficulty, some such setbacks might have been expected. The significant fact was that both educational and agricultural activities were continuing. But in the same month an unexpected development abruptly ended the entire Chonin project.

Chonin's spring fiesta, held yearly in October, attracted many people to the village. Members of the Community Council felt that this would be a good opportunity to raise funds. The school fund was low, and the charitable society of Saint Vincent de Paul was in need of help. The Council decided to run a beauty contest in the school building as part of the fiesta. Five festival queens were to be selected from among the prettiest girls in the village. Each ticket sold entitled the seller to one vote for his favorite, and the five queens would be those whose supporters sold most tickets. A committee formed to run the fiesta included the project coordinator and two members of the Community Council—Senhor G, an active church supporter, and Senhor J, a political representative of the District of Chonin.

On the appointed day Chonin de Cima was in a festive mood. Early in the day people began to arrive from the outlying farms and mica diggings on foot and on horseback. Soon groups of saddle horses could be seen hitched before the little cantinas from which issued sounds of laughter as the men sat over their glasses of rum. Women visited their friends, and the girls in gala attire paraded up and down the main thoroughfare. In the schoolhouse there was great activity as women decorated the walls with boughs and colored paper cutouts, set tables, and prepared food and drinks.

In the organizing committee, however, there was increasing altercation and confusion. The crowd was larger than expected, and the tickets soon ran out. The coordinator, without consulting the committee, began reselling tickets already handed in. "The election of the beauty queens is being subverted!" exclaimed Senhor G and Senhor J. More refreshments were needed than had been expected. The coordinator changed the order of events without consulting the committee. "Unwarranted changes in plans," cried Senhor G and Senhor J.

As the people began to crowd into the school, the coordinator refused to admit men who were dressed in undershirts and ragged trousers and those who he felt had imbibed too freely of rum. "You are insulting our friends; the door must remain open to all!" shouted Senhor G and Senhor J. "They shall not enter," insisted the coordinator. "I have the right to maintain order and the good name of the nucleo."

Tempers rose and words flew. Senhor G and Senhor J were joined by others who opposed the coordinator. He was accused of being an outsider who had been interfering in the affairs of the community. Other members of the nucleo staff were criticized. Some aspects of the program were loudly ridiculed. There was a show of force by Senhor G and Senhor J and their supporters. The coordinator left the school followed by the nucleo staff.

That evening the coordinator held a meeting of the nucleo staff at his home. He insisted that a petition to withdraw the program be signed by the staff and sent to the Executive Committee. This the staff refused to do. Next day the coordinator left. One by one the programs were withdrawn. By the end of the year the Chonin project no longer existed.

At first glance it might appear that this was a capricious incident, something clearly peripheral to the official program, which would have been forgotten after tempers had cooled. With program ends reasonably well on the way to achievement, this disagreement should have had little effect on the overall project. But while the incident itself might appear insignificant, it brought to the surface difficulties related not to program ends but to program means. Something within the project's administration was at fault.

The Administrative Machinery Breaks Down

The administrative organization of the Chonin project had been systematically planned and carefully formed. On the local level its main features were a Community Council made up of community members, a local coordinator, and a plan to work in close cooperation with the project staff.

The Community Council. The Community Council was intended by the program planners as a device for involving the community in a program for improving their own welfare. Too often in the past, they reasoned, similar programs had produced no real or lasting benefits because the local population had simply been the passive recipient of action initiated and carried through by outsiders. The Chonin Community Council was intended as a broadly representative nonpolitical body wherein every segment of the community could make its voice heard and express its wishes to agency personnel. In open discussions it was to arrive at decisions that would reflect the views of the community as a whole, thus serving as a sounding board to the services. In addition, it was to carry out, through the operation of its special committees, specific welfare tasks in the community.

The Community Council was organized in accordance with these ideals. It was composed of landowners and the landless, leaders and rank-and-file, men and women, political "ins" and "outs." During the two years of the project, the chairman of the Council was a local farmer who, although energetic and cooperative, was on the political side which was out of power in the District. Whether he was chosen for this position to prove that the Council was truly "nonpolitical" is not clear, but this choice had the result of alienating the local group in power. Although some of these men were also on the Community Council, they began to obstruct or stay away from the meetings. Since they held positions in the municipio government, their growing opposition did little good in the matter of obtaining local cooperation. The intensity of this political opposition was made apparent in many ways, particularly in the selection of committees. One man who was asked to serve on a committee refused to do so, saying that he would not serve with a man from the opposing party.

In addition, members of the Community Council did not share the program planners' picture of the Council as a voluntary, selflessly civic-minded organization. One day the local coordinator organized a work bee to fence and clean up the schoolyard. The materials were supplied by the agencies. Agency members worked together with local Council members. After the task was completed, the Council members who had participated asked to be paid. When the coordinator explained that this was outside of service obligations and was performed voluntarily, the local people replied, "You are paid by the government to do this, why shouldn't we?"

The Role of the Coordinator. During the course of the Chonin project, the position of coordinator was held by three different men, all Brazilians. The first incumbent was the agronomist who served in the dual capacity of acting coordinator and agricultural program head for the first six months of the project. When he resigned as agronomist, he also gave up his job as coordinator. His appraisal of the situation had led him to the conclusion that the task of coordinating the program by means of the Community Council would be extremely difficult.

The second coordinator assumed the post in July of 1951 after the departure of the agronomist. He was a former schoolteacher and a native of a rural community similar to Chonin. His experience working close to rural Brazilians and his identification with the people of Chonin had led him to believe that rapid change in such a community was not to be expected. He was critical of those technical experts who were pushing forward substantial changes in health, agriculture, and education and introducing new practices and organizations into the community of Chonin. "You just can't push these people around," he would advise. This policy of going slowly satisfied members of the Community Council but displeased the service agencies. After six months the second coordinator was removed from his job by the Executive Committee on the grounds that he was not active enough.

The Executive Committee then looked around for someone who would be committed both to the goals and to the methods of the project. They found him in the third coordinator, an active and aggressive agricultural technician who assumed considerable initiative in advancing the project goals and creating new organizations and methods for realizing program objectives. Among these organizations were a health club, an agriculture club, a football club, a parent-teacher association, and a local school board. Innovations included a cash fund for a school lunch program; money for this fund was to come from voluntary contributions, entrance charges to public functions, and the sale of produce from the agricultural demonstration plots.

Both the pace and scope of the third coordinator's activities alarmed local leaders. The Council included most of the community's leading figures, who were thus in a position to watch the coordinator closely. As he progressively expanded the power of his position, local leaders felt their power proportionately reduced. Moreover, the coordinator failed to use his position to reconcile the opposing political factions that composed the Community Council. Instead of undertaking the difficult job of creating a unified "nonpolitical" civic group from a split and highly partisan body, he let himself become embroiled in political disputes and attempted to play off one side against the other. Local leaders on the Council became jealous of his power and resentful of his political maneuvering. They began a whispering campaign against him which soon spread to include the program as a whole. This growing resentment came to a head at the spring festival.

The Role of the Prefeitura. According to original plans the prefeitura of Governador Valadares was to have played an active part in the total program, sharing administrative responsibility and furnishing what local services it commanded. Early in the program the prefeitura had promised to set up a modern water storage and distribution system for the village, assist in the transportation of materials to the project, improve the roads and repair the bridges in the district, provide office space for the staff in Governador Valadares, furnish an additional schoolteacher, and build a kitchen for preparing school lunches as an annex to the Chonin de Cima school.

Early in the program the prefeitura provided workers to widen the main street of Chonin de Cima and to build a number of drainage ditches. As the program progressed, however, it became evident that prefeitura cooperation would not continue. In fact, instead of expediting matters, these officials became unfavorable to the project. None of their original promises was fulfilled, and even the minimal cooperation necessary to project functioning became almost impossible to obtain. This was particularly evident in the case of road repair. The transportation lifeline of the project was the highway connecting Chonin de Cima with the seat of the municipio at Governador Valadares. A spur highway linking Chonin de Cima with the main highway became virtually impassable during the rainy season, and the authorities made no effort to remedy the situation. In December of 1951, two bridges on the main highway were washed out and were not rebuilt until the following May. Project personnel based in Governador Valadares, particularly the doctor and nurse, had great difficulty in getting through to Chonin de Cima. These transportation problems not only created practical hurdles but lowered personnel morale as well.

The anthropologist had requested the prefeitura to provide four census takers to aid in the background survey of Chonin de Cima and its rural surroundings. This petition was ignored until after the project actually was begun. Only after repeated and insistent requests were the four men provided. However, half way through the survey these men were withdrawn.

Planning Vision and Community Reality

The explosive showdown battle between the coordinator and local authorities at the spring festival was simply the external manifestation of growing tension which finally reached the breaking point. That this tension had been building up slowly but steadily is evident from the series of differences between the Community Council and the local coordinator. It was in the area of project administration, rather than in the specific service areas of health and community improvement, that the project ran aground.

It was originally intended that changes introduced by the service agencies should be lasting, not superficial. To this end program planners made "education" rather than "service" the keynote of their program. The people of Chonin were to participate actively in project activities and through participation absorb and retain the lessons of health and community improvement. In practice there was considerably more service and considerably less participation than planned. Because this was so, the service aspect of the program caused little difficulty. Few people could find cause to object if technicians came to Chonin de Cima and renovated their schoolhouse.

True, the health and agricultural services did encounter difficulties, but this was not particularly surprising. Both had had years of experience in communities similar to Chonin where bad transportation and widespread poverty had made their work hazardous and slow. In the field of health, adherence to folk medicine, native curers, and health practices contrary to the tenets of modern medicine could be expected to change but slowly. Experience elsewhere in Brazil has shown that if modern health services are coupled with health education and maintained in a community for a long enough period, people become accustomed to the new ways and begin to demand these services. Viewed in this perspective, it is evident that the health service in Chonin de Cima carried out its part of the bargain.

The agricultural service ran into difficulties connected with land titles, which blocked the credit program, and with poor roads, which made the use of tractors impractical. However, by the end of the second year both the agricultural and health services had trimmed their expectations and made certain adaptations to existing conditions. They operated on a reduced scale, but they did continue.

The project's administrative machinery, however, was not so easy to alter. The ideals of those who planned the project were built into that machinery. It was aimed to secure the coordination of separate service activities, the cooperation of federal, state, and local governments, and the widest possible community participation. The Community Council and the local coordinator were organizational devices set up to achieve these ends. But they were devices created with an eye to the ideals of the program rather than to the political realities of the local situation. The Community Council was intended as a device for giving all segments of the community an opportunity to share in the planning and execution of the project and to keep project personnel and the people closely apprised of one another's position and ideas. In practice it turned out to be a device for disrupting the political equilibrium of the community.

It was interesting to observe the workings of the Community Council. Meetings would open with the Council chairman describing the activities of the past month, usually explaining at length why objectives had not been achieved. The local coordinator would then suggest lines of action. Some of the local leaders would comment favorably on these suggestions while others would criticize them; members who customarily had not participated in community decisions remained silent. When it came to a vote, however, the usually unchallenged local leaders were often overruled, something new in their experience. In other words, these meetings became contests between the coordinator and the effective political and religious leaders who saw their positions being threatened by a man whom they considered an outsider. The device of the majority vote gave to both the party out of power and to those who had never had power a lever by which they could jointly overrule those in power.

The people accepted the service agencies and their programs more or less as gifts of a benevolent government. But setting up a "nonpolitical" Community Council disrupted the existing pattern of social organization. Important landowners and political and religious leaders who traditionally had made independent decisions concerning community affairs were now asked to sit together with sharecroppers and housewives to plan the future of the community. To them this was an unheard-of procedure. The policy of making decisions free of political and religious considerations cut the ground from under the local leaders who had always made decisions in terms of politics and in relation to religious associations.

The customary pattern called for an organization in which the political leaders of the party in power had complete freedom in decision-making without the countervailing presence of the political opposition. In the Community Council, local officials found themselves in a position where a coalition of three forces—those out of power, the normally disenfranchised, and the project coordinator—were given an instrument to undercut their authority.

The introduction of a Community Council intended to be nonpolitical into a community geared to authoritarian personal rule by members of the party in power was a contradiction which no amount of good will and personal ingenuity on the part of the coordinator could overcome. The search for an effective coordinator was virtually an impossible ideal. Motivated by ideals of cooperative effort, program planners had created a position that only an extraordinary man could have been expected to fill successfully. The coordinator was visualized by the planners as a Brazilian who would be receptive, cooperative, and generally passive in his relationship with the project heads, accepting their values and orders with minimum resistance. At the same time he would be active and resourceful in his relations with the villagers. He was to be active in promoting the goals of the project—goals to which people might be indifferent or opposed. But the decisions reached under his guidance in the Community Council were to be majority decisions, democratically arrived at.

Interestingly, each of the three men who successively filled this position responded to its contradictions in a different way. The first coordinator, after six months of trying to meet the requirements of his job, simply decided it was impossible and relinquished the position. The second coordinator, experienced in the ways of the rural Brazilian community, felt that attempts to bring about rapid change might antagonize the people and efforts to exercise forceful leadership might alienate local authorities. He moved carefully and slowly, but his caution was interpreted by the Executive Committee as inaction, and he was dismissed. The third coordinator pushed the program with force and initiative. The more effectively he operated in terms of program means and objectives, the more antagonism he aroused. The pressure finally reached a critical level, and when the coordinator overreached his authority at the spring fiesta, local leaders pounced upon him, touching off an explosion that blew up the project in Chonin.

IMPLICATIONS

Bright Ideals

Those who planned the Chonin project were guided by ideals based on humanitarian values; they aimed to lessen human suffering and better the conditions of life. What was unique about the Chonin project was the extent to which the ideals influenced not only the ends of the project but its means as well.

The ideals that shaped project ends were those of cleanliness, good health, freedom from ignorance and superstition, technical efficiency, and material progress. It is hard to know without additional research how much these ideals coincided with those of the people of Chonin; this case has not shown that they were rejected. The ideals underlying project means were those of cooperation on all levels, coordinated effort, self-determination and self-help, democratic rather than autocratic methods, efficient organization, and nonpolitical and nonpartisan action. All these ideals were based on a conviction that nothing should be forced on people that they themselves did not want and that newly introduced habits or practices should be enduring. The administrative machinery of the Chonin project was set up to achieve these ideals. The tragedy of the project was that its means were almost entirely a response to a planning ideal and almost negligibly a response to the realities of Brazilian community life.

If as much attention could have been devoted to examining the people of Chonin and their mode of living as was devoted to formulating program policy, chances for success would have been much improved. If greater attention had been paid to the actual conditions of land ownership in Chonin, the agricultural service would not have attempted the supervised loan program. If less attention had been paid to the training of teachers and more to the conditions under which they held their jobs, the educational program might have encompassed different and more feasible objectives.

If less attention had been focused on the vision of nonpartisanship and more on the fact that Chonin was composed of active and conflicting political forces, a different light would have been thrown on the whole concept of a coordinating council. If less attention had been devoted to the vision of a coordinator who would skillfully smooth out differences and reconcile opposition and at the same time be forceful and dynamic, and more to the kind of man realistically available for this position, the role of coordinator would have appeared in a different context.

Much of this important information might have influenced the original planning of the project had the social survey taken place before or during its initial stages. Unfortunately, the survey could not start until the program was well under way, and relevant information collected by the anthropologist and his assistants came too late materially to affect the form or policy of the project in Chonin.

A New Start

Fortunately, the lessons emerging from the premature ending of the Chonin project were learned in time for immediate and useful application elsewhere. Following the demise of the combined project in Chonin, the whole program, including many of the same service personnel, was transferred to the town of Pedro Leopoldo, situated in the same state. Here the program is functioning smoothly and effectively.

Numerous features of the Pedro Leopoldo project are a direct response to the lessons learned in Chonin. In Chonin the project encountered practical difficulties such as depleted soils, absence of legal titles to land, bad roads, and isolation from urban centers. Pedro Leopoldo was selected with an eye to averting such difficulties. It is on a paved highway 40 kilometers from the state capital. It is in a limestone area with rich soil. Lands are legally owned. Proximity to a large city with its markets and urban advantages is helpful both for the agricultural program and for the morale of project personnel. These practical advantages undoubtedly increase the project's chances for success in Pedro Leopoldo, although the Chonin experience shows how material difficulties can be circumvented with effort and ingenuity. However, the most critical obstacles in Chonin were not in the practical but in the interpersonal area.

The most fundamental lesson learned during the Chonin project was the decisive role of political involvement and local organization. There is no local coordinator for the Pedro Leopoldo project, and there is no community council. Coordination is effected by an official in the state capital, insulated from direct involvement in local political intrigue. In place of a community council, the service agencies work directly through the established local authorities and other local leaders. Projects requiring both money and labor from the community as a whole have been successfully carried out through the cooperation of local authorities of the party in power. Chonin was a vivid illustration of the fact that a community council is no universal panacea; it is practicable only where conditions are suitable.

Thus, the project at Pedro Leopoldo has benefited directly from experiences in Chonin, both in the matter of selecting a community and in formulating operating policy. If it fails, it will be for reasons as yet unforeseen.

Lasting Benefits

Despite the fact that the Chonin project was terminated abruptly and dramatically, some of the basic aims of the program were nonetheless achieved. About a year after project personnel left Chonin de Cima, the social anthropologist returned for a four-day visit. He found evidence that the program had apparently produced lasting results.

These results were particularly evident in the field of health. People were continuing to use the new medicines for the treatment of malaria, dysentery, and other common ailments. The health education program had affected health habits in many ways. Some people continued to boil and filter their drinking water. Small wall racks with toothbrushes were a permanent feature in a number of houses. The privy program in particular had caught on. The project left behind it 22 concrete slabs used in privy construction. On their own initiative, local people took advantage of this to construct new privies. In addition, all the privies constructed under project auspices were kept in good repair, a sign that people had not only accepted a new type of installation but had absorbed the new health ideas that went along with it.

Education in the village has changed little. The improvements made on the school premises have remained, but selection of teachers and teaching practices are substantially the same. The agricultural service, even in its reduced form, produced some evident results. Hybrid corn seed, vegetable gardens, and improved poultry breeds have come in, apparently to stay. Many houses now contain the simple but useful types of furniture the home supervisor taught the people to make.

But the most lasting effect of the project perhaps was the awakening of the people to the realization that a fuller and richer life is possible. The poorer people in particular miss the medical service. The story is told that when a sick man comes to Chonin looking for medical service they tell him bitterly, "Go seek treatment from Senhor G!"—one of the men instrumental in killing the program. This creation of a felt need for better health, better education, and an improved level of living is the essential prerequisite for the improvement of rural life in Brazil. Moreover, the experience gained by those who participated in the project has been of inestimable value in putting it on a more solid foundation in its new location.

SUMMARY

The Chonin combined services program was well planned from the standpoint of abstract administrative procedure. The basic philosophy was explicit, program goals were clearly conceived and stated, and the machinery for their implementation was logically developed. But one factor was not clearly recognized, namely, the importance of the established social organization of the community and its relationship to the project. By trying to by-pass the local political organization through a nonpolitical Community Council, the project clashed with the values, personalities, and the traditional structure of the community. Planners neglected to give sufficient emphasis early enough to the actual dynamics of community interaction. Although the difficulties involving the Community Council, the coordinator, and the local political community were seen by some during the first year, they were not seen by enough of the responsible people to impel effective reappraisal and reorganization.

It seems clear, therefore, that the Community Council and its relationships to the coordinator were weak links in the planning process and contributed to the breakdown. The experience of the health service in other parts of Brazil has shown alternative solutions to the problem of gaining local participation. In Pedro Leopoldo such participation has been achieved by working with the existing local organization and its leadership. The task of persuading the people and getting their help has been left to the leaders without the formation of community councils or the appointment of coordinators.

SELECTED REFERENCES

Freyre, Gilberto, *Masters and Slaves*. Alfred A. Knopf, New York, 1946. An English translation by Samuel Putnam of a modern Brazilian classic (*Casa-Grande y Senzala*). A historical study of the development of plantation life in the northeastern coast of Brazil.

Pierson, Donald, *Cruz das Almas*. Smithsonian Institution, Institute of Social Anthropology, Government Printing Office, Washington, 1951. A study of a rural community in the State of São Paulo, Brazil.

Smith, T. Lynn, *Brazil:* People and Institutions. Louisiana State University Press, Baton Rouge, 1947. An exhaustive study of the Brazilian people, their institutions, and history.

Wagley, Charles, *Amazon Town*. Macmillan Co., New York, 1953. A very readable account of life in a small Amazon town.

Race and Class in Rural Brazil. UNESCO, Paris, 1952. An excellent joint study by Wagley and his students of race and class features in northeastern Brazil.

Wagley, Charles, Octávio Gouvêa de Bulhões, Stanley J. Stein, and Carleton Sprague Smith, *Four Papers Presented in the Institute for Brazilian Studies*. Vanderbilt University Press, Nashville, Tenn., 1951.

Case 14

A MEDICAL CARE PROGRAM IN A COLORADO COUNTY

by Lyle Saunders and Julian Samora

In setting up a program to solve a particular health problem, it is important to include the right features and to omit features inappropriate to the situation. It is usually easy to eliminate elements once they are seen to be superfluous, but it takes real ingenuity to isolate the dispensable elements. The history of the modern alphabet is a good example. Alphabetic writing depends on some two dozen true letter-signs and goes back to the cumbersome form of ancient Egyptian writing which involved more than 400 miscellaneous characters for syllables, words, objects, and ideas. It did not occur to the Egyptians to discard all their symbols except the 24 true letter-signs scattered among the rest. It took two thousand years for this realization to be achieved.

Professor Saunders and Dr. Samora record an instance of a medical care program which apparently collapsed under the weight of excessive organizational machinery. Designed to lighten the load of illness among subscribers, the cooperative health association, suitable in other surroundings, proved a dead weight in a setting where people could not see the point of joining an organization, attending meetings, and paying dues. These features are omitted in a revised medical care program now being tried in the same section of Colorado. Here again, as in the case described by Dr. Oberg and Mr. Rios, it took painful trial and error to learn what to leave out.

The reader may conclude that the organizers of the Brazilian project and of the Brazos County plan were foolish not to realize what the authors now make obvious. But if he stops to think how long it took to simplify the alphabet, he may wonder instead how the organizers learned so rapidly that more could be done for community health by introducing fewer organizational devices. —EDITOR

THE PROBLEM

The Failure of a Health Cooperative

On December 1, 1946, a cooperative health association began operation in Brazos County, Colorado.[1] Its purpose was to pro-

[1] The county name and all other local place names used in this case are fictitious.

377

vide medical care and certain minimum health services to the
7,500 rural, mainly Spanish-American people of the county at a
price they could afford.

At the time the Association began to function, auspices were
favorable. The only physician practicing in the county had died
two years before. The nearest available doctors were at Piños, in
another county, 20 miles from the nearest Brazos County community and more than 40 miles from its largest population center.
To use their services meant either a long ride for a sick person or
bringing in a physician for home visits at the usual fee of a dollar
per mile one way. For chronic illnesses and for many acute conditions people relied on the folk medical knowledge of their families
and friends or consulted untrained lay practitioners.

There had never been a public health unit in Brazos County.
Little was known about good environmental sanitation practices
or preventive health measures. Health conditions were far from
ideal. Infant and maternal death rates were high; infectious diseases, particularly tuberculosis, infant diarrhea, upper respiratory infections, and the common diseases of childhood, were
prevalent. Diets were generally poor, and inadequate nutrition
common. There was no regular program of immunization
against specific diseases and many chronic cases went untreated.

The new Association seemed admirably designed to meet the
need for a health program in Brazos County. Its plans were
modest, yet reasonably adequate. It proposed to offer a wide
range of services including examination, diagnosis, and medical
treatment; immunizations and other preventive services; obstetrical and maternity care; minor surgery with indicated short-
term hospitalization; ambulance service including, when necessary, transportation to Piños; prescriptions and such drugs as are
customarily dispensed from the physician's bag. The Association
planned to provide a doctor, one or more nurses, and a health
center to serve as office, clinic, and hospital. It had no grandiose
notions of providing complete medical care, but rather hoped to
give the people of Brazos County enough service to meet their
minimum health needs and to bring persons requiring specialized
equipment or skills into contact with medical personnel and
facilities at Piños and the larger towns to the east.

Plans for the Association had been carefully drawn with the help of experts from the Farm Security Administration and other governmental agencies, some of whom had been involved in a similar program in a nearby New Mexico county where the population, economic and physical conditions, and health problems were like those of Brazos County. When it began operation, the Association had on deposit in the bank a grant of about $42,000 from the Farm Security Administration for construction of a health center and the purchase of equipment and supplies. It had the enthusiastic support of prominent people in the county, including religious and business leaders. A total of 405 member families had paid the first year fee in full and 135 others had each paid $10 and pledged to pay the remainder when a doctor was employed.

Here was what seemed to be a promising situation: a population needing health services and medical care; an apparently sound plan for providing for a considerable portion of their needs at a price within their means; a governmental subsidy for capital outlays to enable the project to get started; free consultation and advisory services from qualified professionals; the active support of prominent local people; and a membership large enough to make the operation economically feasible. Yet the project can fairly be described as a failure almost from the start. The story of that failure is briefly but clearly told in the membership records of the Association for the six years it managed to limp along:

1946–1947	405 fully paid members
1947–1948	287 " " "
1948–1949	90 " " "
1949–1950	60 " " "
1950–1951	25 " " "
1951–1952	1 " " "
August, 1952	0 " " "

Why did the Brazos County Health Association fail? With such preparation and resources, why was the program not a lasting success? What was there in the situation that contributed to the failure of such carefully laid plans? What were the deficiencies in the design or operation of the program that made it unacceptable to the people it was intended to serve? To suggest even partial answers we must know more about Brazos County and its people and the circumstances under which the Health Association came into being.

THE SITUATION

Brazos County Builds and Abandons a New Health Organization

Brazos County

Brazos County is a sparsely settled area of some 1,200 square miles just north of the Colorado-New Mexico boundary. The 6,000 inhabitants (1950 census) live on isolated farms and ranches and in 12 villages located within a 20-mile radius of the county seat, a community of 1,300 people.

There are no industries, agriculture being the principal occupation. The main sources of income are field crops, hay, and livestock. Incomes are relatively low, the median family income in 1950 ($1,245) being less than half that for the state as a whole. The rural level of living index (1940) was 50, as compared with the average of 100 for all counties in the United States. Only a third of the homes have electric lights; one in 20 has a bath tub or shower, and one in 17 a telephone or refrigerator. In 1950 about half the families had radio sets. Two-thirds of the population twenty-five years of age and older have completed five grades of school, but only one in eight has graduated from high school.

Mobility is fairly high, and many people migrate in search of jobs. Family and community ties, however, are strong and people who migrate tend to return to the county.

Brazos County is about 80 per cent Spanish-speaking; 19 per cent English-speaking ("Anglo"); and 1 per cent Japanese-American. Nearly all those in the Spanish-speaking group were born in the United States, most of them in Brazos County. In general, the English-speaking and Spanish-speaking populations tend to live apart, either in separate communities or in separate sections of the same community. Three of the 12 villages are predominantly Anglo; the others, including the most isolated ones, are largely or wholly Spanish-American.

Religious affiliation tends to follow ethnic lines. Most of the Spanish-speaking are Catholic; a majority of the Anglos are Protestant. In religion, as in other matters, Spanish-American communities tend to be highly autonomous, and each builds and maintains its own church, has its own sodalities, and celebrates its own holy days.

The tempo of life in the county is fairly slow. Family and community affairs, agriculture, and religion are the main interests. On Saturday and Sunday people come from the surrounding villages to the county seat, the main trade center, to buy and sell, visit, attend a dance, or see a movie at the local theater. Trading is conducted according to traditional patterns. Most people have charge accounts at the local stores and pay them when they can. Few people operate on a cash basis.

Factional differences are common in the county, and strong feelings can be engendered over minor issues. There is little feeling of unity. Few issues or personalities appear as potential focal points for unifying effort. Loyalties are centered around family, religious, and political groupings. Programs initiated or supported by one group are almost certain to be opposed by another. Politics is a favorite topic of conversation. Elections are always "hot," and patronage is taken for granted by winner and loser alike.

Spanish-Americans

The Spanish-speaking inhabitants of Brazos County are part of a large population in the American Southwest that includes some three million persons. It is a population that is both scattered throughout the Southwest and concentrated in certain areas, like Brazos County, where the Spanish-speaking inhabitants are numerically dominant. The Spanish-speaking people of Brazos County are Spanish-Americans, a subgroup within the larger Spanish-speaking population, whose ancestors have been living in parts of the Southwest since it was first colonized by Europeans in 1598.

The Spanish-Americans have a distinctive culture largely derived from that of sixteenth- and seventeenth-century Spain. Some elements were adapted from Pueblo, Navaho, or Apache Indian groups, with whom the Spanish-Americans have had a long history of contact, and some cultural traits have been borrowed from Anglos who have been filtering into the Southwest in increasing numbers since the early 1800's. But the hard core of the culture is the heritage of Spain as modified during several centuries of relative isolation in a rather harsh environment.

The type of culture and social organization developed by the Spanish-Americans in their long period of isolation is almost perfectly embodied in classical descriptions of the typical "folk society." Population aggregations were small. The common form of settlement was the village, with houses clustered around a central plaza. Beyond the houses and corrals were farm plots and common grazing lands. A subsistence economy based on agriculture was maintained. The economic unit was the family, not the individual, and the fortunes of all members of the community tended to rise and fall together. There was a high degree of isolation from other cultures, and relatively few opportunities for borrowing traits or being stimulated to invention and innovation. There was little division of labor, and most of the village populations were highly homogeneous, everyone having about the same range of knowledge, attitudes, and skills. The technology was simple. Muscles of men and animals provided power. Tools of any sort were few; nearly all were made locally.

Social change was slow. The physical surroundings, social organization, and cultural patterns remained much the same. Traditional knowledge and wisdom were transmitted to others through the informal processes of everyday living. Virtually no one knew how to read or write, or felt any particular need to possess these somewhat esoteric skills. The realm of the sacred shaded into that of the secular, and religion played a prominent part in all important activities. Members of families and communities shared a strong sense of group identification which, however, did not preclude conflicts or disunity between family or community groups.

The principal institutions were the family, the church, and the *patrón* system. Among and within these all the life needs of an individual could be met. For the rare emergencies beyond the power of family or community to handle, there was always the *patrón*, a benevolent authority who claimed certain services and in return served as intermediary with the outside world.

Any problem that might arise could be met with well-tested, familiar community and family resources. No one organized or joined any associations outside of a few traditional groups connected with the church or irrigation. One was born into the group he belonged to; each was a multi-purpose group within which a number of his needs were met.

In many important ways the culturally derived goals, practices, beliefs, and perception patterns of Spanish-Americans differ from those of Anglos, and personality traits are differently valued by the two cultures. Such characteristics as aggressiveness, competitiveness, ambition, initiative, individual responsibility, practicality, efficiency are given lower values in the Spanish-American culture; conversely, the characteristics of conformity, acceptance, resignation, adjustment are valued more highly. Traits that were well adapted to life in the isolated Spanish-American village are less useful at the present time when Spanish-Americans, through choice and necessity, increasingly interact with growing numbers of Anglos.

Spanish-Americans have been a numerical majority in Brazos County since they first began settling there a hundred years ago. The Anglos, however, because of closer identification with the dominant culture of the state and nation and their possession of knowledge, skills, and resources not readily available to the Spanish-American group, exercise an influence in the affairs of the county far out of proportion to their numbers.

Relations between the two groups are rather complex. While there is little or no overt hostility, neither group understands or approves of the other to any appreciable extent. Everyone knows clearly to which group he and everyone else belongs. Some Anglos have adopted a few Spanish-American traits, but not to the point where they consider themselves members of the other group. Through long contact with Anglos, nearly all the Spanish-

Americans have acquired some Anglo traits. A small proportion have gone so far that they think and act much like Anglos and maintain only a peripheral membership in the Spanish-American group.

The Spanish-Americans of Brazos County began to use Anglo medicine long before the Health Association was conceived or organized. About 1887 an Anglo physician came into the county and set up a practice which continued until his death in the late 1920's. He was succeeded by a Puerto Rican doctor who practiced until his death in 1944. Meanwhile, a second Anglo physician set up practice in the county in 1938. In 1942 he moved to Piños, drawing some of his patients from among his former clientele in Brazos County.

Anglo medicine, however, tended to supplement rather than replace traditional practices and lay practitioners. At the time the Health Association was formed, Spanish-Americans were using Anglo medicine less frequently than before because there was no physician readily available. There was no strong feeling against it, nor was there any widespread conviction that Anglo medicine was conspicuously better than their traditional medical ways.

Organizing the Health Association

The idea for a Health Association and first organizational efforts came largely from two men, both Anglos and both professionally concerned with health. One was the regional health services specialist of the federal Farm Security Administration. The other, a professor at a state college, was at that time directing a college-sponsored program at the county seat. Although an Anglo, he had worked for years in the area and was known and liked by a good proportion of the Spanish-American group.

In 1945 the Farm Security Administration specialist visited the county to discuss with the professor a proposal for improving the water supply in a community five miles from the county seat. The two men discussed health conditions in Brazos County, and the agency specialist suggested that the Farm Security Administration might be of help in improving the local health situation. The professor talked to a number of local people, stimulated their interest, and organized a visit to a health cooperative in New

Mexico sponsored by the Farm Security Administration. Those who made the trip were persuaded by their experience that this type of health program was feasible for their county, and two weeks later, after further discussions, the professor and the agency specialist called a meeting to explore the possibility of taking action.

At this meeting, held in the fall of 1945, an organization was tentatively set up and a board of directors elected. Insufficient preparation, disputes among the officers, and general lack of experience in organizing and promoting a long-range program contributed to the early failure of this first attempt. The officers were unable to agree on a plan of procedure, and nothing was done after the first meeting. The idea of an organized local health service remained alive, however, and informal discussions were continued, particularly by the professor and those who had visited the New Mexico association.

Early in 1946 a second meeting was arranged by a county seat service club to reorganize the Health Association. About 50 persons, Anglos or highly Anglicized Spanish-Americans living in the county seat, attended. A second board of directors, including a president, vice-president, secretary, treasurer, and member-at-large, was elected and given the responsibility of formulating plans for an Association. The Farm Security Administration had indicated that it was prepared to make a substantial cash grant for constructing a health center and purchasing equipment if satisfactory arrangements could be made. The directors, working closely with FSA personnel, soon developed a plan for a voluntary health cooperative they felt would meet the needs of the county.

The plan, closely resembling that of the New Mexico health cooperative, proposed an annual budget of approximately $20,000 to cover all operating costs including salaries for a physician, two nurses, a manager, a clerk-receptionist, a janitor, and a cook. Membership was to be on a family basis, each family paying $38 a year. At this rate, 540 families, paying in $20,520 a year, would be necessary to maintain the organization. The physician was to be guaranteed an annual salary of approximately $6,500 based on a dollar a month from each member family. In addition, he was to be free to provide to members services not included in their contract and to engage in private practice among non-members. Sixty-four per cent of his income from additional services to members and from nonmember practice was to go to the Association, which would then pay all his overhead expenses including salaries of assistants, rent, mileage, and the cost of instruments and medicines.

For their membership fee, families were to receive, when needed, physical examinations, diagnoses, and medical treatment; ordinary drugs for maternity home and bed patients; emergency home visits and emergency treatment at the health center; obstetrical care; prenatal and postnatal counsel and care; ambulance service from home to the center and from the center to the hospital at Piños; tonsillectomies and other minor surgery; routine immunizations; venereal disease treatment; and prescriptions. A grant was to be requested from the Farm Security Administration for the construction of the health center, for wells and pumps, and for clinic equipment and an ambulance.

On the basis of these plans a drive for members, sponsored jointly by the service club which had called the organizational meeting and the directors of the Association, was begun in the spring of 1946. At meetings held in every community in the county, one or more of the directors explained the program, answered questions, and attempted to sign up members. The parish priest at the county seat and in his seven missions described the health program from his pulpit and urged his parishioners to become members. He offered the facilities of a church-sponsored credit union to those who could not immediately afford the membership fee. The Protestant minister in one of the Spanish-speaking communities also recommended the Association to his parishioners.

News articles, favorable editorials, and announcements of Association meetings were printed regularly in both English and Spanish in the county seat newspaper. The proprietor of the only theater in the county permitted the directors to talk about the health program between features. A brochure in English and Spanish explaining the proposed program in detail and showing plans for the health center was prepared and distributed. Directors attended meetings of various organizations located in the county seat and in Anglo communities to explain the operation of the Health Association. The radio station at Piños broadcast a series of spot announcements in Spanish.

Although considerable interest was generated, the membership campaign progressed slowly. However, enough members signed in the first weeks to suggest that the goal of 540 might eventually be reached. The directors, therefore, rented a building at the county seat to serve as a temporary office and health center, equipped the office, hired a manager-solicitor whose immediate duties were to keep the office open and to solicit memberships, and began to seek a physician and a suitable site for the permanent health center being designed by the Farm Security Administration.

The Decline of the Cooperative

The membership goal was not reached in June, as had been expected. By September, however, 405 families had paid the full fee of $38 and 135 others had paid $10 each and pledged to pay the remainder when a doctor arrived. On the strength of this showing, the Farm Security Administration granted the Association $41,950 for a building and equipment.

A physician was hired in November, together with all other proposed personnel except a cook. Shortly after the doctor arrived the temporary center was equipped and a station wagon purchased for use as an ambulance. On December 1, the Association began to offer services to its members.

Some difficulties were encountered from the beginning, including the problem of finding suitable housing for staff members. Nevertheless, the Association functioned fairly well for the first six months. During this period, however, certain problems appeared which contributed to the eventual decline of the organization.

It soon became apparent that most members were uninterested in the nonmedical activities of the Association. The first annual meeting was scheduled for February, 1947, at which time incumbent officers were to report on the affairs of the Association and new officers were to be elected. The meeting was called and well publicized, but the 30 members necessary for a quorum were not present. A second meeting was called two months later, but again there were not enough members present to conduct business. It was not until July that the first annual meeting was held, and then it was possible to get enough members together only because the Association was on the verge of collapse and vigorous efforts were being made to save it.

A second problem was that of insufficient members. At no time during the history of the Association did paid-up memberships total over 405, although 540 were required for solvency. Of the original members, 135 had paid only $10. Few of these completed their payments. Some took advantage of their temporary membership to obtain needed medical work and then permitted themselves to be dropped. One member, for example, paid his deposit, then had all his children immunized and their tonsils removed. After this he refused to continue his membership payments. In general, those who had not paid the full fee were given three months' service and then dropped. But the doctor's salary, pegged to the membership, kept shrinking as the number of members decreased.

By June, 1947, the membership problem was so serious that the doctor talked of leaving when his one-year contract expired. Faced with this situation, the directors decided that if the first annual meeting could not be held by July 20 and the membership could not be brought up to 540 they would dissolve the Association and return the unexpended portion of the Farm Security Administration grant. A prospective loss of more than $30,000 was apparently a considerable stimulus, and the service club that was instrumental in organizing the Association joined forces with the newspaper and local businessmen in the county seat to launch another intensive drive for members. By the July 20 deadline, membership had climbed to 544, but nearly half represented contributions of $10 and pledges to pay the balance.

Another persistent problem was fee collections. The physician was called upon to provide members with services not covered by their Association contract and for which he was permitted to charge extra. In addition, he gave service to many nonmember patients. According to their agreement, the Association and the physician were to share all these extra fees. But it turned out to be almost impossible to collect for extra services. In a typical month, for example, statements totaling some $2,000 were sent out, while payments of only $190 were received.

When the first annual meeting was finally held on July 20, a new board of directors was elected, and the physician, heartened by the apparent success of the membership drive, announced that he would stay another year. About this time, too, plans and specifications for the health center were completed and bids called for. However, when the bids were opened some months later, all were found to be too high, building costs having increased since the plans were drawn, and revision of the specifications became necessary.

The membership drive of July, 1947, did nothing to put recruitment on a firm basis, and the number of members continued to decline. Again many who paid $10 and pledged the remainder did not complete their payments. In the absence of further intensive recruitment efforts, few additional families joined. By late 1948 membership had dropped to 90. It was impossible to get members together for an annual meeting for any year following 1947, and the board elected at that time continued to serve until the Association failed. Discouraged by the lack of interest, they made no further special efforts to drum up membership. In 1948 the physician resigned. However, a successor was appointed within a month. In 1949 membership dropped to 60. Meanwhile, the directors had managed to get their building plans revised, but by the time new bids were received building costs had again increased. It was thought that it might be possible to get other federal funds to match the $34,000 remaining from the Farm Security Administration grant, but the lowest bid on the revised plans was $85,000. The county commissioners instituted a mill levy that raised $10,000 and a wealthy individual promised financial help, but the directors were reluctant to take any action without being absolutely certain of having all the money they needed. So nothing was done, and the Association continued to occupy its temporary rented building.

After 1949 the membership continued to decline. In 1950 there were 25 members. During 1951 one determined family remained loyal to the cause. In August, 1952, the last membership expired.

The Farm Security Administration funds remained in the bank. The equipment, the rented space, and the station wagon continued to be used by the physician, whose practice was both extensive and lucrative. People were using and paying for Anglo medical care. The Health Association, however, was dead. But the desire for medical service was not.

In the summer of 1953 a group of Brazos County citizens— again largely from the county seat—met, elected a new board of directors, and started a new Health Association. Only local people were involved in the initiation of the new project, although it should be noted that their action coincided with the beginning of a specific interest in Brazos County and its problems by the State Department of Public Health and the medical school of the state university.

Among the first activities undertaken by the new board was a drive for funds for a new health center building. By contacting nearly everybody in the county, the board raised the equivalent of $25,000 in pledges of labor, materials, or money. This, plus the unexpended portion of the Farm Security Administration grant and the $10,000 raised through special taxation, supported the construction of the building, which was nearing completion in July, 1954. The pay-in-advance phase of the program has been abandoned and a plan for medical care on a fee-for-service basis is being worked out. At the time this case study was written, matters were still largely in the planning stage, and it was too early to tell whether the new organization would be more successful than its predecessor.

The Causes of Failure

The Question of Finances. In seeking reasons for the failure of the Brazos County Health Association, the one that comes most readily to mind—and one that some might consider a sufficient explanation—is that joining the Association involved a greater economic burden than families could or would assume. However, many factors indicate that this is not the whole story, and indeed may not even be an important part of the story.

It is true that the people of Brazos County are not economically well off in comparison with the total population of the state of

Colorado. Their median income is less than half that of the state population, and many of them live in poverty. For people on this economic level, $38 a year, particularly when it must be paid in a lump sum, is a lot of money. On the other hand, 1945 to 1953 were years of relative prosperity in Brazos County. Economic indices were well up and there is evidence that these were better times than the people had known for some years.

More immediately pertinent is the fact that even as the Association declined county people were privately paying considerable sums for medical care—and to the same physicians who would have treated them had they been members of the Association! The Association, it will be remembered, contracted to pay a salary of about $6,500 a year to the doctor hired. But the first physician netted $10,000 in his first year and approximately $20,000 the second, and his successor is reported to have earned between $20,000 and $30,000 annually in recent years. Certainly many patients paid considerably more than $38 per year for the services they received. The people of Brazos County were buying medical care *as they felt a need for it*, but they were buying it outside the Association and as individual families, not as members of an organized group.

If the failure of the Brazos County Health Association is not attributable to economic causes, what were the reasons? Causes may be sought in two general areas: cultural differences between those who initiated the project and those whose cooperation was needed to keep it going; and differences between Anglo and Spanish-American patterns of relationship and behavior which made the Association unacceptable to any but the most highly acculturated Spanish-Americans. Stated simply, the means provided by the Association were not those traditionally and characteristically used by Spanish-Americans in this area to meet their health and medical needs. There was little in the Association's way of operating that conformed to their familiar, time-tested ways of dealing with sickness; there was much that was unfamiliar, and from their point of view, irrelevant. From an Anglo point of view, the health situation in Brazos County was bad, and the Association a good means for improving it. To the Spanish-Americans the health problem seemed less serious and the means of improvement less desirable. Their perception of the seriousness of the problem and the value of the solution was not such as to provide strong motivation for joining the Association, particularly when the same medical service was available under an alternative, and for many a more attractive, arrangement.

Insiders and Outsiders. It is probably significant that the original impetus for the Association, the form of the organization, and its formal leadership during the first year of operation were all largely provided by persons who were strangers or Anglos or both. The Farm Security Administration representative was an Anglo who had never lived in the county and was not well known there. The professor, who probably did more than anyone else to instigate the project and who remained an active behind-the-scenes force throughout its history, was an old resident of the county, but an Anglo. He was known and liked by many Spanish-Americans, but when the chips were down and lines drawn he was regarded by the Spanish-Americans as "one of them" rather than "one of us."

The Health Association was introduced to Brazos County by the following process: a federal agency with an established program and operating policies saw Brazos County as a likely arena for action. A professionally trained county resident, alert to local "needs" and "problems," found in the agency program an instrument for dealing with some of those needs and problems. The resulting plan of action conformed to a pattern already familiar to and acceptable by the federal agency. It provided for a large grant of funds to serve the triple purpose of motivating local people to act, making it possible for them to act rapidly, and making sure that the action would take a form acceptable to the agency. The agency workers also provided the idea for a type of machinery, a somewhat standardized kind of health organization, which they believed could be instituted by local people and would operate to their benefit. The plan was thus largely Anglo in origin and conception, formulated by Anglos in terms of their own values and imposed on the people of Brazos County through the motivating influence of a grant of money. It was not a plan that would have been formulated by the Spanish-Americans themselves.

The board of directors responsible for the inauguration and first year of operation of the Association was democratically selected, but at a meeting attended by no more than 50 persons, mostly from the county seat. The man elected president was Spanish-American, but he had been in the county less than two years, being a faculty member at the same institution as the professor. When, during his presidency, factional differences arose over whose land would be purchased for the health center building, an old resident of the county circulated a petition to remove him from office on the grounds that he was not a property owner. The vice-president, a woman, was both Spanish-speaking and an old resident, but in Brazos County a woman's place is in the home. The secretary was both a newcomer and an Anglo, and the treasurer, while an old resident, was also Anglo. The only board member who was genuinely representative of the county's Spanish-American population was the member-at-large. The manager hired by the Association was Spanish-American, but he was new to the county and divided his time between the Brazos Association and the similar organization in New Mexico. The physician was a newcomer, an Anglo and a Protestant who was more interested in treating people for regular fees than in the mechanics of the Association as such, and who devoted a considerable portion of his time to his rather lucrative nonmember practice.

Thus, from the point of view of the average Spanish-American, the Association was an organization of outsiders to which he owed neither responsibility nor loyalty. The local people who did devote intensive effort to the Association were mainly the most highly acculturated members of the Spanish-American group— business and professional men, politicians, the newspaper editor —and thus more responsive than the average person to the Anglo point of view and the motivating power of the Farm Security Administration's $42,000 grant. A few were less acculturated individuals who saw in the situation an opportunity for leadership status.

Anglo and Spanish-American Ways. Procedures followed by the Health Association differed markedly from traditional local practices. In the first place, membership in the Association meant that to get medical care a person had to engage in a series of apparently irrelevant activities—attending meetings, discussing policy, electing officers, formulating and following a set of by-laws, paying dues. This approach is familiar in Anglo culture where objectives are customarily achieved through formal organizations created for specific purposes. It was much less familiar to the Spanish-Americans of Brazos County who came from a background in which there were few special purpose organizations and who were accustomed to dealing with sickness, as with almost everything else, directly and personally. Meetings for discussing and resolving matters of public interest were common enough. However, these meetings dealt with matters of immediate concern which were settled, if at all, by the pronouncements of respected elders or by overriding one or another of the rival factions. There was little group experience in devoting a continuing series of meetings to the same set of problems; nor were people familiar with the kind of individual give and take, collective effort, continual compromise, and the delegation of authority and responsibility necessary to the effective functioning of an organization like the Health Association.

Health, in the tradition of the Spanish-Americans, was an individual or family matter. The focus was on the individual case, and the afflicted person was brought directly into contact with available resources for treatment and care. The more roundabout approach to medical care of the Association found little in the culture of the Spanish-Americans to support it.

Second, leadership practices of the Association were at variance with familiar cultural patterns. The Association was managed by officials selected by popular vote in accordance with the Anglo democratic tradition. Although the Spanish-Americans in Brazos County, like those in other parts of the Southwest, have long participated in the Anglo political system, the right and obligation of individuals to vote for leaders of their choice is an Anglo and not a Spanish-American concept. In the Spanish-American tradition political action was dominated by men and was authoritarian rather than democratic. Traditional leadership was exercised through the religious, family, and *patrón* institutions, and a man became a leader because of who he was rather than his personal characteristics.

Neither the persons selected as leaders for the Association nor the method of selection were in line with traditional ways. No Anglo, non-Catholic newcomer, or woman could come to occupy an official position through the old selective process except through highly unusual circumstances. Yet of the nine persons most influential in the early stages of the Association, all but one possessed one or more of these alienating characteristics.

Closely related to the leadership factor is the authoritarian manner in which affairs in general were traditionally managed within the Spanish-American culture. Achieving objectives through a system involving committees, directors, quorums, majority rule, and equal voting rights is an Anglo pattern. In the Spanish-American tradition decisions were made by the few and accepted by the many. Age, sex, family position, community standing were what determined whether one commanded or obeyed. These are still determining factors in parts of Brazos County, even though, on the surface, other factors may seem to have supplanted them.

The Association was set up in the traditional Anglo organizational pattern; it was nonpartisan, nondenominational, and democratic. But the people who belonged to it have long been highly denominational, fiercely partisan, and authoritarian. These differences contributed substantially to the Association's failure.

A third important principle underlying Association practice that was not in conformity with traditional Spanish-American ways was that of paying in advance for protection against need. This idea is quite familiar to Anglos who characteristically live for the future. It is much less familiar to Spanish-Americans, who are more exclusively oriented toward the present. In matters of health this means that if one is sick today, the sickness should be treated now. If one is healthy today, there is little need to be concerned about what may happen tomorrow.

Paying in advance for an anticipated illness makes little sense to people whose time orientation is to the present rather than the future. Much better to use the money for something which gives satisfactions now and worry about illness when it arrives. As one member said when asked why he did not renew his membership, "Last year I paid thirty-eight dollars and no one in my family was sick!" He felt he had lost or wasted his money, since he did not receive any services for it. An Anglo would feel that he had been "protected" during the period his membership was in force, even though he obtained no direct benefit. From the Spanish-American point of view, money paid out for sickness which never comes is money thrown away. This attitude toward time helps to explain why many families who could have obtained a considerable amount of care for a relatively small investment paid out much more in fees for private medical service than membership in the Association would have cost.

Information Without Understanding. The Association was further weakened by the fact that many members never fully understood what the Association was, how it worked, what was expected of them, or what they were entitled to. A study was made of members of the health association in New Mexico, also serving a predominantly rural Spanish-American population; at the end of a full year of membership only 3 per cent of those interviewed had any clear understanding of the purpose of the organization, about 17 per cent had a fair understanding, and 80 per cent knew little or nothing about the organization to which they belonged. Less than half could name one or more of the board of directors, and more than a fifth did not know that the organization had such a board.

While comparable data are not available for the Brazos County Association, the situation was undoubtedly similar. The idea for an association did not evolve out of grass-roots discussions of health problems, but rather was presented, fully grown, in a series of public meetings. The average layman probably got his first and only information about the Association at the organizational meeting or by listening to his priest describe the Association and its program. People signed up not because they understood the plan and approved it. They were either persuaded by the status or the promises of those selling memberships or by the support of the priest, or because friends and neighbors were joining and it seemed the thing to do. The fact that so many membership pledges were not fulfilled indicates either that these people all changed their minds after signing up, which is unlikely in so large a group, or that they joined for some reason other than conviction and understanding.

Personal contact with one's relatives and friends is the traditional Spanish-American way of acquiring information. Information about the Association, however, was disseminated by other means: newspaper stories and radio programs, printed brochures, posters, and speeches and announcements wherever people gathered. These means were probably of doubtful efficacy, so that information reaching the general population was frequently incomplete and occasionally wrong. Consequently, some who joined the Association did not know or care enough about the Association to continue their membership; others were unpleasantly surprised to find that all medical care was not included in their contract when they were billed for extra services. Since Spanish-speaking people throughout the Southwest have a reputation as good credit risks, a possible explanation for the large proportion of uncollectible bills was the fact that members could not understand why they should be charged when they had already paid a full membership fee.

The Brazos County Health Association, then, was largely designed by Anglos and in accordance with Anglo notions of how health problems should be handled. Its original impetus came from two Anglos, and members of the board of directors who guided organization were either themselves Anglos or were largely oriented toward Anglo ways. In its emphasis on formal organization, democratic procedure, and the prepayment principle, the Association represented an approach diverging considerably from traditional ways of treating sickness. The great proportion of the Spanish-Americans of the county probably had no clear understanding of the Association or its program, and few recognized the existence of a general health "problem" demanding some sort of collective effort. In these circumstances, the fate of the Association is not surprising.

IMPLICATIONS

The kind of situation that developed in Brazos County is neither isolated nor, in its broader aspects, unique. The same pattern of events is familiar wherever one people offers medical and health services to another. It is a pattern that usually leads to wasted effort, broken hopes, and impaired relations because it so frequently includes the imposition or intrusion of alien ways upon a people who can neither understand nor accept them.

Throughout the Southwest, Anglos in a variety of situations are offering medical care and health service to Spanish-speaking people, many of whom share a substantially different culture. An overwhelming proportion of those who offer Anglo medical care are themselves Anglos. What they do and why they do it are so obvious and right to them that it needs no further justification. The small proportion of native professionals in medicine and related fields have had a long exposure to Anglo practices and values and for the most part are highly Anglicized. Consequently, most health efforts involving the Spanish-speaking group are predicated on Anglo assumptions, values, and goals and are therefore likely to be unacceptable to some of the Spanish-speaking people. This is equally true in the case of private practitioners and public health personnel, as well as the cooperative Health Association.

In the field of health, as in other fields, action programs cutting across cultural or subcultural lines must, if they are to be accepted, conform to the existing perceptions, beliefs, attitudes, and practices of the group they are to affect. Furthermore, if such programs are to have any chance of continuing after the initial organizing impetus is withdrawn, they must permit the pursuit of culturally meaningful goals through culturally acceptable means.

The Brazos County Health Association, along with the New Mexico health cooperative and numerous other health programs in the Southwest, satisfied neither of these conditions. Many aspects of the Association's program were at variance with traditional Spanish-American ways of dealing with sickness. It was an imposed program; it violated established leadership practices; it ran counter to the accepted method of dealing with sickness on an individual basis. A whole set of seemingly irrelevant actions— joining an organization, attending meetings, paying fees, voting, and the like—became attached to the treatment of sickness and became a condition of participation in the new arrangement. While the Association's major goal, better health for Brazos County, was probably acceptable in the abstract, such related subgoals as the maintenance of an organization, the development of preventive procedures and attitudes, and the building of a health center were not meaningful or important to many local people.

The implications of the Brazos County case go far beyond the county, the American Southwest, or our national boundaries. In many parts of the world, professional and technical experts from the United States and technologically advanced nations of Europe are working to develop programs of agriculture, industry, education, and health in areas inhabited by people culturally different from themselves. Such efforts, unless guided by a general awareness of the influence of culture and a particular knowledge of the cultural traits of the recipient population, will certainly produce frustration and wasted effort for the implementing group while failing to benefit or even harming subjects of the program.

It is not easy to be critically self-conscious of one's own cultural preconceptions. It is not easy to be objective about goals invested with profound cultural meanings; nor is it easy to modify familiar methods of operation which have worked in other circumstances. But unless this difficult reevaluation is undertaken by those who plan, organize, and implement programs of technical change in cross-cultural situations, the experience of the Brazos County Health Association will be repeated time after time in other settings and under other names.

SUMMARY

A cooperative health association designed to provide certain minimum services to its membership was organized and began functioning in 1946 in Brazos County, Colorado, an area inhabited primarily by rural Spanish-Americans. Vigorous membership campaigns twice succeeded in obtaining the 540 members necessary to keep the Association solvent, but the support thus won was half-hearted and the membership sagged as soon as the organizing impetus was withdrawn. The failure of the Association, which ceased to function in 1952, can be explained by the fact that its inception, organization, promotion, and management were the work of persons not culturally representative of the majority of the county's population, and that the program itself contained many elements incompatible with traditional practices and beliefs.

A new effort to provide medical care for the people of Brazos County has recently been undertaken. It is still Anglo in conception but embodies substantial modifications of the original plan. The new attempt incorporates features which bring the program more in line with local beliefs and practices, and it is hoped that it will receive more popular acceptance than was accorded its predecessor.

SELECTED REFERENCES

Fergusson, Erna, *New Mexico:* A Pageant of Three Peoples. Alfred A. Knopf, New York, 1951. One of the few available good studies of Spanish-Americans.

Kibbe, Pauline, *Latin Americans in Texas*. The University of New Mexico Press, Albuquerque, 1946. Dealing largely with Mexican-American and Mexican people rather than Spanish-Americans, this book is a fine source of information on socioeconomic conditions among the largest Spanish-speaking population in the Southwest.

McWilliams, Carey, *North from Mexico:* The Spanish-Speaking People of the United States. J. B. Lippincott Co., New York, 1949. One of the few books which attempt to deal with the entire Spanish-speaking population of the Southwest.

Mead, Margaret, editor, "The Spanish-Americans of New Mexico, U.S.A.," *Cultural Patterns and Technical Change*, United Nations Educational, Scientific, and Cultural Organization, Paris, 1953. Although quite brief, this section provides considerable information about specific cultural patterns of the Spanish-Americans.

Saunders, Lyle, *Cultural Difference and Medical Care:* The Case of the Spanish-Speaking People of the Southwest. Russell Sage Foundation, New York, 1954. Dealing with the larger group of which the Brazos County Spanish-speaking people are a part, this book is essentially a much expanded development of the point of view presented in this case.

Tuck, Ruth, *Not with the Fist*. Harcourt, Brace and Co., New York, 1946. Mainly about Mexican-Americans in California, this is one of the most sensitive accounts of Spanish-speaking people in the Southwest ever written.

PART VI
COMBINING SERVICE AND RESEARCH

Case 15

MEDICINE AND POLITICS IN A MEXICAN VILLAGE

by Oscar Lewis

In writing about the community and the health officer, Dr. George Rosen urges us "to recognize first of all that the community is a power structure. Somewhere it has a locus of authority. There are people in it who decide what many other people shall or shall not do, how they shall live and work, and many other fundamental matters." Any new venture in the health field will stand or fall partly on its merits and partly on its implications for strengthening or weakening the prevailing pattern of power. This has been documented in Dr. Kimball's case study of an Alabama community and in the Brazilian study by Dr. Oberg and Mr. Rios. In yet another form, it is again exemplified in Dr. Lewis' case study.

Dr. Lewis relates a troublesome episode that formed part of the field experience upon which his book, Life in a Mexican Village, *is based. The importance of the present study rests on what it reveals about overt and covert aspects of the power process. It reviews the intricate maneuvers by which a psychological research project was played off against a medical service originally set up in response to popular request. For instances of other programs combining research and service activities, the reader is referred to the Canadian study by Dr. John and Dr. Elaine Cumming, the Thai study by Dr. Hanks and his associates, and the Wellesley case study by Dr. Naegele.—*EDITOR

THE PROBLEM

Villagers Stop Using a Local Clinic

Shortly after arriving in the Mexican village of Tepoztlán in 1943, our community research team began to meet with the heads of families in various parts of the settlement to make ourselves known and to explain why we were there. Although our primary objective was to study village life rather than to change it, the villagers took advantage of these introductory occasions to direct attention to their pressing problems. They pointed out that their lands were becoming increasingly sterile, that for lack of water they could raise only a single crop a year, that they needed another school, and that there was no doctor in their village. One dignified, elderly Tepoztecan expressed the general attitude when he said, "Many people have come here to study us, but not one of them has helped us."

At the same time the Mexican government, through its Department of Health and Welfare, was concerned over the problem of resistance to modern medicine in some of the rural areas. They wanted to know more about the reasons behind the apparent lack of confidence in modern doctors and the difficulties encountered in trying to win the villagers away from native *curanderos*.

Acceding to the wishes of both the villagers and the government, we decided to set up a small medical clinic in Tepoztlán. The villagers had made it clear that if they were to cooperate by satisfying our research aims, they would expect something practical in return. They had expressed a need for improved medical service, and the clinic appeared to be a good answer to the problem. Federal officials similarly declared themselves more willing to cooperate with us if some of our research work was designed to throw light on problems faced by the government. The Department of Health and Welfare was reluctant to furnish a doctor solely to perform examinations in connection with purely theoretical research on personality development, as we had requested, but readily agreed to send a doctor to treat patients of the proposed medical clinic in Tepoztlán. The Department also became very much interested in our suggestion that the doctor experiment by discussing disease and cure with his patients in terms of native concepts, rather than ignoring these as "unscientific," as a method of establishing rapport and winning confidence.

The plan to establish a clinic thus appeared to answer expressed needs of both local and government people and to provide a way for us to obtain the active cooperation of both these groups. Arrangements were made to obtain the facilities for the clinic, and a doctor was sent by the Mexican Health and Welfare Department. The clinic was only one part of a broader program of services made available to the villagers at their behest. In addition, two agronomists and four social workers were brought in to serve the villagers. Little or no opposition was encountered to their work and to the research itself.

During the first week, in early February, the clinic had 11 patients and after about two months, this number increased to 35. Then abruptly, in April, patients stopped coming, and the clinic came to a complete standstill. What lay behind the failure of the clinic? Why should attendance cease so suddenly and completely in the face of an expressed need by both the government and the villagers? To find the answers, we must understand the social structure and the people of Tepoztlán: their resources, hopes, fears, and attitudes toward authority. Because the medical service program was only one part of our team's activities and because the parts became linked in devious ways, it is also essential to explain the psychological phase of our research and the response it engendered.

THE SITUATION

A Requested Service Is Ensnared in Political Intrigue

Tepoztlán and Its People

Tepoztlán is an ancient highland village of about 3,500 people 15 miles from Cuernavaca, the capital of the state of Morelos, and 60 miles south of Mexico City. Since 1936 it has been connected by a paved road to the highway running between Mexico City and Cuernavaca and has daily bus service. Tepoztlán is located just above the malaria area and is considered one of the most healthful spots in the state of Morelos, with one of its lowest death rates. However, this is a relative matter. The average rate of infant mortality for the period 1930 to 1940 was 102.3, and the general mortality rate for the same period was 20.2.

The village includes peasants, artisans, and shopkeepers, but over 90 per cent of the 853 families earn their living from agriculture. Most of the land is mountainous, forested, and depleted. Less than 15 per cent of the total land area is arable and only a single crop of corn is harvested each year. Some own their agricultural plots or have rights to certain parcels of the public land which remain with the farmers as long as they continue to work them. Other farmers must till the poor soil of the stony hillsides belonging to the community and free to anyone who wishes to cut and burn away the trees and bushes every two or three years in order to plant corn and beans. Rapid erosion prevents the poor-land farmer from using the same hillside clearing year after year.

Both Spanish and Nahuatl,̕ the native Indian language, are spoken in the village. About half of the people are bilingual, the other half speaking only Spanish. More than 40 per cent of the adults are illiterate. There are two schools in the village attended by more than 500 children.

The village is divided into seven *barrios*, each with its patron saint, internal religious organization, festivals, and a plot of land worked collectively by the men of the barrio to provide for the upkeep of the chapel. There is considerable esprit de corps among barrio members who act as a cooperative unit on some occasions. The barrio is a more meaningful unit to many villagers than the official governmental divisions of the village into political wards. In addition to the seven barrio chapels, there is also a large central village church with a resident Catholic priest.

The village has changed in important ways since the Revolution. These changes may be summarized as follows: a rapid increase in population; some improvement in modern health services, threatening the position of the curanderos; a rise in the standard of living and in the aspiration level of the people; a decrease in the number of peon and landless families (formerly these constituted the bulk of the families); the growth of a greater variety and specialization of occupations; a decrease in the use of Nahuatl and a corresponding spread in the use of Spanish; a rise in literacy and the beginnings of newspaper reading.

In sharp contrast to the rapid changes which have occurred in other aspects of life, there has been no comparable improvement in the agricultural techniques and capacities of the village. This has given rise to a dilemma; on the one hand, there is a rapidly increasing population and a higher aspiration level, while on the other hand, there is a growing sterility of the land, decreasing yields, and progressive difficulty in satisfying newly felt needs.

Setting Up the Clinic

Once we had decided to set up a medical clinic, we began to plan its organization. At first we considered the idea of setting up a temporary clinic to last only for the duration of the assignment of the doctor provided by the Department of Health and Welfare. Later, however, at the suggestion of the Department, we decided to establish the clinic as a village cooperative. The cooperative form of organization was being encouraged by the federal government at that time, on the assumption that it was in accord with native tradition. We also believed that a cooperative would be more useful in that the doctor might be kept on by the village itself long after we had left and the doctor's original assignment expired. Moreover, we viewed this enterprise as an experiment in setting up a democratic institution in a village in which the tradition of democracy was practically absent, and as a test of the readiness and ability of the Tepoztecans for such an organization.

The plan for the cooperative was fully explained to the local authorities in Tepoztlán, especially to the mayor of the municipality, and it seemed to meet with his interest and approval. When a doctor was finally obtained from the Department of Health and Welfare, the mayor was asked to call a meeting of the entire community to introduce the doctor and to discuss plans for the cooperative. He promised to call such a meeting but never did. The members of our mission thereupon visited many of the families in each barrio, and a meeting of the villagers was arranged. A Tepoztecan band was hired to create a fiesta atmosphere, for we had already learned that practically the only occasion that will bring Tepoztecans together is a fiesta. More than 160 Tepoztecans attended the meeting. This was a good turnout for the village, considering their general lack of confidence. The organization of the cooperative was discussed, and many Tepoztecans participated in the discussion.

It was decided to charge a membership fee of one peso, and 25 centavos a month thereafter. In addition, members were to pay one peso to consult the doctor, and this would include free medicines. The money collected was to form a fund for the purchase of medicines and other supplies and for paying the rent of the doctor's office. The ultimate objective was for the cooperative to be self-supporting, even to the extent of paying for a doctor if it had to. It was hoped that the six-month period for which the doctor was assigned by the Department of Health and Welfare would give the cooperative the opportunity to accumulate the necessary funds to carry on independently.

It was believed by the staff and borne out by the consensus of the first meeting that the barrio provided the most logical basis upon which a cooperative organization could be built because it was the primary cooperative unit in the social organization of the village. As already indicated, each barrio has its own patron saint, its chapel, its own festivals, and a plot of land which is communally worked by the men of the barrio to provide for the upkeep of the chapel. Fiestas were traditionally organized on a barrio basis, and in recent years participation in sports events has been on a similar basis. Thus, the few cooperative activities in the village were barrio activities. Furthermore, the barrio chose its own ceremonial officials in a fairly democratic fashion, whereas the village officials, though nominally elected, were in practice chosen by the governor of the state of Morelos. In organizing the cooperative on a barrio basis, we were therefore attempting to tie it to a geographical and social unit which still retained some of its indigenous cooperative traditions.

At the mass meeting a central village committee of seven members was elected, one from each barrio, and provisions were made for the election of barrio committees consisting of three persons each. These local committees were to be charged with recruiting members in their barrios and with popularizing the cooperative. The meeting ended on a hopeful note, and the central committee promised to get right to work organizing the barrio committees. But at the first scheduled meeting of the central committee, only three members appeared, and this was symptomatic of what was to follow. After three weeks, only three of the seven barrio committees had been organized.

In the meantime, the doctor furnished by the Department of Health and Welfare arrived in Tepoztlán. A room in a house on the central plaza was obtained as an office. Essential equipment and medicines were purchased out of the first funds collected by the cooperative. Although no nurse was available, the social worker attached to the community research project assumed some of the nursing duties and accompanied the doctor on home visits. In addition to his clinic duties, the doctor worked in a research capacity with another part of the program, but he remained on call at all times for clinical services.

In line with our intention that the clinic serve a research function in addition to its service activities, it was planned that in addition and prior to the usual physical examination of each patient, the doctor should also use forms that called for the following kinds of information: a textual account of the history and causes of the diseases from the patient's point of view; whether the patient visited the curandero; the diagnoses and therapy of the curandero; the fees paid, and so on. The doctor was expected to utilize this information wherever possible in establishing rapport with the patient. Furthermore, it was hoped that in this way it would be possible systematically to obtain important data on native concepts of disease and therapy, and by comparing the diagnosis of the patient and the curandero with that of the doctor, to understand better the rationale behind native concepts.

Since funds from the cooperative came in slowly, the facilities of the clinic were never quite adequate. In addition, the first doctor furnished by the Department of Health and Welfare was a young, unmarried man whose previous experience was limited and had been confined to urban areas. Neither by training nor temperament was he particularly well fitted for the sensitive and demanding task of treating the people of a rural Mexican village. After a month, he was replaced by an older doctor with more experience.

However, our initial difficulties in getting a suitable physician and adequate equipment did not appear to trouble the prospective clients of the clinic. During the first week, as already indicated, the doctor had 11 patients, and subsequently the figure slowly increased to 35. Then quite suddenly, patients ceased to come altogether. For all intents and purposes, the clinic was through.

It would be tempting at this point to attribute the demise of the clinic to the inadequacies of its doctors and physical facilities and to look no further to find reasons for its downfall. But such an explanation would be partial at best. In the first place, the drop in attendance was abrupt and complete, not the gradual falling off one might expect to result from cumulative dissatisfactions.

Second, as we shall see, there are good reasons for believing that much the same thing would have happened even if the service had been excellent and the physical facilities exemplary. Although we cannot discount completely the effect of dissatisfaction over the quality of the clinical service, it will become apparent that other forces at work in Tepoztlán exerted greater influence. To discern the nature of these forces we must look to the general climate of the village, particularly the medical and political climate.

The Medical Climate of Tepoztlán

The trial clinic on the central plaza of Tepoztlán was not introduced into a medical vacuum. On the contrary, it found itself within a milieu of well-established medical beliefs and theories of disease and within a network of traditional practitioners whose curative techniques reflected these beliefs and theories.

There are three kinds of health practitioners in Tepoztlán—curanderos, *mágicos*, and "el doctor." Curanderos are the most numerous and are primarily women. They are visited most frequently and charge small fees of 25 or 50 centavos. There are two mágicos, men who may use the herb remedies of the women but also resort to spiritualism and magic and are feared for their great power. Their fees are higher, ranging between one and ten pesos. The curanderos and mágicos are, of course, Tepoztecans. However, "el doctor" is an outsider who has taken up residence in the village. He poses as a doctor but has no professional training. He charges fees as high as 100 pesos. Curanderos are sometimes paid in corn or other produce. This is one of the very few remnants of the old barter economy and indicates how closely the curandero system and the native economy were integrated. With the increasing dominance of a money economy there is now more cash available, and some families visit the doctors in Cuernavaca.

There was no resident doctor in 1943, but the villagers had had some previous experience with doctors and modern medicine. Two young Mexican doctors had spent six months each in the village in fulfillment of their training requirements for the doctor's degree. Public health teams had visited the village frequently since 1936 to administer injections against infectious diseases;

some Tepoztecans had visited the federal Public Health Station in nearby Cuernavaca, and a few of the local midwives had received some instruction from public health nurses.

For the majority of people, however, indigenous folk medicine as practiced by curanderos is still the dominant form of medicine. Thus, the traditional remedies for "evil eye" and "fright" involve a combination of folk beliefs, ancient herbal lore, and Catholic practice. A child is believed to be the victim of the evil eye if he comes home crying and very much disturbed. An egg is broken into a glass and if a long eye-shaped spot appears on the yolk, the person responsible for putting the eye upon the child is a man; if the spot is round, it is a woman. The child's clothes are changed and he is "cleansed" with a soiled kerchief or shirt if the guilty person was male, and with an apron or shawl if a female. Some children are cured by being cleansed on their foreheads, with the tongue making the form of a cross.

"Fright" is an illness which leaves children sad and pale; it is cured by women who can "lay the shadow" that afflicts them. These curanderos keep a supply of powdered cedar, palm, and blessed laurel which they throw on the forehead, breast, wrists, palms of the hand, nape of the neck, and into the nostrils of the sick child. While this is being done the woman prays the Credo, and at the end holds the child's head and cries out that the shadow should withdraw and that the child no longer need be frightened. Some cure fright by having the priest read the gospel over the child in the presence of the child's godparent of the same sex.

The most celebrated healer in Tepoztlán is one Rosalino Vargas, known as Don Rosas. He is also believed to be a powerful sorcerer and is feared by many of the villagers. Some people claim to have seen him riding through the village at midnight wearing a long black cape, with sparks issuing from his eyes and mouth. Don Rosas, who often uses the fear he inspires to his own advantage, has several enemies, at least three of whom made attempts to murder him in recent years. Don Rosas is wealthy and has a flourishing practice. He has seven female assistants; there is much gossip to the effect that these women are his paramours who sleep with him in turn, one for each day in the week. Don Rosas' loyal clientele insist that the seven women help him treat the sick and perform a series of mysterious devotions which he practices nearly every night.

The technique employed by Don Rosas on his patients contains an interesting combination of Catholic, pagan, and possibly African elements. He does not deal directly with a patient but gets information concerning the nature of the illness through an assistant who questions the patient. After the conference the patient is taken to a room which resembles a chapel in that it has an altar and images of saints. The patient is seated on a chair close to a heavy curtain behind which sits Don Rosas. The visitor is given an image of a saint to hold while the curandero prays and goes into a trance. When he is "as if dead" an assistant wafts incense smoke toward him and he begins to speak, as though from a deep sleep, telling what illness the patient is suffering from. Whether or not a cure is possible, is determined by a glass of water which has been placed among the images near the incense burner. If the water turns white there is hope for a cure, if black there is none.

If a remedy is possible, Don Rosas then points out the necessary steps to protect the individual and his family from the enemy who is provoking the symptoms. The patient must drink a sweet-sour tasting liquid, prepared by Don Rosas and stirred with a metal cross. The patient then pays two pesos for the cure but first must cleanse himself with the bills in the parts of his body which give him pain, and leave the money on the altar. Before leaving, the patient is given additional medicines to take each night and is generally advised to cleanse himself with very hot herb applications. More medicine is given as needed without charge and the patient is advised that the medicine must never be placed on the ground since it would lose its potency. Some patients need several consultations, all of which are conducted in the same manner, before they feel well again.

Although he does not hold any official municipal position, Don Rosas is a tremendous power in Tepoztlán because of his prestige and renown as a curer. There is little doubt that the introduction of a medical clinic in the center of his own community did not escape his watchful eye. Nor did it escape the notice of others in positions of power who did hold office. While the medical aspects of the clinic were of paramount concern to local health practitioners, its organizational aspects attracted the watchfulness of local political officials.

The Political Climate of Tepoztlán

The village of Tepoztlán is the largest of eight villages that comprise the municipality of Tepoztlán. It is the seat of the municipal government and as such is the most important administrative and political center of the municipality. The municipality of Tepoztlán is one of 27 municipios of the state of Morelos. It is governed by the state constitution which provides for "free municipios," local governments elected by popular vote.

The municipal government consists of the following officers: mayor, syndic, comptroller, secretary, treasurer, police chief, subpolice chief, justice of the peace, his secretary, and a porter. In addition, there are eight councilmen, each representing one of the wards of the village. The four major officials—mayor, syndic, comptroller, and justice of the peace—are elected by popular vote for a two-year period. The other officials are appointed by the mayor in agreement with the syndic and comptroller.

The duties of the major officials are determined by state law. Their manner of functioning depends upon their personalities. A meek mayor will serve only as a figurehead and allow the syndic and secretary to run the government. An aggressive mayor may take over the functions of the other officials. As executive officer, the mayor is the official representative of Tepoztlán in dealings with the outside. His signature is necessary for most correspondence and official acts. He sets the fines for infractions of the law; in addition, villagers often bring their private difficulties and family quarrels to him.

By far the greatest number of tasks falls to the secretary. He is generally the most literate of the officials. He opens and closes the government offices six days a week, signs all correspondence, attends all public functions, maintains the records of the municipio, advises the other officers of the state law, keeps the mayor informed of all complaints, and attends to all complaints and requests for certifications.

According to the law of the state of Morelos, Tepoztlán is supposed to be a free and autonomous political and administrative unit. In practice, however, the municipio appears more as an administrative dependency of the state governor. It is he who makes most of the municipio's major decisions, and decides local conflicts. There are no well-organized political parties in Tepoztlán; rather there are a number of loosely organized factions. This makes it necessary for every candidate for political office to play politics skillfully to obtain sufficient support from the unorganized electorate. Any recent incident or situation in the public eye is enlisted to further one's political fortunes. Municipal elections command much public attention and are bitterly fought.

When the medical clinic was established early in 1944, local politicians were looking ahead to the municipal elections in November. The mayor especially was worried about his position, since he had been temporarily jailed a short time before by the state governor for practicing nepotism. The comptroller, who had been appointed mayor pro tem, was most reluctant to relinquish this office when the mayor was released and ready to regain his post. Two councilmen with their eye on higher office had formed an "Education Committee" to espouse the construction of a new school and were hostile to the newly appointed principal of the existing school.

It was into this atmosphere of political intrigue and jockeying for power that the clinic happened to be introduced. It intruded directly or indirectly into the sphere of interest of important and influential figures in Tepoztlán—Don Rosas, the mayor, the comptroller, the Education Committee, the school principal, and others. Since none of these could claim credit for introducing this new public service and since its presence distracted the people from the coming elections and served as a reminder of how little the local officials did for the village, the clinic became the object of their attack. Each in his own way examined our project as a whole to find something that presented a vulnerable front for attack. They found it in the testing program.

The Attack on the Testing Program

When we arrived in Tepoztlán, we brought official letters to the principal of the school from the Minister of Education and the Director of Education in Cuernavaca—letters which recommended our project and asked for all necessary cooperation. We met with the principal and school staff to explain the purpose of the testing program and to describe briefly each of the tests. We also explained that each child to be tested would first be examined, fully clothed, by our doctors to determine the existence of any physical defects that might affect the psychological responses. The teachers and principal all expressed interest in the program and willingness to cooperate.

Among other things, the testing program included administration of the Rorschach test. In this test a standard series of figures resembling large ink blots printed on cards are shown to subjects. Since the blots are abstract in form, each subject can interpret them as he wills, much as one "sees" things in drifting clouds. We arranged to have four women of our staff give the various tests daily in the mornings. Since each selected child had to be tested four times, we were careful to space the tests so that no child was tested more than once a day. All of these tests were individual and had to be administered privately. There were no classrooms available for our use, so we had to do the best we could out of doors. The principal set up four tables for us in the courtyard of the school. The spot was by no means secluded, since six of the classrooms had windows and doors which faced it. At the open end of the court were a number of banana trees, behind which were the toilets. Thus, the court was seldom without passersby, and we were rarely alone.

For four months our investigation in the school and in the rest of the village proceeded smoothly with many manifestations of good will and cooperation on the part of the villagers. Then, quite unexpectedly, in April the principal of the school put an abrupt stop to all the testing, claiming that a small group of men and women had accused our workers of asking the children immoral questions and had threatened to stone them if they did not leave the village at once. The municipal authorities, without consulting us, had begun an "investigation" of these rumors and were calling witnesses and questioning them in such a way as to create more suspicion and to spread the gossip throughout the village.

The accusations were specifically as follows: that the testers were showing indecent pictures to the children; that the testers were taking the children off alone to the banana grove for the purpose of undressing them; that the doctor was undressing the girls for physical examinations.

This turn of affairs was a serious threat to the entire project. We set to work at once to investigate. We visited the principal of the school and went over each test in detail with him and with his staff. They all declared that the tests were in no way objectionable and that the accusations were unfounded. The principal explained that a mother had come to the school to tell him that her husband had forbidden her children to return to school because he thought they were losing too much time as a result of the testing program. The principal had asked her to send her children back and he promised to end the testing. In checking the chronology of events, we learned that the principal had ordered the testing program stopped two days before the mother appeared at the school.

The principal went on to say that a few days after he was visited by the mother, a committee of 12 men and women came to the school to protest against the "immoral" tests which we were giving their children. The leaders of this group were members of the Education Committee, the bitter enemy of the school that had been attacking the principal ever since he had arrived in Tepoztlán. After visiting the school, the Committee went to the town hall, where they persuaded the mayor to institute an investigation.

We spoke with the two councilmen who were the leaders of the Committee and showed them the tests. They agreed that they were not immoral but stated that this was no proof that our workers were not asking other questions not included in the tests. They said they were of the opinion that the tests were too complicated and too advanced for so backward a people and were bound to be misinterpreted by them. This device of citing ignorance of the people as a reason for rejecting innovations was frequently used by the conservatives in the village. We urged them to put a stop to the mayor's "investigation," but they refused. A talk with the mayor was equally unsuccessful. He was continuing the investigation with enthusiasm, evidently impelled by motives of his own. He turned a deaf ear to our explanations and was noncommittal during the interview. The municipal secretary, one of the few Tepoztecan women to hold this post, was a religious fanatic and was much disliked in the village. She had a great deal of influence over the mayor and was conducting the investigation for him.

That evening we were visited by a man who introduced himself as "Antonio Lopez, a Christian, and a friend of the Tepoztecans." He had a marked military manner, clicked his heels, and spoke with a German accent. He said he was a friend of one of the leaders of the Education Committee and wished to warn us that he did not like the work we were doing in Tepoztlán. He said that, although it was true that for the present Mexico and the United States were friendly, he was of the opinion that the situation would not last long and that the people were suspicious of our motives. In the course of our conversation, he also lamented the fact that education was no longer in the hands of the church but said that, too, might be changed in the future. We later learned that this man was part German and had been educated in Germany. He was a Synarchist and four years before had been ordered out of Tepoztlán by the state governor because he was behaving like a Nazi agent.

Synarchism is a well-organized political movement, the Mexican brand of Fascism. Although it has received the support of and worked closely with Nazi and Falangist elements since its inception, it is nevertheless a grass-roots movement with a large peasant base. In 1943 the strength of the Synarchist membership was estimated at well over a million. Tepoztlán was marginal to the regions of Synarchist concentration, but nearby towns had suffered from Synarchist-inspired uprisings in protest against the government program of conscription.

We appealed to a state senator who was a native of Tepoztlán and who happened to be living in the village at the time. He offered to help us, and we arranged to go to the state governor with him the following morning. The governor was not in Cuernavaca, and we had to speak to his aide. We told him our story, and he was satisfied with our explanations. He wrote a strong letter addressed to the mayor of Tepoztlán stating that our study was a Mexican government project and had the full approval of the governor of Morelos. He added that the accusations against us were unfounded, and ordered the cessation of the investigation. He also asked the authorities to detain Antonio Lopez and to bring him to Cuernavaca for questioning. We were encouraged by the cooperation and friendliness of the governor's aide and thought that the whole matter would soon be cleared up.

We returned to Tepoztlán and presented the letter of the governor's aide to the municipal secretary, since the mayor himself was not in, as usual. Her response was that the investigation would continue, that Lopez was not in the village (although we had seen him), that in her opinion Lopez was a friend of the Tepoztecans, and that nothing could be done to molest him.

We learned that day of the manner in which the village investigation was being conducted. The head of one of the local families working with us received a peremptory order from the mayor to present himself at the town hall within a half-hour. He was asked to tell what immoral questions the project social worker who lived in his house was asking. This man's daughter, aged thirteen, was taken into a room by the woman secretary and was asked, "Is it not true that the workers are asking you bad questions?" When the girl denied this, the secretary told her not to be ashamed and to speak to her as a woman. She said, "Is it not true that the doctor undressed you? What bad things did you talk about in the banana grove?" With such procedures, the secretary succeeded in aggravating the situation and in arousing more people against our work.

With the cooperation of the state senator, we arranged a hearing at the town hall with the two councilmen for the following day. When we arrived, we found the room filled with people— about 25 women in addition to the two men. We knew that it was impossible to have a calm hearing with these women and suspected another maneuver on the part of the local secretary and the mayor. However, we had to proceed. We took the names of all the women present and found that not one of them had a child who had been tested by us. We then read the questions of our tests, and one of our workers made a moving speech, which seemed to calm the women. However, the secretary brought in a surprise witness, a girl of twelve, whom she had succeeded in intimidating. The child was frightened, tense, and on the verge of tears. She stated that we had asked her the questions we had been accused of asking (she repeated those mentioned above), and her words once more aroused the women in the audience. We produced the test of this particular child and wanted to read her responses, but the secretary shouted that no one wanted to hear the immoral answers and that we would read only the good things and leave out the bad. The women began to shout and some began to cry.

The mayor then arose and said that it was clear that we were not wanted in the village and that under no circumstances should we continue with our work. We answered that this group was only a tiny minority of the village and did not represent the true village opinion. We asked the mayor to call a meeting of the entire village so that we could demonstrate the sentiment of the people; he agreed to call a larger meeting for the following Sunday. As the meeting began to break up, the secretary asked to see the Rorschach cards which we had shown earlier to the women without comment from them. The secretary said she had seen things in the cards which proved her point and that she would like to show them to those present. She thereupon began to point out the sexual organs and phallic symbols which she "saw" in almost every one of the ten amorphous designs—this, in spite of the fact that there were men present. It is interesting to note that claiming to see sexual objects in the cards occurred very rarely in the 125 Rorschachs given to children and adults in Tepoztlán. By her actions, the secretary unconsciously revealed her own personality and helped to explain her behavior. This demonstration naturally agitated the women further.

We left this meeting with a feeling that things were going from bad to worse. However, we were later visited by a group of Tepoztecans, who said that they were very much ashamed of the way these people were behaving and said that the same thing happened time and again whenever an attempt was made to improve the village. We decided to see the governor, but again he was inaccessible, and we proceeded to Mexico City to advise Dr. G, director of the Inter-American Indian Institute and sponsor of our project. Dr. G pointed out that cultural missions in the past had run into similar or more serious difficulties in the villages. Dr. G and the senator thereupon conferred with high government officials who gave us a letter to the governor of Morelos, and we set out for Cuernavaca to see him.

Our interview with the governor was both a surprise and a disappointment. At first he said that he had never heard of our project. We made the necessary explanations and told him of our recent difficulties. He thereupon said that the United States owed Mexico a great debt because of our imperialistic history and that Americans should be more "loyal" to Mexicans than vice versa. Americans do not understand Mexicans and cannot get along with them. In connection with Antonio Lopez, he observed that Nazi doctrine, "because of its belief in order and authority," had a much greater appeal to the peasants than did our American democracy. We left the meeting with the realization that we could expect nothing from the governor. However, he said he wanted to send his aide to the planned meeting on Sunday.

Upon our return to Tepoztlán, we were again visited by the group of friendly Tepoztecans. They came to advise us against attending the Sunday meeting and suggested that the proper procedure would be to have the governor call the two councilmen to Cuernavaca for a talk and a cooling-off period, charging them with defamation of honor. We agreed with them but said we did not want to use such methods. Furthermore, it was too late for us to prevent the meeting. The group then offered to bring about 200 men and women to the meeting to support us. At their suggestion, we agreed to accompany them to the governor's aide before the meeting in order to present him with their point of view.

This man, probably advised by the governor, spoke to us in a very different manner during this second visit. He declared before our committee of Tepoztecans that he had never heard of our project nor of the Inter-American Indian Institute and scolded us for not informing his office of our mission. We reminded him that we had presented the governor with a letter from Dr. G and had received an acknowledgment of the same, and that we had been accompanied at the time by the senator, who also introduced us. The governor's aide flatly denied all we said and asked his clerk to look up the letters in the file. I reminded him that we had a letter written by him on our behalf addressed to the mayor of Tepoztlán. The clerk said the letters were not in the file but that she would look again.

Encouraged by this, the governor's aide continued to berate us and said that in all probability we did not know how to get along with Mexican peasants. He said that as technicians we probably were not sufficiently *simpático* and that we should have known that our tests and ink blots were bound to suggest sexual and immoral symbols to rustic people. The clerk had by this time found the letters in question, and the governor's aide changed his tone a bit. However, his performance had a depressing effect on our Tepoztecan friends, who had believed that we had the strong support of the government, and the situation was quite embarrassing. The governor's aide said he would attend the Sunday meeting and would settle the entire matter for us. Although the governor's aide, the senator, and the school principal all promised to speak in our favor and defend our work on Sunday, we were by this time skeptical of promises and awaited the meeting with curiosity but with little hope.

The Sunday meeting drew only about a hundred persons, in spite of the fact that the mayor and his assistants visited every home in the village to persuade the residents to be present against us. Of the hundred, the majority were friendly to our project. However, the same 25 women and the two hostile councilmen grouped themselves about the speakers and were the only ones of the assembly who could make themselves heard. There were very few other women present because, as we were told later, no decent woman would attend such a meeting. The rest of the village had the impression that only those who were against us were supposed to come.

All three speakers, the governor's aide, the senator, and the school principal, made ingratiating speeches full of demagogic promises and without a word in our defense. The governor's aide said he was proud of these mothers who defended their children with such zeal and that he would see that the testing program would not continue. He urged the people to be patient, as we were winding up our work and would soon leave the village. The senator avoided the subject of our project entirely, while the principal sought to gain the good will of the village by stating that as soon as he heard we were doing indecent things he stopped the testing immediately for, above all, he was eager to guard the children entrusted to his care. Our friends, who had gathered there to speak for us, thought that it was useless to do so in view of the attitude of the main speakers, so not a good word was put in except by ourselves.

Shortly after the meeting, we were visited by a delegation from the organization of the poor-land farmers, who had supported us throughout our difficulties, and by a delegation of those who worked the communal lands. They spoke with great feeling and said that we were the objects of a political intrigue. They said the women did not represent more than a small minority and that they were widows or spinsters, because no man would permit his wife to behave in so scandalous a manner. They asked us to stay on and continue our work in Tepoztlán, and they believed that the whole thing would blow over in a few weeks and that no one would molest us. They offered to circulate a petition and get 600 signatures to convince us that we should continue our beneficial work. We agreed and asked them to address it to Dr. G and the Institute. In a few days, they brought us about 200 names, saying that they could not get any more because the mayor had heard of what they were doing and began to threaten the people who signed.

As a result of this affair, our entire testing program was temporarily suspended. Our research staff continued to interview informants and devoted themselves to writing up their backlog of material. Little by little, however, we increased our activities and succeeded in giving more tests in the homes. When assignments of our research workers ended and they had to leave the village, they were given warm send-offs by their Tepoztecan friends, departing for their homes elsewhere in Mexico loaded with gifts and with invitations to return.

What Lay Behind the Attack

What lay behind the attack on the testing program? The mayor, the secretary, the school principal, the two councilmen on the Education Committee, and others who openly denounced the program justified their opposition on the grounds that the tests were immoral. Some of those who opposed the program may sincerely have believed this, but there is ample reason to believe that other reasons were of equal or greater importance. We have already seen that there were a number of highly influential people in Tepoztlán who saw in the clinic a threat to their own position and that there were others who saw the presence of active outsiders as an opportunity to advance their own political interests.

In the former category the outstanding person was Don Rosas, Tepoztlán's most eminent curandero. In spite of the power and prestige he enjoys, Don Rosas cannot help see the gradual and inexorable advance of modern medicine into rural Mexico as a threat to his position. Opening the clinic in the central plaza of Tepoztlán placed his enemy on his front doorstep; the very first patients to visit the clinic were those whose ailments had not responded to treatment by the curanderos. Although Don Rosas himself did not play an active part in the various meetings where the hostility of the villagers to the program was expressed, he was an active influence behind the scenes. Not only did he agitate the mayor, the secretary, and others, but he was directly responsible for the rumor that indecent pictures were being shown.

When the clinic was first established, it was immediately seen by Don Rosas as a threat, and one to be eliminated by any means. But he was too clever to risk an open attack on a venture that was patently humanitarian and had already received the support of a substantial number of villagers. Casting around for the best strategy, he hit upon the testing program as the logical target. The purposes of psychological testing were difficult for many villagers to grasp. Moreover, the pictures shown on one of the tests were highly ambiguous in form and subject to all sorts of interpretations. Don Rosas made a trip to Mexico City and there purchased a set of pornographic pictures. Upon his return he showed these pictures around the village, telling the parents,

"*These* are the pictures they are showing your children! *This* is what they call science!"

Don Rosas was not the only influential figure in Tepoztlán who saw the clinic as a threat. Its inception was a danger signal to the mayor, and through him to the state senator and state governor, all of whom had already been alerted to the disruptive potentialities of the research team by a previous incident.

We had been in Tepoztlán one month, when a committee of poor-land farmers appealed to us to aid them in a boundary dispute with a neighboring village. The communal land was involved and if the dispute was lost, 200 families might face destitution. In spite of the fact that communal land was in question, neither the mayor nor the senator was doing anything about the case. The poor-land farmers claimed that these two officials were acting on the orders of, or out of fear of, the state governor, who they said had an interest in a large cement factory which obtained its fuel from the forests located on the disputed land. The committee had come to us because we happened to have an attorney on our staff. We explained that we could not help them officially or appear in court for them, but that our lawyer could advise them privately, as a friend. We made this decision because many of the families involved had been cooperating with us in our study of family life. Also, we felt that the dispute was a real threat to a large group of Tepoztecans and to the entire village. An investigation convinced us that their claims were just, and we felt obligated to do what we could. The word got around, and apparently the state governor and the senator, as well as the mayor, interpreted our decision as strengthening the hand of political forces opposed to the established powers.

When the clinic was set up, people began to say that the project members were doing more for their welfare than their own mayor was doing. This was ample grounds for mobilizing the opposition of the mayor, already made wary by the communal land incident. Don Rosas would have had little difficulty in persuading the mayor to direct the power of his office against the program. Perceiving the service activities of the project as a threat to their interests, Don Rosas, the mayor, and the governor instigated or supported feeling against the project.

Another group of influential figures decided to capitalize on this resentment, once aroused, to further their own political fortunes. Municipal elections were to be held in a few months. In addition to the mayor, who hoped to exploit public indignation over "immorality" to gain reelection, one of the two councilmen who headed the Education Committee was hoping to become mayor and promoted resentment for similar reasons. These two men became the spearhead of the attack on the project.

The opposition of the school principal was related to the activities of the Education Committee. The principal, newly appointed to Tepoztlán, was being opposed at every turn by the Education Committee. This group charged the principal with being immoral and a Communist, because he allowed special dances to be given in the school for the purpose of raising funds. The Committee had opposed innovations in the school and was engaging in obstructive activities. Our presence provided further grounds for fighting the school.

The eagerness of the principal in stopping the testing program without consulting us or investigating the charges could have been attributed to his fear of the Education Committee. However, he had ordered our workers out of the school before a single complaint had been made. One of the teachers told us that the principal, in an effort to ingratiate himself with the Education Committee and represent himself as a defender of morality, went to them with accusations against us, which they eagerly took up and carried further, since they had been looking for some grounds for attacking our project. Arranging the visit of the mothers to the school and the town hall was their way of carrying out plans to persuade the mayor to conduct an investigation and to arouse the village.

The actions of the Education Committee were also tied to Antonio Lopez, the Synarchist organizer. He had succeeded, years before, in converting the two councilmen who headed the Education Committee. At one time these men had openly proclaimed themselves as Synarchists, but recently had ceased doing so although they still were intimates of Lopez. These men had branded our group "an imperialist mission," and their anti-U. S. sentiments provided further incentive for their opposition to us.

In brief, our well-intentioned efforts to win the cooperation of the villagers by helping them solve some of their problems were interpreted by several local figures as a personal threat.

By advising the poor-land farmers we unwittingly were helping the faction out of power; by establishing the clinic we were implicitly reproaching the "do-nothings" in power. The testing program, whose purposes were only vaguely comprehended and only indirectly beneficial to the people, provided a vulnerable target, and it was here that hostility aroused by the introduction of the medical clinic could be played out.

The strategy was effective. The loudly expressed indignation of the officials and a small but vocal group of villagers succeeded in intimidating the rest of the people for a period of time. The clinic languished and we made no attempt to reestablish it. The testing program was stopped in the school but continued quietly in the homes; in the six months that followed, the research program was carried out without further disturbance.

Cooperatives, Individualism, and Politics

We have already seen that inadequacies in the facilities of the clinic had little bearing on its failure. In fact, one might speculate that the clinic would have aroused even greater opposition had it been medically more effective. If so humble an example of modern medicine could provoke disruptive antagonism, a well-equipped clinic, better able to meet the needs of the villagers, might have posed an even greater threat to those in power.

It is also possible that less opposition would have been aroused had we not decided to organize the clinic on a cooperative basis. We have already given the rationale for deciding on the cooperative type of organization. Had we known then what we found out later, we would have reconsidered our decision. However, the very fact that we acted as we did set into motion events that gave us additional insights into the culture of Tepoztlán.

The Mexican Revolution had far-reaching effects upon Tepoztlán. It succeeded in breaking down the rigid social class distinctions which once existed in the village and imbued the people with a consciousness of their rights as individuals. The strong individualism of Tepoztecans manifests itself in their social and economic institutions. The biological family is the more or less self-sufficient and independent economic unit. Social relations between families and even close relatives are formal and distant. Land is owned individually, and even the communal lands are worked individually. Work exchange is uncommon; wage labor prevails in intra-village relations. Occasions upon which either men or women cooperate in their daily tasks are few. Before the Spanish conquest more than 400 years ago, there existed a system of cooperative labor called *cuatequitl* which was used for the building of village public works, but it was never a purely voluntary organization and has now almost completely disintegrated.

Practically the only occasions upon which the Tepoztecans have shown either a willingness or capacity to work together has been in connection with their fiestas and when their communal lands were threatened. But even in regard to the latter, there is growing disunity. In the land dispute previously described, only those individuals whose interests were directly affected took measures to protect themselves.

Another reason the cooperative form was not appropriate to Tepoztlán relates to the great complexity of social, economic, political, and religious cleavages among the villagers. There are landless peons and wealthy farmers; literate and sophisticated merchants of the central plaza and illiterate and primitive farmers of the outlying barrios; the sons of the families that dominated Tepoztlán prior to the Revolution and the very Zapatistas who overthrew them; the fanatic believers in the old Catholic religion as practiced in Tepoztlán with its elements of paganism, and a Protestant sect which has succeeded in winning almost an entire barrio as adherents; sympathizers of Synarchism on the one hand and sympathizers of the left-wing labor movement on the other. In addition to all this, within many families there are differences between the younger and older generations which reflect the rapid changes taking place in the village.

IMPLICATIONS

Our experience in Tepoztlán suggests a number of more general problems concerning the comprehensiveness of village research and improvement programs, the type of doctors suitable for work in rural areas, the role of local organizational patterns, and the significance of the local balance of power.

Combined Programs

From the standpoint of our research aims, it seemed desirable to provide the services of a medical clinic to gain good will and cooperation. Conversely, the psychological testing program seemed warranted, quite apart from its value as a social science research tool, as one means of understanding the people's attitudes and behavior in order to have a better basis for predicting the outcome of health and betterment programs. Thus, a combination of research and service programs held out the promise of better results than could be expected from either activity alone. At the same time, each was capable—as it turned out—of arousing overt or covert opposition which could be directed against the other. It might be argued that a limitation of activity in the village would expose a smaller flank for attack. The merits and handicaps of mixing research and service are difficult to assess apart from the particular situation. Even in a specific case, as in Tepoztlán, the fact that one course of action encountered trouble does not necessarily imply that an opposite course would have been more successful.

A more positive stand can be taken on the issue of whether a medical care program would thrive better if it were introduced by itself or if it were made part of a more comprehensive improvement program. While it is possible that a more general approach might threaten more interests and thus incite a more general counter attack, it is also clear that even a very limited program of modern medical care such as was attempted in Tepoztlán would have great difficulty sustaining itself so long as the villagers remain as poor as they are. Even the modest fee of one peso charged by the cooperative proved too much for many. Financial means is not the whole answer, but it is a necessary element in the totality of factors affecting the success or failure of a medical service clinic. The spread of modern medicine hinges, among other things, on increasing the income of the villagers and is related to the larger problem of raising the standard of living by increasing purchasing power. This in turn requires an action program wider than health improvement by itself.

Introducing Modern Medicine in Rural Mexico

Despite their high degree of acculturation, the majority of Tepoztecans are not ready to give up their curanderos. However, they are ready to consider the doctor an alternative, especially in cases of chronic or serious illnesses. This was clearly shown by the fact already mentioned that the doctor's first patients were persons who suffered from chronic illnesses which apparently had not responded to the treatment of the curanderos. Because of this circumstance the doctor begins with a handicap. Unable to produce miraculous cures in these far-gone cases, he loses prestige.

There is a great lack of confidence in doctors, partly because so many of them display an attitude of superiority toward native concepts of disease and often ridicule native beliefs and practices. Indeed, the Tepoztecans, as well as the doctors, are keenly aware of their different conceptual worlds. This is undoubtedly a serious obstacle to the spreading of modern medical practice and unless the gap between these two distinct levels of explanation is bridged, progress will be very slow.

A few examples from Tepoztlán will help to make this clear. According to Tepoztecans, there are "hot" and "cold" diseases, just as there are "hot" and "cold" foods. A mother who is convinced that her child is suffering from a hot disease brought on by the adultery of her husband, knows that the child needs a cold medicine. If she goes to a curandero, she tells him that the child is suffering from a hot disease, but if she goes to a doctor she says nothing. If the doctor's medicine does not improve the child, the mother attributes it to the fact that the doctor did not understand the nature of the illness and gave the child a hot medicine instead of a cold medicine.

On the other hand, if the curandero does not effect a cure, her explanation is of a different kind. She now believes that the heat of the disease was so great that there was no medicine cold enough to counteract it; her faith in the curandero and distrust of the doctor continue. In the case of the illnesses supposedly caused by humors or spirits of the air, most Tepoztecans are reluctant to visit a doctor because of their conviction that doctors do not understand either the cause or the cure of such diseases.

Governed by their own interpretation of illness, people in the village approach modern doctors with distrust, realizing that they do not fully understand certain classes of illness, such as those due to evil humors or those related to the hot-cold distinction. It is, therefore, important for the doctor to become familiar with the native concepts and to utilize them as a psychological means of gaining confidence. The job of establishing rapport and gaining confidence under these conditions is no easy one. It demands a doctor who has the zeal and spirit of a missionary and some understanding of the relativity of cultural values.

Aside from factors of personality and of understanding local beliefs, the ability of a doctor to gain confidence and prestige depends upon his technical skill in making accurate diagnoses and effecting cures. While it is unfair to generalize about the quality of Mexican rural doctors as a whole, our impression from personal experience is that they are poorly trained and equipped and show little enthusiasm for work in the villages. Considering the conditions under which rural doctors must live and work in Mexico, it is probable that this phenomenon is more widespread. There is little incentive for the superior doctor to leave the city and go to rural areas. At best, few are willing to undergo the hardships of rural life with its isolation and lack of comforts and diversions; in addition, salaries are low, opportunities for advancement are few, and there is little permanency of assignment. As a result of these conditions, rural doctors are frequently recruited from those of inferior abilities and this in turn makes it more difficult to win over the Indian villager to modern medicine.

Local Organizational Patterns

Any attempt to revive or establish a "democratic" institution, such as a cooperative in a community that has lived for years under an authoritative system, must take cognizance of the profound effect of this conditioning to authority upon the psychology of the people. The lack of personal initiative and village spirit found in Tepoztlán may be attributed to this conditioning. Our experience made it clear that chances for success would have been better if we had operated according to current organizational practices. Had the doctors been brought in to set up a private clinic rather than a cooperative, there might have been less difficulty. Previous attempts to set up cooperatives in other activities had met with similar or more drastic difficulties. In 1930 Tepoztlán organized a Forestry Cooperative for the production and sale of charcoal. It lasted only a few years, for the village divided into hostile political factions. The officers of the cooperative were suspected of stealing funds, the president was murdered, and the cooperative dissolved. A more recent cooperative to run the bus line between Tepoztlán and Cuernavaca also is rent by dissension and violence.

The results in Tepoztlán lead to the conclusion that the introduction of modern medicine should not be attempted through the mechanism of cooperatives in regions where a long-standing cooperative tradition is lacking. The more general lesson is that programs, to be practical, are not to be devised according to an ideal organizational model, however much this model may appeal to program planners, but must take account of the organizational pattern familiar to the people of the particular community.

Entrenched Power

Those who enter a community to engage in an action program must recognize the implications of the fact that they are not entering a power vacuum. In every human community there exists a network of relations between individuals. It is to the interest of many of these individuals to maintain this system of relationships. Any group of outsiders moving into a community will be seen by some as potentially disruptive, even if they plan no action. If they do plan action, whatever positive measures they undertake, no matter how benign, will be perceived by some community members as a threat to their own status and interests.

It is tempting to attribute the antagonism of these people and their obstructive activities to the fact that they are wicked people, opposing common good because of selfish motives. Even if this were so, the frequency of such obstruction makes it reasonable to anticipate its occurrence and to be able to cope with it realistically.

It may appear to some that the downfall of the clinic in Tepoztlán can be attributed simply and directly to the personal antagonism of Don Rosas. Already worried that his power and position of privilege would be undermined if modern medicine got a foothold in the village, he immediately viewed the clinic as a competitor and resorted to unscrupulous methods to bring about its downfall. This is undoubtedly true, but can the clinic's downfall be simply attributed to the personal villainy of one man?

Don Rosas' actions were motivated by the fact that he belonged to a profession that was being slowly crowded out by newer and more modern techniques. There is no reason to believe that any of the other curanderos in the village felt differently about the clinic. But since Don Rosas was more powerful than the others, he was in a better position to do something about his antagonism. Rather than an evil individual, Don Rosas can be taken as a symbol of the traditional practitioner everywhere who is being deprived of his status and importance by the advance of modern medicine.

But aside from the threat to traditional medicine, we have seen that Don Rosas was not alone in opposing the clinic. In fact, virtually every established political figure in Tepoztlán—the mayor, the school principal, the councilmen, the secretary, and others— had or found reasons for sabotaging the clinic. If we are to attribute personal villainy to Don Rosas, we must do the same for the whole of Tepoztlán officialdom. And we must also include the governor and senator of the state of Morelos. Rather than conclude that this just happened to be a particularly corrupt regime and expect the next one to be different, it would seem more rational to consider this state of affairs as something inherent in the culture of Tepoztlán and, in fact, of many communities.

Instead of explaining the attack on the medical clinic in Tepoztlán as the unscrupulous work of a fortuitous aggregation of villains, it would be more realistic to regard it as a special case of a general response to the introduction of any new enterprise into an established community. Whenever the activities of an outside group—health team, research project, or any enterprise affecting the pattern of interpersonal relations within a community

—are perceived by those in power as threatening their position, they will attempt directly or indirectly to undermine the efforts of that group.

SUMMARY

When our research team came to the Mexican village of Tepoztlán to study its culture and its people, the residents asked us to help them in a practical way, pointing out that they lacked a doctor, among other things. The Mexican government supplied a doctor for a six-month term, and we helped the community establish a medical cooperative that might be able to persist as a going concern even after we left the village. Despite the fact that the cooperative seemed to meet an expressed need and despite its initial success as judged by attendance, the clinic quite suddenly lost patronage and was abandoned.

Compared with carefully planned, government-sponsored health and medical programs in underdeveloped areas, our small-scale endeavor which grew out of the needs of a research project was clearly a minor, almost amateur, effort. Nevertheless, this case study highlights a number of principles and problems to be found in most attempts to introduce modern medicine into so-called backward areas of the world.

This case throws light upon the dynamic forces at work in a peasant community which, on the surface, appears simple and static. It shows quite clearly that the success or failure of a medical program depends on many cultural factors besides the competence of doctors and the quality of services. The major obstacles encountered in the Tepoztlán case were these: readiness to distrust innovations and a generalized lack of interest in changing local ways of doing things; inadequacy of economic resources, even the one peso fee being too high for many villagers; lack of rapport between doctors and patients resting on the doctors' ignorance of native illness concepts and an attitude of superiority; continued faith of the villagers in their local curanderos; finally, and perhaps most important, readiness of local interest groups, headed by the leading curandero, to view the medical cooperative as a threat to their power.

SELECTED REFERENCES

Gruening, Ernest, *Mexico and Its Heritage*. Century Co., New York, 1928. An excellent overall history of Mexico tracing the major social, economic, and political events since pre-Hispanic times.

Lewis, Oscar, *Life in a Mexican Village:* Tepoztlán Restudied. University of Illinois Press, Urbana, 1951. A comprehensive description of village life with an analysis of the changes which have occurred since Robert Redfield's earlier study of 1926–1927.

Redfield, Robert, *Tepoztlán:* A Mexican Village. University of Chicago Press, 1930. A pioneer study of a Mexican village especially good for the detailed description of the fiesta cycle.

Tannenbaum, Frank, *Mexico, the Struggle for Peace and Bread*. Alfred A. Knopf, New York, 1950. A concise survey of Mexico's sociology, politics, economics, and psychology by a leading historian who has had almost three decades of familiarity with the country.

Whetten, Nathan L., *Rural Mexico*. University of Chicago Press, 1948. A comprehensive description and analysis of rural Mexico, which provides an excellent background and frame of reference for the understanding of a particular village like Tepoztlán.

Case 16

A NUTRITIONAL RESEARCH PROGRAM IN GUATEMALA
by Richard N. Adams

Public health and medicine push forward on two fronts at the same time —service and research. The first study in this volume, for example, describes a program for improving the diet of a South African population; this service program makes use of existing nutritional knowledge. At the same time, research specialists in other places are striving to increase the store of scientific information on the effect of specific nutritional elements on human growth so that health workers in Africa and elsewhere eventually can offer their communities still better services. The present study by Dr. Adams concerns a program of nutritional research that was carried out in Guatemala.

*The experimental design required that school children in each of several villages receive a different combination of nutrients and submit periodically to examinations to determine their nutritional status. When one of the communities threatened to withdraw prematurely from the experiment, Dr. Adams was called in to discover the cause of trouble and overcome the resistance. As the study indicates, he found many sources of difficulty, including dissatisfaction with a medical clinic which had been instituted as a service adjunct to the nutritional research program. Curiously, elimination of short-run services in this community contributed to the survival of an experiment which, along with others if its kind, may lead to the improvement of community health programs in the long run.—*EDITOR

THE PROBLEM

Locating Sources of Antagonism to an Experimental Feeding Program

In the years since the end of World War II, public health activity in Latin America has increased substantially. Support from the World Health Organization and the Pan American Sanitary Bureau has made it possible to expand existing projects and to institute new ones. Among these new projects was an experimental program undertaken by the Nutritional Institute of Central America and Panama, known as INCAP (*Instituto de Nutrición de Centro América y Panamá*). The officials of INCAP felt that a

435

critical weakness of some of the older Latin American health projects lay in their failure to recognize the relevance of local social and cultural conditions. Many programs had been carried out in communities whose way of life was very different from that of the professional people who staffed the projects, people who frequently lacked the insight into local culture necessary for effective work in these communities.

Late in 1950 research workers in Magdalena, a small farming village in the Guatemalan highlands, reported to INCAP headquarters that their nutritional research project involving school children had run into considerable difficulty. Villagers were becoming increasingly antagonistic to members of the field team; rumors had been circulated that the project was pursuing subversive political purposes; parents complained that their children were being harmed. Some subjects of the program failed to keep appointments, and worse, extremists threatened to have the field team expelled from the village.

In an effort to meet this crisis, INCAP sent an anthropologist to Magdalena. Project workers told him that the villagers were unwilling to cooperate, but they found it difficult to point to the reasons for this attitude or to specify the sources of resistance. The anthropologist was faced with the task of answering this question: What was behind the antagonism of the villagers to a fact-finding program intended for their own benefit?

THE SITUATION

Conducting Nutritional Research in a Rural Community

In 1950, before the anthropologist joined the staff, INCAP had initiated a project of providing food supplements to school children in five Indian villages in the Department of Sacatepéquez. The project was part of a program to determine what supplemental food elements, if any, were needed to improve the local diet, which appeared to be deficient in animal proteins. Certain identical measures were carried out in all five villages. In each community the school children were divided into groups, usually two or three in number, and these groups were provided with regular daily nutritional supplements or placebos.

This feeding program required that the children be brought together at a certain time each day and be given food supplements under the supervision of a trained member of the field team. In some villages a midmorning snack was also given to determine the nutritional value of additive vegetable proteins. At periodic intervals it was necessary to give each child in the program a physical examination in order to gauge results. The most important items of information obtained from these examinations were height, weight, and blood data. At the initiation of the project and at suitable intervals, a more complete examination, including x-rays, was given.

When INCAP began its work, the program director recognized that positive cooperation by village authorities, school officials, parents, and school children would be necessary if the project was to be carried on long enough to produce scientifically valid results. Absenteeism by the participating school children had to be kept at a minimum. To help achieve these ends, INCAP had employed a Guatemalan social worker with training and experience in the United States and Guatemala. She tried to encourage cooperation by organizing various community activities.

As a further step in gaining community cooperation, INCAP had set up a medical clinic in each of the trial villages. It was felt that providing this service in an area where medical resources were scarce would enhance the value of INCAP in the eyes of the villagers and induce them to cooperate more fully with the nutritional research program. The clinic service provided a full-time nurse, who remained in the village the better part of each day. In addition, a doctor visited the village two or three days a week to see cases referred by the nurse or the social worker. The nurse and doctor were instructed to treat only those cases that could be handled by the facilities of the clinic. More serious cases, such as those involving complicated examinations or surgery, were to be referred to the departmental hospital in the city of Antigua.

In January, 1951, when the anthropologist joined the INCAP program, the experiment was proceeding satisfactorily in four of the five participating villages. In Magdalena, the fifth village, the program's existence was threatened, as already indicated, by the growing recalcitrance of the villagers. INCAP personnel working in Magdalena at that time included a nurse, who made daily visits to the INCAP clinic; the project social worker, who spent the major part of her time in this particular village; and a doctor, who visited the village periodically. When the anthropologist joined the program, it was decided that he should carry out his research work independently and not become associated with the service activities of the social worker. It was felt that involving too many people in these activities would increase chances of misunderstanding. The anthropologist was placed in overall charge of the social worker, but the latter remained responsible for carrying on her own field activities.

This arrangement worked out well. The social worker consulted regularly with the anthropologist, discussing her current and projected activities. The anthropologist, on his part, concentrated on obtaining background information on the economy, social organization, beliefs, and values of the Indians. The social worker, the nurse, and other temporary personnel helped to collect these data. As information was gathered, a picture of the general culture of the village was drawn. On the basis of this information, decisions were made concerning policies and methods to be adopted by the clinic team and the social worker.

At only one point in the program was it found necessary to diverge from this procedure. This occurred, as will be related, when the entire INCAP team was suspected of being involved in nefarious political activities. Aside from this incident, however, the separation of research and action functions worked smoothly and proved well adapted to the needs of the INCAP project.

The Magdaleño Way of Life

From the point of view of the anthropologist, the program in Magdalena was regarded as a meeting ground of two cultures. The personnel of INCAP came to Magdalena as Central and North Americans with goals characteristic of their occidental culture. Public health, nutrition, and scientific experiment are important concerns in this culture; they are not important in Guatemalan Indian culture. The Magdaleños, for their part, carried on their customary daily life—maintaining their homes, growing maize and beans for consumption, making charcoal for cash income, and the like. Understanding some of the basic features of this way of life will supply insight into the reasons for the antagonism of the villagers to the INCAP program.

Despite the fact that each Indian village has its distinctive features, Magdalena is fairly representative of the numerous villages in the Guatemalan highlands. The chief interests of the Indians lie in three principal areas: their individualistic economy, their family life, and their religious activities.

The family is the basic economic unit. The members of each household work for that household alone, and there is little cooperation between family units in the production of maize and other economic goods. This economic independence of each family is highly valued by the villagers. Just as the household is the center of economic life, it is also the center of social life. The greater part of a person's time is spent with his family. Except when village or religious matters are pressing, evenings are spent at home. During the day the men, like farmers the world over, labor in the fields or are off working to earn extra money. The women visit among themselves, but this is usually done only when there is some legitimate reason. After the family, the village is the next most important unit of organization. Municipal service is an acknowledged requirement for all adult males. Age provides the ordering of authority, and among those of the same age-group, experience is the criterion for leadership. As one grows older and proves his qualifications in increasingly difficult civic tasks, he is given greater and greater responsibility in the managing of community affairs.

Religion plays a pervasive part in the life of the villagers. Aside from the family and village, an important feature of social organization is the system of religious associations. These associations are maintained in order to sponsor the fiesta of a particular saint or holy day. While the formal religion and religious activities are predominantly European Catholic in their origin, there are many attitudes and less formalized beliefs which may be traced to the Maya heritage of the villagers. One should not conclude from this dual origin, however, that religious beliefs and practices in Magdalena are a hodgepodge of unrelated elements. The elements of the contemporary religion of Magdalena have been fairly well coordinated into a single religious system and outlook on the world of men and spirits.

A "westerner" might brand many beliefs of the Guatemalan Indian as magical, superstitious, or irrational. Because of this the westerner, including professional public health personnel, finds it easy to criticize the Indian for practices that appear strange and unreasonable. On analysis, however, one frequently finds that these apparently odd beliefs have a real logic behind them—that they are a part of a systematic but different way of looking at the world. To conceive of having more than one way of looking at the world, the reader need only be reminded of the findings of theoretical physics; there, a universe difficult of comprehension has been described in the language of mathematical logic. Similarly, the language and ideas of the Guatemalan Indian define for him a world the outsider may find difficult to comprehend.

Viewed through the eyes of the Magdaleños, INCAP's experimental nutritional project could appear as an attempt by a specialized branch of western society to interfere with their lives and their customs. It became the job of the anthropologist to look at the activities of the project personnel from the perspective of the villagers and in terms of the beliefs and values shaping their observations and judgments of the world around them. The ultimate objective of his efforts was to make the INCAP program appear acceptable to the villagers by locating areas of misunderstanding and distrust arising from friction between the two different cultural traditions.

Investigation disclosed that each instance of difficulty arose out of the interplay between the cultural practices and beliefs of the villagers and those of the project personnel. The attention of the anthropologist was focused primarily on village culture, but he also found it necessary to direct attention to those aspects of the project itself that contributed to the resistance. The following sections will review four aspects of village culture that played a part in the overall difficulties. Subsequent sections will discuss problems involving the organization of the research project. The four aspects of village culture were: (1) the existence in the village of opposing factions; (2) anti-Communist sentiment, which became directed at project members; (3) a belief that taking blood samples made one susceptible to illness; (4) a rumor, based on local beliefs, that the children in the program were being fattened so as to be sent away and eaten.

Village Factionalism

One of the first problems to become evident involved the social organization of the village. The social worker had noticed that people in one section of the village seemed to resent her activities more than those in the other. Although she was aware that the people of one section considered themselves somewhat different from those of the other, she did not regard this as particularly significant. When she began her work, she had made friends wherever possible, paying little attention to where they lived. She tended to make more friends in one section simply because the people there seemed more hospitable.

It soon became apparent that this difference between the two sections of the village was of considerable importance. These sections are called *barrios*, as in many Latin American communities. A barrio is a geographical subdivision of a village or town similar to wards in American cities. The nearest North American equivalent is the term "section." We refer to "the other side of the tracks" as a section of town; we say that over in "that section" they do things in such and such a way. The barrio, however, is more clearly delineated; everyone knows exactly where his barrio stops and the next begins. Furthermore, each person is aware of being a member of a given barrio. Barrios are usually named, and the people who live in a barrio are referred to by the barrio name.

Just as people who live in different "sections" of town are thought to behave somewhat differently from those who live elsewhere, so the members of different barrios are thought to have slightly different characteristics. In Magdalena the two sections were known as the Upper Barrio and the Lower Barrio. The terms "Upper" and "Lower" referred to their respective positions on the side of the hill on which Magdalena is located rather than to relative social ranking, although the members of each barrio tended to look down on their opposite numbers. Upper Barrio members were much more conservative than those of the Lower. While all members of the Upper Barrio belonged to the

Catholic Church, there were a number of Lower Barrio families who had been converted to Protestantism, and even some who professed no religion.

Even in everyday customs, the members of the Lower Barrio considered themselves more progressive; they made less use of the Indian language and of certain features of the Indian woman's costume. The Upper Barrio people, for their part, tended to regard the residents of the Lower Barrio as "pagans" who showed little respect for religion or traditional customs. In recent years the Upper Barrio has remained with the conservative element of the country's population and has supported conservative candidates in the national elections; the Lower Barrio has supported liberal and radical candidates. At the time of the study, this meant that the Lower Barrio was progovernment and the Upper was antigovernment.

In making friends wherever she could, the social worker had become more closely associated with the Upper Barrio. This process was circular; as she made more friends in one barrio, she became simultaneously less acceptable to the other. The object of the INCAP work was to gain the cooperation of the entire village, not merely of one barrio. When the full significance of the barrio rivalry became clear to the anthropologist, he advised the social worker to cultivate residents of both barrios, thus weakening the feeling that the project was concerned with only one. She began to divide her time more evenly between the two barrios and became less and less identified with one. This had the favorable effect of lessening the resistance in the Lower Barrio.

The Accusation of "Communism"

Public health personnel working at the community level are frequently faced with problems that stem from national political conditions. Such issues may become so explosive that the worker is compelled to leave the field until the political furor subsides. When the INCAP program became involved in such a situation, it was impossible to withdraw without jeopardizing the experimental research.

In 1945 Guatemala ended a thirteen-year period of dictatorship. Following an interim period of confusion and reorganization, a constitutional presidency was established. At first, the new government sponsored many liberal measures and welfare activities, such as the establishment of a social security institute and a school of social work, the expansion of public health work, and the participation of the government in INCAP. The liberal atmosphere that pervaded the country coincided, however, with fights against Communism in other parts of the world. Guatemala attracted some Communists who had been pushed out of other countries and who tried to influence the Guatemalans. The conservative element in the country became more and more identified with anti-Communists, and progovernment forces were joined by the pro-Communists.[1]

Antagonism between anti-Communist forces and the progovernment people, who allowed Communists to work unmolested, reached a critical point in 1951. Anti-Communist propaganda increased, and demonstrations against Communism were staged in many cities and towns. In Magdalena this issue served to unite even the two barrios against a common foe. Anti-Communist activity, however, was much more widespread in the antigovernment than in the progovernment barrio. Signs were posted on gates and houses of the Upper Barrio reading, "We are anti-Communist! We are for Jesus Christ!"

As the wave of anti-Communist feeling rose, it became apparent that the Indians suspected INCAP of being a Communist organization. The personnel of the field team were received with increasing coldness by many villagers. A rumor was spread that the social worker, nurse, doctor, and anthropologist were Communists who had come to gain control over the children and interfere with the community.

To the Magdaleños spreading the rumor, there was clear and persuasive logic behind this accusation. Anti-Communists had insisted that the government was teeming with Communists and hence was communistic. From this it was reasoned that any organization or individual connected with the government must also be communistic. It was well known that INCAP, although an international organization, worked closely with the Guate-

---

[1] Editor's Note: Since this case study was written, the government of Guatemala has again changed hands, the conservative anti-Communist forces gaining control.

malan Ministry of Public Health; consequently, INCAP too must be communistic. A further conclusion followed from this reasoning; since INCAP was communistic, and Americans worked with INCAP, Americans must be also.

The Indians' concern with Communism was very real. While few had any understanding of international Communism, anti-Communist propaganda in Guatemala stressed certain relevant aspects of Communism. The propaganda focused on land, family, and religion. These three elements form the basis of the Indian way of life. Economically, the Indian is a small capitalist. Those who do not have land want some, and those who do have land consider their property the foundation of their lives. The anti-Communists said Communism would take the Indian lands. The family is the most important social unit, and the alleged Communist intent to destroy the family appeared to the Indian to threaten the basis of his life. The propaganda also pointed out that Communism is anti-Catholic. Most Indians of Guatemala are Catholic, and the open hostility to Communism by the Church made it clear that to be Catholic was to be anti-Communist.

With the villagers ready to see the threat of Communism everywhere, it was not surprising that the INCAP program was made a scapegoat. Quite apart from the Communism issue, the activities of the project workers were difficult for the villagers to understand, and therefore suspect. Provided with the rationale for branding the project communistic, the stage was set for trouble.

The crucial nature of this problem made it necessary for the anthropologist to join forces with the social worker in effecting a solution. Anti-Communist feeling had become so intense that the program in Magdalena might have collapsed if immediate steps had not been taken. The social worker was instructed to visit all her friends with the following information: (1) INCAP was an international, nonpolitical organization; it had no interest in, or connection with, the political parties or activities of Guatemala or any of the other member states. The employees of INCAP had varied political beliefs but none was communistic. (2) Americans were especially anticommunistic; this could be easily demonstrated since at that very time the Americans were fighting against

Communists in a place called Korea. While making visits, the social worker discovered some of the paths by which the rumors were being spread. Using this information, the anthropologist traced the rumors to their principal propagators. He talked with these men at some length, making the same points as the social worker and telling them bluntly that the rumors they spread were not only false but actually a help to the Communists.

These steps were crude and direct but evidently served the purpose. The rumors died down, old friends began to warm up, and little more was heard of the matter. Some months later the annual election for mayor provided a test as to whether the issue had been handled successfully. In this election, the town split in the usual way, the progovernment barrio nominating one candidate for mayor, and the antigovernment barrio another. At election time, the issue of Communism arose again. The conservative barrio called the progovernment barrio communistic, but at no time during the hectic days of the election was there any suggestion that the label "Communism" was being attached to INCAP or members of the field team.

It may be mentioned that the efficacy of the tactics used in Magdalena was later confirmed when the rumor that INCAP and its personnel were communistic arose in another of the five experimental villages. Here, however, no social worker or anthropologist was in the field, and there was no method to combat the rumor. Although some knowledge of the social structure of the village was available, this was of little help. Ultimately, INCAP had to remove its program from this community because of the intense hostility mobilized against it.

Beliefs About Blood

The two preceding sections have underscored the importance of understanding those aspects of village life that concern formally organized groups—aspects which can be called "structural" factors. It is equally important, however, to understand the attitudes, beliefs, and values of those who belong to these groups— aspects that can be called "cultural" factors. Such understanding is especially important where two different systems of beliefs and values come in contact with one another. The next two sections indicate how divergences in beliefs and values between villagers and field team led to problems and misunderstanding.

INCAP's periodic physical examinations of the school children in Magdalena included taking blood samples. The field team realized that the Indians were somewhat reluctant to allow their children to submit to this process, but since resistance was not especially marked at first, little attention was paid to the matter. At least some of the INCAP medical personnel assumed that Indians could be expected to react queerly to modern medicine, and that this was just another manifestation of their "ignorance." However, as the program developed and subsequent medical examinations became necessary, the Indians became increasingly reluctant to allow their children to submit to the blood-taking. Some families encouraged their children to evade the examination, while others flatly forbade them to comply.

At one point, some parents became so concerned over an approaching medical examination that they began to withdraw their children from the feeding program. When questioned, they said that they were getting tired of the project's repeated attempts to take blood from the children. It became evident that unless remedial measures were undertaken the Magdaleños would ask the entire project to leave town. Searching for a solution to this problem, the anthropologist concentrated his research on the problem of blood and the strong resistance to blood-taking. At the same time, he requested the director of INCAP to postpone further blood-taking until more knowledge was available.

Conversations were held with many villagers on the subject of blood. Gradually it became clear that there was a basic difference between occidental and Guatemalan Indian ways of thinking about blood. When a "westerner" cuts his hand, he tries to stop the flow of blood, cleans the cut, and allows it to heal. Once a scab is formed or the cut is nearly healed, he thinks little more about the incident. For the Guatemalan Indian, however, a cut is a serious matter. As he understands the functioning of the human body, blood does not come back into the system once it has been lost. If blood is lost, it is lost for good, and the individual is permanently weaker. In essence, blood is conceived as non-regenerative.

Oddly enough, this fact had already been suspected by some of the project medical personnel, but they had failed fully to perceive its effect on attitudes toward blood-taking. One informant told the anthropologist that the villagers simply could not understand why doctors who claimed to know how to make people well went around intentionally taking the blood of little children, thus making them weaker. Weakness made one more susceptible to illness, so that blood-taking was the reverse of what doctors should be doing. This informant concluded that doctors could not know very much about making people well. Another informant provided a very graphic demonstration of how the loss of blood leaves a smaller total quantity of blood in the system. Some years before, he explained, he had severely cut himself in the leg with his cutlass. The wound bled for many hours and he felt very weak afterward. Later he noticed a depression in his hand; he concluded that this depression or hole appeared precisely where the lost blood had come from. To demonstrate, he stretched out his hand so that fingers and thumb were spread and extended back. When he did this, there appeared on the back of his hand, below the thumb and next to the wrist, a distinct hollow between the two tendons. This hole, he explained, did not exist before he had cut himself. The reader who wishes to make this demonstration is likely to find that he, too, can create such a depression in his hand.

Once it became apparent that local beliefs about blood constituted a serious hindrance to the conduct of the program, two steps were taken to counteract the effect of these convictions. The first was to insist upon greater care by INCAP personnel in taking blood. Carelessness in taking more blood than was required had been reported. There was also the problem of getting the blood from the field to the laboratory in Guatemala City so that it would not be spoiled by standing too long before being examined. The amount of blood that could be processed in one day was discussed with the laboratory technicians, and it was found that by adequate planning all the samples from Magdalena could be handled in two days. Previously, three, four, or even five days had been spent collecting blood samples in the village. With these measures taken care of, field personnel were instructed to take half of the blood samples on one day, and the other half on the following day. In this way, there was less time for the Magdaleños to think about the examination and for feeling to arise against it.

This step, however, was merely a preliminary one. The second step was to get the Indians to permit the taking of blood samples despite their beliefs about blood. To do this, a cue was taken from the Indians' own thinking. Since blood was considered a measure of weakness or strength, and since weakness or strength predisposed a person to be sick or well, it would follow that blood could also be a measure of whether a person was sick or well. Accordingly, the social worker began to explain the necessity for taking blood samples in terms of finding out whether the blood was sick or well. If a person had sick blood, he needed curing; if he had well blood, this was also important to know. As in the case of the Communist rumor, the social worker devoted much time discussing this with her friends throughout the village. Gradually, hostility toward blood-taking subsided. The social worker was allowed more than two months in which to spread the new rationale for blood-taking. When the next physical examination was given, there were only murmurs of discontent. Some months later, INCAP was agreeably surprised to learn that a request for adult volunteers to give blood samples for information on prevalence of venereal disease had yielded more than 40 samples. Examinations of some of these were unsuccessful, and volunteers even agreed to provide a second sample.

The Fear of Being Eaten

Tied in with ideas about blood was another belief which created a major problem for the program. In conversations with the Indians the social worker frequently heard something about "taking the children to the United States," or about "how they eat children." It became apparent that there was a widespread fear that the INCAP program was designed to fatten the children so that they might be sent to the United States and eaten. The blood-drawing was said to be part of this scheme; it was a test by which INCAP could decide whether the children were fat enough for shipment.

Field studies indicate that the fear that children will be eaten is a fantasy theme common to a large portion of the Indian population in Guatemala. A woman in another highland village is quoted in the literature as declaring: "They say that people in the United States don't die. When they get old they become young again. But I don't know whether this is true. They also say that when Americans have five or six children they will eat one or two, because there are so many people. How terrible to eat people! Perhaps it isn't true. They say that they put the baby in an oven and toast it well and eat it." The same writer states: "One of the most insistent symbolic themes [in that village] is the fantasy of being devoured. . . . It is hardly an exaggeration to assert that imagined dangers classically present themselves in cannibalistic shape."[1] One of the UNICEF (United Nations International Children's Emergency Fund) teams in Guatemala also encountered evidence of this idea. In many communities where UNICEF had been providing milk for the children, it was frequently mentioned that the children were being fattened in order to send them to the United States or Russia for eating.

An idea common to communities having little contact with each other is apparently a very old one and one that is deeply ingrained in the cultural heritage. Simply denying that such beliefs are true and asserting that they are not supported by known facts has little effect. The strength of such beliefs rests on the fact that they are traditional modes of explaining events that appear threatening. There is one characteristic of this belief, however, which made it relatively easy to cope with. While the fear that children would be eaten is probably an ancient idea, its extension to the INCAP program was necessarily recent. The aim was not to eradicate the belief, but to dissociate it from the activities of INCAP. It seemed reasonable that the belief could be detached from INCAP as easily as it had originally been attached. This turned out to be true. The social worker and the anthropologist discussed the matter with informants with whom they had good relations in order to determine how the idea was related to other cultural themes. At the same time a field worker observed a mother threatening a recalcitrant child that he would be eaten if he did not behave. Other parents were questioned about this,

[1] Paul, Benjamin D., "Symbolic Sibling Rivalry in a Guatemalan Indian Village," *American Anthropologist*, vol. 52, April–June, 1950, pp. 214–215.

and it became evident that such threats were widely used as disciplinary measures.

After a few weeks of probing, the matter was approached directly. An INCAP worker driving into the city with one of the influential men of the village asked him if he would be interested in visiting the INCAP laboratories to see the processing of the blood. He expressed immediate interest and was shown through the laboratories. The technicians explained exactly what the blood was examined for in each stage of the processing. At the same time the field team began discussing the issue with their friends in Magdalena, pointing out that INCAP was in no way connected with sending children away and that the blood samples were not used to see if the children were fit to eat.

The demonstration plus the talk about town seemed to work. The anthropologist was talking with a group of men after a prayer session when the man who had visited the INCAP laboratory decided to tell what he had seen. The men asked him critical questions but gradually became convinced as he answered each one. At no time thereafter did the field workers hear any more of the "cannibalistic fantasy," except as it was occasionally brought up jokingly. There is no reason to think that the belief could not again be attached to INCAP or to some other agency, and if it should, it would have to be dealt with again.

The Dubious Value of Special Services

Up to this point, attention has been focused on aspects of local culture that contributed to misunderstandings between the villagers and the project personnel. But it is important to note that aspects of the project—its organization and the attitudes and attributes of its members—can also create difficulties. This section and the next will show how factors inherent in the project itself affected the attitudes of the villagers.

As research in Magdalena continued, an unexpected situation developed. The clinic service, originally established to promote cooperation, seemed to be causing more trouble and discontent than good feeling. Of the various complaints made to the social worker, fewer and fewer had any relation to the feeding program but were directed instead against the clinic or some phase of the medical service. One reason for this dissatisfaction had to do with differences between the villagers and the clinic personnel in their conception of the nature of disease.

It became apparent that the Magdaleños' ideas about health and sickness were quite at variance with the methods practiced by INCAP's clinical personnel. Furthermore, INCAP clinicians were unaware that there was any systematic difference in beliefs; they tended to ascribe the Magdaleños' reactions to superstition, ignorance, or stupidity.

But the difficulties caused by this mutual lack of understanding were aggravated by a factor of equal importance having to do with the organization of the clinic. INCAP was able to offer only limited clinical facilities. It was not equipped to carry on full-scale public health work but had planned to offer service for less severe cases. To the Indians, for whom hospitalization was something to be avoided at all costs, the doctors seemed to be refusing service to all but the least difficult cases. As a result, their estimation of the medical personnel dropped seriously.

Later in the program, it became necessary for administrative reasons to reduce the clinical services still further. Since the clinic seemed to be a source of trouble, there was no reason to be disappointed over this turn of events, and, indeed, the decrease in clinic service brought no complaints from the villagers. In fact, it seemed that the less medical activity there was, the more the villagers were willing to cooperate.

This situation points to a number of factors to consider in program planning. In the first place, it is doubtful whether it was wise to establish the clinic. INCAP was not equipped to furnish extensive medical service, and the Indians' medical problems could be handled adequately only on a fairly broad scale. Second, there is evidence that medical personnel need real indoctrination before they can deal effectively with people holding beliefs about the nature of sickness and curing extremely divergent from their own. Finally, when working in areas like rural Guatemala, it would appear wise to concentrate on the main goals of the program. If the object of a project is to carry on nutritional experiments involving supplementary feeding for school children, the project should be designed to achieve this goal; it should not include complex adjuncts to complicate the overall situation.

Another set of events serves to illustrate this latter point. Early in the program, the social worker had organized a number of community activities in the belief that they would create interest in the general program. She had initiated a municipal chicken coop, promoted the acquisition of a pig by the school children so they could breed better hogs, and sponsored "social nights" at which prizes were given and movies shown. The anthropologist could not see how these projects helped in achieving the primary goals of the project and recommended their gradual removal. He advised the social worker to spend more time with the families of the community and encouraged her to carry on minor research projects in order to widen her understanding of the people and enable her to interpret what she observed in a larger context. It was not that such features as a chicken coop, a breeding pig, or social nights were bad; rather, they did not appear to aid in achieving the goals of the project, and the villagers did not associate them with INCAP. They seemed a waste of energy and an unnecessary expense.

Once it became apparent that these auxiliary projects hindered rather than helped the total project, the clinic also appeared unnecessary. There was no evidence that the loss of these extra projects bothered the people. The feeding program in the schools continued with little difficulty, and no one seemed to care whether there was a breeding pig or not.

Friction Among Project Personnel

In addition to factors already mentioned, developing friction between staff members impaired the efficiency of the clinic. Villagers claimed that they were not treated well by the staff; even good friends of project personnel stopped using the clinic and thought up excuses for their reluctance to see the doctor.

One of two project nurses visited Magdalena for a few weeks and then was replaced in the village by the other nurse. This alternation impaired communication between the social worker, the doctor, and the nurses. To complicate the situation further, it so happened that the doctor and the social worker disliked each

other. One nurse sided with the doctor and the other with the
social worker. Consequently, when the nurse favoring the doctor
was in the field, neither she nor the doctor would pay much attention to the cases brought to them by the social worker; and when
the other nurse was in the field, the doctor was skeptical of cases
brought by either the nurse or the social worker. These difficul-

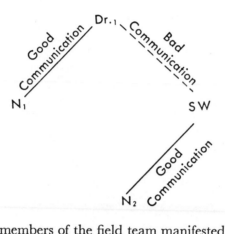

ties between members of the field team manifested themselves in
many ways. It was almost impossible to get the doctor and the
social worker to agree on the use of the transportation facilities;
the nurse who sided with the doctor constituted a special problem
since she was dependent upon the social worker for the daily ride
to and from Magdalena.

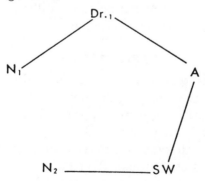

The situation was partly rectified when the anthropologist
joined the field team. The social worker was placed under his

direction, and the communication relay was completed by the addition of an extra person, but it was still cumbersome and inefficient. The problem was not adequately solved until a different doctor and nurse joined the field team. With these substitutions, a more adequate communication circuit was established, and many of the disagreements between personnel disappeared.

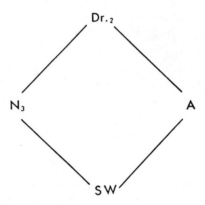

Although this situation was only one of the factors that contributed to the troubles of the clinic, it points up an important lesson. Lack of adequate intraorganizational communication, no matter what its cause, can hinder a project just as surely as problems that stem from the community. In this case, it was interpersonal conflict that hindered communication, but other factors can produce the same result: language difficulties, class differences, or poor organizational structure.

IMPLICATIONS

The problems that arose during the INCAP program in Magdalena illustrate many significant issues in the field of public health. On the surface these may appear to have particular meaning for work in foreign cultures. Upon reflection, however, it should be evident that they are as relevant to public health work in western culture as elsewhere. To realize this, one need merely accept the proposition that public health and medical personnel manifest certain subcultural differences from the people with whom they work; these subcultural differences can produce problems quite as complex as those raised by the more obvious differences between western and Indian culture.

Necessary to effective work in any culture is a systematic knowledge of the social organization, attitudes, and beliefs of the people. The ideas about blood and the "cannibalistic fantasy" that caused difficulties in Magdalena were part of Guatemalan Indian culture; one would hardly expect to encounter the same notions in sophisticated sections of New York City. There are, however, comparable beliefs to be found in the numerous ethnic, cultural, and religious minority groups in the cities and country areas of the United States. Each culture has its own peculiar characteristics that may be relevant to any given program. It is of the utmost importance to study systematically the cultures in which work is to be done in order to deal intelligently with problems that may arise.

Knowledge of the organizational form of both the sponsoring agency and the local community is important in our own as well as in foreign cultures. While we can assume that we have more initial knowledge of our own immediate culture than of a culture like that of Magdalena, the assumption of too much knowledge in either case is dangerous until the general structure of the societies in question has been delineated through study. In Magdalena, even though the field workers knew of the existence of local barrio organization, its relevance to the program was not recognized until study was focused on it.

While the need for understanding a local culture is generally recognized, the importance of systematic knowledge of the sponsoring organization is frequently overlooked. The particular difficulties that arose in Magdalena because of communication difficulties between various members of the field team might have been alleviated had the members themselves been aware of the consequences of their actions, or had the administration been conscious of the problems involved.

A conclusion that seems to run counter to experience in the United States arises from our description of the confusion caused by the presence of the clinic in the town. Public welfare workers in the United States often conceive of their job as being one of changing many things at once. Programs of sanitation, public health clinics, preventive programs, and other projects may be conducted simultaneously on the theory that new habits will come as an integrated unit. In Magdalena it was evident that the presence of the clinic, as well as the projects sponsored by the social worker—social nights, the chicken coop, and the breeding pig—served not to aid the formation of new habits, but rather to confuse public understanding of the specific goals of the program. In more general terms, we may phrase this as the "importance of limited objectives." The specific goal of INCAP in Magdalena was to establish the school feeding program. To aid in achieving this end, the clinic and social work activities were set up. Study made it clear that the additional projects were distracting and not helpful to the achievement of the main goal. To what degree one should limit his objectives depends both upon the nature of the project and the nature of the community. If one wishes to promote change, the generalization might be made that the more different is the subject society from the sponsoring society and the less the two understand each other, the more limited should be the objectives of the program.

The difficulties raised by the issue of Communism in Magdalena can arise in almost any part of the world where technical aid is under way. Whether it can be handled elsewhere in the same manner as it was handled in Magdalena is impossible to predict without specific knowledge of the local situation. The Magdalena case shows, however, that it is necessary for the field worker to keep in touch with the basic issues of the times. An Indian village that seems isolated may actually be in a ferment over problems stemming from vital issues of the day.

SUMMARY

This case study has shown that many of the problems that arise during the course of a research program using human subjects can be solved successfully if adequate knowledge of the culture of both the subject population and the project personnel is available and is applied. Anthropological research disclosed that growing resistance to a program of nutritional research in the Guatemalan highland village of Magdalena could be attributed to six sources: (1) The project had become too closely identified with only one of two opposing factions in the village and had thus alienated the other. (2) By a logical train of argument, but one based on erroneous premises, the project had become identified with the Communist movement and had become the target of intense anti-Communist feelings. (3) The villagers assumed that blood, once lost, could not be regenerated, and thus opposed the taking of blood samples as a practice that would promote illness. (4) Local conceptions had induced the belief that the purpose of the nutritional program was to fatten the children so that they could be sent away and eaten. (5) Resentment by the villagers over the limited services of a small-scale medical clinic affiliated with the research project spread to the rest of the project. (6) Friction between project personnel was sensed by the villagers, aggravating feelings of dissatisfaction. Identification of each of these factors made it possible to devise effective means for dealing with them.

As a final note, it should be observed that while systematic study was required to isolate and define the problems involved, the ways in which the problems were handled were frequently not "scientific." The application of knowledge is still in great part an art; it can be done well or badly, and the result can be effective or chaotic. The fact that social science can and should be used in study and analysis must not obscure the fact that dealing with human beings is still a human problem.

SELECTED REFERENCES

Adams, Richard N., "Un Análisis de las Creencias y Prácticas Médicas en un Pueblo Indígena de Guatemala," *Publicaciones Especiales del Instituto Indigenista Nacional*, Publication no. 17, Guatemala, 1952. An analysis of medical beliefs and practices of the people of Magdalena, together with suggestions on how contemporary medical practice may be adjusted for greater success.

Gillin, John, *The Culture of Security in San Carlos:* A Study of a Guatemalan Community of Indians and Ladinos, Middle American Research Institute, Publication no. 16. Tulane University of Louisiana, New Orleans, 1951. The Indians of this eastern Guatemalan town are acculturated to about the same degree as those in Magdalena. The book includes data on local medical beliefs and practices.

McBryde, F. Webster, *Cultural and Historical Geography of Southwest Guatemala*, Institute of Social Anthropology, Publication no. 4. Smithsonian Institution, Washington, 1947. Although the area concerned does not specifically include Magdalena, it is not far removed, and the volume does give an idea of the variation of Guatemalan Indian economy.

Oficina Sanitaria Panamericana, "Publicaciones Científicas del Instituto de Nutrición de Centro América y Panamá," *Boletín de la Oficina Sanitaria Panamericana, Suplemento no. 1*, Washington, 1953. This is a collection of papers on nutrition published by INCAP. For most of these, cross references are made to original versions in English.

Paul, Benjamin D., "Symbolic Sibling Rivalry in a Guatemalan Indian Village," *American Anthropologist*, vol. 52, April–June, 1950, pp. 205–218. This study includes a description of the "cannibalistic fantasy" in another Indian community located in the same general highland region.

Tax, Sol, editor, *Heritage of Conquest*. The Free Press, Glencoe, Ill., 1952. This is an attempt through a series of summarizing topical papers to bring initial synthesis into the extensive ethnographic materials available on the Indian cultures of Guatemala and Mexico; see especially chapters 3 through 10.

REVIEW OF CONCEPTS AND CONTENTS

At one time people believed that the sun rose every morning and set on the opposite side of the world every evening. We now know that this common-sense view is a geocentric illusion. In point of scientific fact, the earth is a relatively small body that spins on its axis and rotates around the sun. Most of us accept this new view on faith. We can grasp its meaning by setting aside the direct testimony of our senses and imagining that we look out at the world from the vantage point of the sun. The entire earth would be only a whirling speck from this solar observation post, just as the entire sun is only a small, if conspicuous, feature in the panorama of the earthly spectator.

Most of us are not astronomers, however, and find it inconvenient to abandon our customary geocentric perspective. Although we accept what science tells us about the sun and the universe, we file this knowledge in a corner of the mind. For most practical purposes, our world is still a fixed plane bounded by a circular horizon. For us, the sun still rises predictably in the East and literally sinks in the West. We can consider this familiar image illusory, not real. But "reality" often depends on one's purpose and perspective. We could as well argue that the layman's view of the heavens is the real thing and that the sun-centered model is a scientific "illusion" that serves useful but specialized purposes.

Naturally enough, professional health workers tend to see the world revolving around health. They find it technically rewarding to order their universe this way, just as astronomers prefer to see the world revolving around the sun. Health is an important subject no matter how one looks at it; to the common man, health is as critical as the sun. But like the sun, health is usually just part of his daily vista; it is seldom the point around which everything else revolves.

Any specialist has a unique point of view which sharpens his perception within a restricted area of interest. For this benefit he pays a price; he finds it hard to recapture the unspecialized way of seeing things. The health professional is no exception to this rule. With health at the center of his perceptual system, he often finds it difficult to view health as laymen customarily perceive it. This may not matter much if he remains in the laboratory or acts as a technical consultant. But if he wishes to work effectively with groups of people he must overcome his trained incapacity and learn to see health from the standpoint of the man in the community.

It would simplify matters if personal and community health could be isolated and treated apart from the complexities of social existence. But the case studies in this book have shown again and again that this cannot be done. Health practices and health ideas penetrate deeply into the domains of politics, philosophy, etiquette, religion, cosmology, and kinship. However, an exhaustive listing of all the facts and forces impinging on the progress of a health program is neither possible nor necessary. Some selection must be made. By what selective screen may the more relevant points of information be sifted from the rest? Rather than attempting to absorb an endless mass of material and risk losing sight of the forest because of the many trees, health workers would do well to adopt a way of looking at the community that gives some coherence and depth to the array of observable details. No one frame of reference can fully serve this purpose, but the concept of culture fills part of the need.

If correctly understood, the concept of culture can provide an organizing frame for encompassing the details that make up the life of a community, and it can help the specialist assume the viewpoint of the man in the street. Explicitly and implicitly, the concept of culture has recurred throughout the case studies; it may now be examined more systematically. How does it relate to such concepts as society and race? How does culture affect perception, communication, and the process of altering health habits?

Society and Culture

Some kinds of animals live predominantly solitary lives. Some form loose aggregations for protective or other purposes. Still others form true societies; these are social animals in the full sense of the term. The most conspicuous examples of social animals are humans and certain species of insects. In evolving their own modes of social organization during relatively recent times, humans have apparently duplicated some of the general features that have been characteristic of insect societies for many millions of years.

A survey of the arts and occupations found among bees, ants, and termites quickly reveals that they, too, have their forms of agriculture, dairying, and animal domestication. They have aggressive warfare, slavery, and organized defense. They have child-care services and sanitary corps for ridding the community of wastes. And they have systems of communication for effecting cooperation and responding to changes in the external situation. Specialization of labor among society members and dedication of the individual to the common welfare ensure efficiency of effort. The members promote the survival of the social system, and the system promotes the survival of individual members. In these broad respects, insect societies resemble human societies.

Unlike humans, the social insects operate their complex organization mainly by means of inherited impulses. Should all the members of an ant community perish, for example, except one fertilized female, the lone survivor would be capable of rebuilding the entire social edifice in all its original complexity within the span of a few short generations. A society of humans could not similarly recover from catastrophe if all humans suddenly disappeared except one adult couple organically intact but innocent of knowledge and all other social learning. Even if these two beings, bereft of the qualities we call human, could miraculously manage to survive and leave progeny, they could not conceivably regenerate a society remotely resembling any now known to us. According to all we know of human history, it would take tedious thousands of generations to rediscover the ways and wisdom needed to run any human society now in existence. This is because humans, unlike insects, order their lives and interpersonal relations largely by means of socially acquired signals.

Children of the hypothetical survivors would be born with vocal cords, appetites, and brains as part of their normal biological heritage. But without benefit of any social heritage, they would have no language to speak, no idea of what foods to eat, and probably no thoughts. In short, they would have no culture. For culture, to cite an early and now classical definition, "is that complex whole which includes knowledge, belief, art, law, morals, custom, and any other capabilities and habits acquired by man as a member of society."[1]

Ants likewise are members of society, but having no culture and needing none, they do not acquire their habits and capabilities from social interaction. Most of their capabilities are built into their bodies at birth. Man, too, is born with instinctual drives. Compared to those of other animals, however, his instincts for the most part are diffuse rather than specific, providing little guidance for the particular way he should respond to a particular environmental stimulus. Perhaps all social activity is ultimately powered by biological energy, yet the particular organizational form of any given society of humans—whether it is characterized by clans or castes or trade associations—is not the product of genetic forces but of the extraorganic agency we call culture. Man is unique among animals by virtue of the fact that his society is essentially regulated by cultural rather than inborn directives.

Whereas insects achieve specialization by modifying their bodies, men do so by modifying their environment. Certain members of an ant colony have powerful jaws for crushing seeds that other members can bring in but cannot crack; certain members convert their bodies into honeypots to meet the colony's need for storaging food. To achieve similar ends, humans manufacture machines and vessels. Thus, technology, as a part and product of culture, takes the place of anatomical specialization in animals. Two other distinctions between social insects and humans deserve mention—differences in the duration of infancy and in the mutability of societal structures.

Immature members do not contribute to the maintenance of insect society; in fact, they impose a burden upon the adults. After a relatively brief period of youth, ants and termites tend to

---

[1] This statement was made by E. B. Tylor in 1871. However, culture can be and has been formally defined in a hundred ways. The worth of a definition depends on the purpose it serves. For a thorough-going review and analysis of the many definitions of culture, see Kroeber, A. L., and Clyde Kluckhohn, Culture: A Critical Review of Concepts and Definitions. Peabody Museum of American Archaeology and Ethnology, Harvard University, Cambridge, Mass., 1952.

live amazingly long and active adult lives. In contrast, maturation is slow in humans; about a third of the total life span is consumed in growing up. To become useful members of human society, children need to absorb skills, attitudes, assumptions, values, and all the other cultural "capabilities and habits acquired by man as a member of society." This slow process of conscious and unconscious learning—sometimes called enculturation—is facilitated by a lengthy period of physical and emotional dependence on parents, teachers, and other enculturating agents of society.

The other distinction concerns stability of social structure. Many forms of society are found among insects. The social systems vary in pattern of specialization, mode of subsistence, method of communication, and other respects, just as human societies vary. Among insects, different social types correspond to different biological species. All colonies of the same species have the same type of society. Species differentiation goes back millions of years. Since the biological type is responsible for the social type, societal differentiation among insects likewise goes back millions of years. The societal structure is thus remarkably resistant to change. By comparison, human societies are very plastic. Different groups of the identical human species are guided by different cultures and live in correspondingly different kinds of societies. Social and cultural patterns are subject to perceptible changes from one generation to another. Were this not so, trying to improve community health habits would be a waste of time.

The terms "culture" and "society" are not identical. They refer to distinguishable realms of phenomena. In nature, societies can and do exist in the absence of culture. Animal society appeared on earth long ago; culture much more recently. Just as society presupposes living organisms, so culture presupposes society and cannot be found in the absence of society. Among humans, society and culture are interdependent; each can exist only in terms of the other. Whether something is called social or cultural is often arbitrary when concern is with the human community and not the biological community in general. Where emphasis falls on the ideas shared by a group, the frame of reference is usually cultural. Where emphasis is on the group that shares the ideas, the frame of reference is usually social.

Although the distinction is critical for some purposes, the terms "cultural" and "social" are often used interchangeably, thus standing for the more cumbersome term "sociocultural." In America, anthropologists favor the word culture or cultural, and sociologists the word society or social where choice permits. A much more critical distinction, too often ignored, is the difference between the organic level of phenomena and the extra-organic or sociocultural level. Confusion can be averted by distinguishing clearly between the concept of race and that of culture.

Race and Culture

Man's capacity to have culture depends on the unique nature of his physical endowment, but this does not justify the conception that behavioral differences among groups of men are largely due to racial differences. A traveler going from one region of the earth to another notices that groups of people vary in bodily type, dress, language, and other ways. Since these various manifestations often strike the observer simultaneously, he easily assumes that they all go together "naturally," just as whiskers, purring, and night vision naturally go together as characteristics of a cat.

But in humans, it is important to distinguish between biologically derived and socially derived traits. Populations that remain separated from others of their kind for enough generations gradually develop distinctive physical features through the operation of such biological processes as mutation, selection, and adaptation. These processes presumably played an important role in bringing the contemporary races of man into being. Human populations that remain apart for a long time tend in addition to exhibit diverging social features. However, the two types of distinctive characteristics, biological and social, while often associated, are not causally related.

The races of man constitute a single species and, despite appearances, the similarities far outweigh the differences. The races overlap and grade into each other. So-called race mixing has gone on for so long in human history that it must be considered a cause as well as a consequence of racial distinctiveness. Virtually all scientific evidence indicates that in humans racial "purity" is a mythical concept.

Scholars are far from agreed on how to classify mankind racially, some recognizing three major racial divisions (Caucasoid, Mongoloid, Negroid), others defining more or different races. Most classifications are based on appearances—skin color, type of hair, stature, head contour, shape of the nose, and so on—but it is difficult to determine whether features that strike the eye are biologically basic or only superficial. A sounder classification may emerge when geneticists learn more about gene composition. The discovery of differences among populations in the frequency of blood-group genes represents a good beginning in this direction.

In simplest terms, a race is a population or group of people sharing a certain set of innate physical characters. Since populations unquestionably vary in their physical makeup, it has been argued that some races are superior to others. At bottom these claims rest on selective perception and the projection of ethnocentric judgments. It has also been argued that racially distinct groups differ in mental ability and therefore in their degree of civilization or capacity to absorb instruction. There is no good evidence, however, that the processes of perceiving, remembering, or thinking are influenced by racial differences. Nor is there any sound basis for believing that groups of mankind differ in their innate capacity for intellectual or emotional development. Purported group differences in intelligence quotients generally reflect the inadequacy of the testing instrument rather than of the tested population. Human groups do differ in their thinking and the conclusions they reach, but the variation is normally not a measure of intelligence or the capacity to reason. The difference is due to the varying climate of assumptions into which people are born and not to the inherited physical differences which happen to distinguish one group from another.

Humans learn much from formal and purposive instruction, but they store much of this learning below the threshold of consciousness. Moreover, much learning takes place without awareness of the process. Because they deliberately instruct children in certain skills, adults easily overlook the fact that considerable inculcation occurs by innuendo, involuntary example, and unintended imitation. The sounds and rules of language can be explicitly taught, but in all cultures the appropriate patterns of speech—pitch, rhythm, accent, connotations, word order, and other features—are communicated mainly by unconscious instruction and unconscious learning. What is true of language holds for most other aspects of culture—their existence and transmission are largely taken for granted by the people concerned.

Thus, social habit systems resemble instinctive reflex responses. Both categories of behavior appear fixed and automatic to the naive observer, who therefore tends to overestimate the influence of heredity and underestimate the effects of social learning. Instinctive behavior is automatic but not all automatic behavior is instinctive. The blurring of this distinction is attested by the loose way in which the term "instinctive" is popularly used, as in the expression, "he instinctively reached for his holster." The word "breeding" now refers to upbringing but derives from the same root as the word "blood," as though manners were transmitted through the blood stream. Popularly, we still speak of blood as the agent of hereditary transmission, although we now realize scientifically that heredity is determined by genes arranged like beads on chromosomes within the nucleus of every body cell.

Until recently we had no science of genetics, and it was plausible to assume (incorrectly) that acquired characteristics could be inherited. If a baby could inherit the sunburn acquired by its parents, as scholars once supposed, why could it not inherit the language spoken by its parents? The processes of social transmission and biological transmission were not well distinguished. Akbar, the sixteenth-century Mohammedan emperor of Hindustan, became curious when he heard that Hebrew was the original language of mankind and that children would speak it automatically if they were taught no other language. To test this claim, Akbar reportedly had a group of infants isolated with deaf mutes as nurses, only to find a few years later that the children communicated by gestures, like their nursemaids. It is otherwise with animals. A young cowbird hatched from an egg laid in a warbler's nest, for example, accepts food and shelter from its foster mother, yet at maturity its flight calls and mating songs are typical of its parasitic kind, not of a warbler.

Culture and Perception

Man lives in a double environment, an outer layer of climate and terrain and natural resources, and an inner layer of culture that mediates between man and the world about him. Through culture, man transforms his habitat, constructing tunnels and towers and respirators, wearing clothes, and reconditioning the air. He not only revises but interprets his outer environment, assigning significance to events according to rules of observation and response implicit in the prevailing culture. One of the functions performed by culture is to serve as a subtle and systematic device for perceiving the world. Since cultures vary, perceptions of the world vary correspondingly.

Most of the culture that an individual incorporates into his person during the slow process of socialization antedates the individual's birth and begins to shape his perceptions long before he stops to question whether his is the only way of viewing things. Ordinarily this question does not even arise unless he has occasion to observe the behavior of people from another culture or social stratum, and even then the easier course is to regard unfamiliar practices as quaint and picturesque or as evidence of error and ignorance.

In some societies people make no distinction between the colors blue and green, comprehending both in a single term. Mistakenly seeing this as "confusion," some observers reached the conclusion that the people were deficient in analytic ability. A reverse situation has also been observed: some groups distinguish several colors where we recognize only one. This was interpreted, not as a mark of superior analytic capacity, but as an indication of limited ability to make abstractions. Ethnocentric bias thus can lead to the use of a double standard of comparison.

Actually, no issue of intellectual competence is involved. Classifications are not intrinsic to the materials classified but are imposed by the perceivers. They are projected upon the panorama of experience like a grid thrown upon a complicated photograph to guide the eye and aid communication. But the source of the guidelines is often so well concealed in the cultural background that the viewers perceive the grid as part of the panorama itself. Color perception is a good illustration.

A comparative study of 60 distinct American Indian groups, based on reactions to color cards, revealed that no two cultures divide the spectrum in the same way. While the average member of any society can discriminate and describe a multitude of shades and tints, the number of standard colors recognized in a group's language ranges from three to eight, our own six-way system (red, orange, yellow, green, blue, violet) falling near the center of the range. A wave length which in one system lies at the dividing line between two colors falls in the middle of a color band in another system. Thus, shades we call blue or violet can belong to five different color categories in another system, that same system treating our red and orange as one color.[1] We may think our classification corresponds to the "natural" division of the chromatic scale, but our claim is no better grounded than that of any other group, equally unaware of its particular cultural bias.

Repeatedly we find that one culture distinguishes what another combines and combines what the other distinguishes. Cultures classify many "spectra" of experience other than the color continuum. Equally subject to varying classification are such ranges of experience as tastes and odors, aches and pains, emotional states, the sounds of speech, the daily cycle, the annual round, the life career, and countless other conditions and occurrences.

A group's mode of classifying experience may seem arbitrary to an outsider. But cultural classifications are seldom random or capricious; they are usually affected by environmental circumstance and cultural interest. People do not bother to make discrimination in matters that do not concern them, and they make fine discriminations in matters they consider important. Where we are content with one word for snow in general, the Eskimo have separate terms for snow on the ground, falling snow, drifting snow, and snowdrift.[2] The Zulus put blue and green together but

[1] Ray, Verne F., "Human Color Perception and Behavioral Response," *Transactions of the New York Academy of Sciences*, vol. 16, December, 1953, pp. 98–104.

[2] Boas, Franz, *The Mind of Primitive Man*. Rev. ed. Macmillan Co., New York, 1938, p. 211.

carefully differentiate many shades of brown in keeping with a strong cultural interest in cattle and their variation.

As a perceptual device, the culture of any group does more than segment the spectra of experience. It also connects specific segments of one spectrum with corresponding segments of another, the system of correspondence varying with the culture. Each culture has its own way of organizing experience. The Pueblo Indians of the American Southwest, for example, connect colors and cardinal directions. They recognize six directions, including up and down, associating each with a particular color. Songs and ceremonial objects repeatedly affirm the connection between north and yellow, west and blue, south and red, east and white, above and speckled, below and black. These symbolic associations enrich art and drama and establish common understandings within the group. However, they can also impede communication between groups, as shown by the following example.

The Chinese, like others, distinguish right and left, but they differ in the kinds of symbolic associations they traditionally make. The left is associated with east, the male force (*yang*), springtime, and the place of honor. This linkage posed a problem for some translators of the New Testament when they came to the statement that Jesus is seated on the right hand of God. Unwilling to violate holy writ by shifting Jesus' position, they stuck to the literal text but at the cost of creating the impression that someone other than Jesus occupied the place of honor on the left.[1]

Medical as well as missionary communication is complicated by disparities of classification and association, as attested by nearly every case study in this book. Communities vary in their manner of segmenting the gradient of health and illness and in the kinds of phenomena to which these states of health are assumed to be connected. The dividing line between normalcy and illness shifts from one group to another and the categories of sickness are as subject to cultural variation as the color series.

Thus, the mestizo population of coastal Peru and Chile divide systems of medicine into two classes, scientific and popular, and

[1] Wright, Arthur F., "The Chinese Language and Foreign Ideas" in *Studies in Chinese Thought*, edited by Arthur F. Wright. University of Chicago Press, Chicago, 1953, pp. 300–301.

diseases into five major categories: obstruction of the gastro-intestinal tract, undue exposure to heat or cold, exposure to "bad air," severe emotional upset, and contamination by ritually unclean persons. Household remedies are appropriate for all classes of sickness. Scientific doctors may also be consulted, but only for illnesses assigned to the first two categories. For the last three classes of illness only household remedies are deemed appropriate; if these fail, a folk specialist is sought. Mestizos patronize clinics and doctors for other matters but not for maladies popularly ascribed to air, upset, or ritual uncleanliness. For these disorders the doctor's remedies are judged ineffectual or actually harmful, since the doctor does not "know" these illnesses and does not "believe" in them. Because the symptoms are similar, tuberculosis sometimes masquerades as "fright" and so remains inaccessible to the doctor or the health center. More successful than the doctor as an innovator of modern medicine is the druggist, who accepts and understands both modern and folk medicine.[1]

In Chile the public health nurse likewise is more effective than the doctor in bringing modern medical concepts to the people, as Dr. Simmons asserts in Case 12, since she is more familiar with the local idiom and less inclined to express disdain for popular medical ideas. In Case 15, Dr. Lewis explains that the separate conceptual worlds of doctor and villager in Mexico constitute "a serious obstacle to the spreading of modern medical practice and unless the gap between these two distinct levels of explanation is bridged, progress will be very slow."

The problem of reconciling divergent systems of perception arises wherever those who confront each other belong to separate nations, different social sectors of the same country, separate institutions in the same community, or different disciplines within the same team. Of course, more than divergences of perception are involved. Differences of aims and interests may also be present, as Dr. Naegele cautions in connection with his Wellesley study (Case 11) and as the essays dealing with power and politics demonstrate (Cases 10, 13, 15).

[1] Simmons, Ozzie G., "Popular and Modern Medicine in Mestizo Communities of Coastal Peru and Chile," *Journal of American Folklore*, vol. 68, 1955, pp. 57–71.

Recognizing the differences does not necessarily dispel them, but this is often a necessary preliminary to realistic collaboration. It is relatively easy to perceive that others have different customs and beliefs, especially if they are "odd" or "curious." It is generally more difficult to perceive the pattern or system into which these customs and beliefs fit. The source of the difficulty lies not only in the process of perception but in the nature of cultural patterning.

The Patterning of Culture

In any community, most people are quite unaware of the cultural regularities that recur in their various acts of perceiving, thinking, evaluating, and doing. But the systematic features of culture are just as discoverable as the principles of grammatical order that governed every spoken language long before grammarians discovered the existence of regularities and correspondences in speech.

As part of the process of becoming a member of his society, the individual learns what might be called the grammar of his culture the same way he learns the grammar of his language— inductively and unconsciously. The regularities and symmetries of a culture are so pervasive as to seem nonexistent to the participants. This does not mean that they are unimportant. In fact, some students of human institutions assert that the most significant thing to know about a society is what it takes for granted. Social scientists have used many terms for describing cultural coherence or patterning, but whatever the term may be, the emphasis generally falls on the arrangement of the cultural elements rather than on the elements of belief and custom as such.

Influenced by the patterning implicit in their culture, individuals perceive a certain orderliness and predictability in the social and physical world about them, but when they encounter people who order their experiences differently, the two patterns seem to interfere with each other. One system of organization seems to dissolve or fragment the second system, so that the other group's ways of behaving and thinking appear as an illogical patchwork. Members of the alien group seemingly separate what belongs together, while combining unrelated phenomena, like the

Thai practitioner's use of the same remedy for both rheumatism and distress over the disappearance of a husband (Case 6).

Where the average layman tends to take this impression at face value, accepting it as evidence of the alien group's ignorance or inferiority, the person with an awareness of patterning will be challenged to "make sense" out of apparent chaos and to look for linkages, implicit premises, and other principles of order. Of course, all cultural systems have loose ends, and the degree of social and cultural integration varies according to the rate of social change and other circumstances. Hence, searching for system does not always yield results, and overzealous expectations may even lead the student of culture to perceive patterns that are not present. At the same time, patterns that rest in the background will scarcely appear spontaneously to the man who fixes his attention exclusively on foreground phenomena. Although concepts can never substitute for accurate and detailed field observation, an awareness of cultural patterning is an indispensable guide to intelligent observation.

A characteristic shared by the contributors to this volume is a perception of patterning and a successful search for meaningful linkages. In Case 1, the writer is not content to note that a woman may not drink the milk of her husband's cattle and to reiterate the common explanation that "this is our custom." He proceeds to link milk taboos to the kinship system and the deep symbolic significance of cattle, relating the latter in turn to problems of soil erosion, agricultural shortages, and dietary insufficiency. In Case 2, the authors are not satisfied to report that interviewing showed popular notions of mental illness etiology to be unsystematic and mutually contradictory. They examine their data from another perspective and discover that the test results and the reactions to their educational program fit together in a functional rather than a rational frame of reference.

In Case 3, the writer begins his field work where another evaluator might have ended, namely at the point of assembling the statistics on the number of housewives who had begun to boil water on their own initiative, those who did so as the result of the hygiene program, and those who continued to drink their water without boiling it. The varied reasons for adopting or failing to adopt new health habits fell into place only after he was able to bring the respective patterns of diet and health beliefs, socio-economic organization, and daily routines into relationship with one another. In Case 4, the author retraces his attempts to perceive cultural linkages and to abstract patterns from a succession of particular medical experiences. The accent on pattern continues in like manner through the rest of the case studies, ending with Dr. Adams' counsel that a systematic study must be made of any culture or subculture in which health work is to be done.

Innovation

Like everything else in nature, the culture of any group is subject to constant change. Even without stimulation from the outside, the culture is gradually altered by a succession of minor but cumulative modifications made by nameless individuals. Occasionally someone in the society makes a conspicuous discovery or invention but this is the exception rather than the rule.

Whenever people from different cultures meet they tend to borrow cultural items from each other, and borrowing usually accounts for most of the specific elements in the culture of any group. Linton has estimated that there is probably no culture extant which owes more than 10 per cent of its total elements to inventions made by members of its own society. He points out, for example, that an American worships a Hebrew deity in an Indo-European language, buys a paper with coins invented in ancient Lydia, and reads the news of the day imprinted in characters invented by the ancient Semites upon a material invented in China by a process invented in Germany.[1]

When the interest focuses on the elements that are borrowed rather than on the borrowers, the term "diffusion" is frequently used. Thus, the notion of "hot" and "cold" foods and their relation to health and illness, a system of belief common to much of contemporary Latin America, apparently diffused from some place in the Old World, judging by resemblances to the humoral

[1] Linton, Ralph, *The Study of Man.* D. Appleton-Century Co., New York, 1936, pp. 324–326.

theory of medicine of the ancient Greeks. It is possible that the Greeks only modified and transmitted a system of medical beliefs originating at a more distant point, perhaps in Asia.

The history of culture shows that communities and nations accept only some of the elements available for borrowing. Moreover, the borrowed idea or practice is usually reinterpreted and modified to fit the particular environmental and cultural framework. Thus, cattle husbandry diffused into many parts of the world from some point in the vicinity of the Near East, but cattle have been put to different use and assigned different meanings in China, India, native Africa, and the Occident.

Programs which seek to alter health practices and attitudes constitute efforts to change the local culture; and health innovations are just as subject to selective acceptance and modification as are any other offered or available innovations. Acceptance or modification is not a random process but depends on how the new item or idea is perceived by the potential recipients, how it accords with their values and assumptions, and whether it is consistent with their system of social relationships. It also depends on the social status of the innovator and the implications of that status for the various segments of the community.

Some "resistances" can be reduced by changing the approach or by altering the organizational form of the sponsoring group or agency. But sometimes neither of these tactics suffices to overcome the resistance. In such instances it may well be that the attempted changes challenge established beliefs or practices which are more fundamental to the stability of the particular social or cultural system than is evident at first inspection.

All cultural systems define codes of interpersonal conduct. They all have ways to reward conformity and to punish deviation that exceeds the limits set by the system, although it must be recognized that behavior considered normal in one society or circumstance may not be tolerated in another. Social control can be effected by positive sanctions such as prizes, approval, and promotions, and by negative sanctions such as ridicule, ostracism, and legal punishment. An individual who will not discharge his normal social responsibilities imperils the stability of his fellows, as well as the equilibrium of their social arrangements and the validity of the communal values. The offender can be banished as a witch or defined as a mental case and segregated in a hospital.

As the first two case studies, respectively, show, new programs of tuberculosis management or mental health education may unwittingly collide with customary sanctions for safeguarding social and psychological equilibrium. A Zulu patriarch withheld consent to hospitalize tubercular members of his household until the doctor retracted a suggestion that his married daughter had brought the disease into the home. According to Zulu tenets of disease transmission, this suggestion could mean only that the daughter was a witch, an accusation that would force the father to turn against her. Another instance reported by Dr. Cassel, but not included in his case study, illuminates the social-sanction aspect of witchcraft accusations. An old man seriously ill with a cavity in the lung failed to avail himself of modern drugs but made a surprising recovery after a native diagnostician found that the patient was the victim of witchcraft perpetrated by the old man's profligate son and insolent daughter-in-law. Indignantly, the sick man evicted the witches from his household, thereby eliminating the source of intolerable domestic friction, yet leaving the father blameless for the drastic act of disinheriting his oldest son.

Witchcraft accusation is one means of fixing blame when misfortune strikes. However, we may also regard it as an effective method, at least in some instances, of coping with socially disruptive behavior. Hospitalizing the mentally ill may perform a similar function in our own communities, as the authors of the Prairie Town study contend. Like witches, the insane are defined as radically different from the normal and shunned as dangerous and contaminating. Most mental patients are not actually dangerous. But they do endanger morale and social solidarity. In Prairie Town and among the Zulus, and in many other communities as well, intangible dangers of this sort are dramatically rephrased as physical dangers. In part, the people of Prairie Town maintain their own mental balance by exaggerating the imbalance of the mentally ill. When an educational program, aimed at improving attitudes toward the ill minority, threatened the equilibrium of the majority, the community became unco-operative and hostile.

One detects a curious circularity of cause and effect in these cases. A person is put in a hospital because he is mentally disturbed. In turn, the fact that he has been hospitalized tends to stigmatize him as "mentally ill" and to jeopardize his chances of regaining a foothold in society. On the surface and according to Zulu belief, some individuals are antisocial because they are witches. In point of fact, some individuals seem to be labeled witches because they are antisocial. Although the parallels should not be pressed too far, the similarities between the African and Canadian cases emerge in the degree to which we delve beneath manifest belief and behavior to find the latent functions they perform.

Of course, social and psychological functions are not indissolubly linked to particular social forms. The management of group anxiety or the exercise of social control does not necessarily depend on social isolation of the mentally ill or on a belief in witches. Such attitudes and beliefs are subject to eventual change, as history shows. But until the community accepts substitute devices for discharging the same functions it will tend to exhibit the kinds of resistances encountered in Prairie Town.

To work effectively with people, we must not only be able to see the world as they see it, but must understand the psychological and social functions performed by their practices and beliefs. These functions are not always evident to the people themselves.

Résumé

The principle that health programs should "start with people as they are and the community as it is" applies both at home and abroad. It is equally applicable whether the goal is to persuade Peruvian housewives to boil their drinking water or to convince the citizens of Seattle to accept fluoridation. The principle itself is no longer novel; its validity is generally acknowledged by professional workers in the fields of public health and preventive medicine. The problem is how to implement the principle. The real challenge is to discover just where particular groups of people stand; a willingness to meet them must be matched by a knowledge of the meeting place.

Each group has its own social, as well as physical, environment. Contrary to popular assumption, social groups cannot readily be placed on a unitary scale of "progress" ranging from naive to sophisticated or from "lower" to "higher" stages of civilization. The social environment of a group, like its physical environment, is the product of numerous historical and situational factors. The social organization, common understandings, and modalities of behavior that constitute the social environment of a particular community cannot readily be divined at a distance or revealed by a magic formula. They must be studied to be understood.

An important aid to understanding the community and its reaction to a medical problem or health program is the concept of culture with its accent on pattern and function as well as on the specific items of belief and practice. The threads of health and illness are woven into the sociocultural fabric and assume full significance only when perceived as part of the total design. Each study in this book is a case in point.

CONTRIBUTORS

RICHARD N. ADAMS, Anthropologist, World Health Organization, has done ethnological research in Peru and all the countries of Central America, and applied anthropological work in Guatemala, El Salvador, and Panama. At present he is completing a three-year survey of Central American cultures.

G. MORRIS CARSTAIRS is Deputy Director of a Medical Research Council Unit attached to the Royal Bethlehem and Maudsley Hospital, London. A psychiatrist with training in social anthropology, he carried out research on culture and personality in Rajasthan, at first as assistant to Mrs. Gitel Steed of Columbia University and later as Rockefeller Research Fellow from Cambridge University.

JOHN CASSEL is Associate Professor of Epidemiology, School of Public Health, University of North Carolina. After completing his medical education in Johannesburg, he joined Dr. Sidney L. Kark for training at the Institute of Family and Community Health in Durban, and for more than five years worked as Medical Officer in Charge of the Polela Health Centre in Natal.

ELAINE CUMMING, who was trained as a sociologist at Harvard University, has served as a research worker with the Psychiatric Services Branch of the Province of Saskatchewan in Canada. She is now doing research in Nova Scotia and is affiliated with Cornell University.

JOHN CUMMING was Senior Psychiatrist at the Saskatchewan Hospital in Weyburn, Saskatchewan until recently. A medical graduate of the University of Toronto, he received special training in social science at Harvard University, and currently holds an appointment at Cornell University.

FRANCIS L. K. HSU is Professor of Anthropology, Northwestern University. Born in North China, he studied at the University of Shanghai and received his doctoral training at the University of London. He has done field work in China's Southwest and Hawaii, traveled extensively in India, Burma, and Europe, and served on the faculties of Columbia and Cornell Universities.

Solon T. Kimball, Professor of Education at Teachers College, Columbia University, is a social anthropologist who has done community research in Ireland, among the Navaho Indians, and in Massachusetts, Michigan, and Alabama. He has been head of the Community Organization Section, War Relocation Authority, and Chairman of the Department of Sociology and Anthropology, University of Alabama.

Jane Richardson Hanks, who acted as Associate Director of the Cornell Research Center in Bangkok, Thailand, has taught anthropology at the University of California and at Bennington College. She has made field studies of the Kiowa Indians of Oklahoma and the Blackfoot Indians of Alberta.

Lucien M. Hanks, Jr., is a psychologist on the Faculty of Social Science at Bennington College. During World War II he worked in Ceylon and Burma for the Office of Strategic Services, and more recently held the position of Research Associate in the Southeast Asia Program of Cornell University.

Oscar Lewis, Professor of Anthropology at the University of Illinois, has made comparative studies of rural life in American communities and of peasantry in Mexico, Cuba, Spain, and India. He has served as Social Scientist with the United States Department of Agriculture and as Field Representative in India for the Ford Foundation.

McKim Marriott, Social Anthropologist and Indologist, spent several years studying villages in the Aligarh District of northern India. Formerly a Junior Research Anthropologist in the Institute of East Asiatic Studies, University of California, he is now making field studies of communities in peninsular India as a Fellow of the Ford Foundation.

Kaspar D. Naegele is Assistant Professor of Sociology in the Department of Economics, Political Science, and Sociology at the

University of British Columbia. In addition to working on the Wellesley project for several years, he has taught sociology at Harvard University and the University of Oslo.

KALERVO OBERG, Anthropologist, International Cooperation Administration, Rio de Janeiro, has had ten years' experience studying culture and ethnology in various regions of Brazil, first for the Smithsonian Institution and more recently for ICA (formerly FOA). He has done ethnographic work in Alaska and Africa, and has served as Economic Analyst in the United States, Ecuador, and Peru.

José ARTHUR RIOS is Researcher, Division of Health Education, Serviço Especial de Saúde Pública, Rio de Janeiro. He received sociological training at Louisiana State University, and was formerly Coordinator of the National Campaign for Rural Education in Brazil.

JULIAN SAMORA, Associate Professor of Social Science at Adams State College of Colorado, is now on leave to do research at the University of Colorado Medical School on the sociocultural characteristics of patients. He has lectured at Fisk University, the University of New Mexico, and Michigan State College.

LYLE SAUNDERS is Associate Professor, Department of Preventive Medicine and Public Health, University of Colorado School of Medicine. He was formerly Assistant Professor of Sociology at the University of New Mexico, and at present is Consultant to the Division of General Health Services of the United States Public Health Service.

DAVID M. SCHNEIDER is Assistant Professor of Social Anthropology, Harvard University. Formerly he taught at the London School of Economics, and he has carried out field work on social structure and personality on the Micronesian Island of Yap, as well as among the Mescalero Apache Indians of New Mexico.

OZZIE G. SIMMONS is Lecturer on Social Anthropology, Harvard School of Public Health. He has served as Director of the Institute of Social Anthropology in Peru and as Cultural Anthropologist with the Division of Health, Welfare, and Housing of the Institute of Inter-American Affairs in Santiago, Chile.

J. MAYONE STYCOS is Associate Professor of Sociology, St. Lawrence University. He has worked as Research Associate of the Bureau of Applied Social Research, Columbia University; as Co-director of the Family Life Project, University of Puerto Rico; and as Field Director of the Jamaican Family Life Project, University College of the West Indies.

EDWARD WELLIN spent three years in Peru as anthropological researcher and consultant, first for the Division of Medicine and Public Health of the Rockefeller Foundation and later for the World Health Organization. He is now receiving special training at Harvard School of Public Health.

INDEX

INDEX

492   HEALTH, CULTURE, AND COMMUNITY

354, 368, 372; psychological, on school children, 300–301, 309, 415–416, 419–420, 423, 426
Research team, 48, 155, 164, 211; role of, 182–183, 288–289, 314–316
Richards, Audrey I., 41
Rio Doce Valley, Brazil, 349
Rios, José Arthur, 349, 377, 403
Ritual: for ancestors, 19; role in curing, 112–116, 142, 169; surgery and injection as, 116, 134
Rockefeller Foundation, 72n, 73
Rorschach test: in Tepoztlán, 415, 419, 421, 423
Rosen, George, 3
Rumors: about programs and personnel, 52, 95, 415–416, 443–445, 448–450

Saint Vincent de Paul, Society of, 363
Samora, Julian, 377
Sanctions, social, 474–475
Sanders, Irwin T., 294
"Sang" (disease concept), 159, 168
Sanitation: and cholera epidemic, 139–143; ideas about, 20, 132, 139–143, 378; personnel, 170, 327, 361–362; programs, 71–102, 170, 327, 361–362; proposals, 273, 283; state of, 20, 26, 45, 75, 190, 378
San Lucero, Chile: municipality, 327–328; staff of health center, 326, 329
Santiago, Chile: San Lucero Health Center, 325–347
Sarasan, S. B., 235
Saunders, Lyle, 377, 400
Scabies, 123
Schistosomiasis, 357
Schneider, David M., 211, 235
School of Sociology and Political Science of São Paulo, 354
Schools, 9, 46, 166, 167, 308–314, 328, 360–361, 406, 415, 416; as communication channels, 139, 175, 179, 184; health role, 136, 139, 162, 163, 170, 171, 172, 286, 313, 342, 349, 354, 360–361, 436–437; teachers, 163, 181, 312, 360–361
Schwartz, Morris S., 321
Scotland, 111, 131
Self-survey of health: Talladega, 269–270
Sex roles: male-female spheres, 17, 20, 27, 28, 29, 36, 37, 76, 97, 208, 219–222, 231, 246, 276, 281, 301, 393; relative status, 7–8, 36, 196, 201, 205, 229; sex standards, 7–8, 138, 193–195, 197–199, 200–201, 203, 206, 230–232; sexual restrictions, 124–125, 141
Shame, 83, 84, 119, 206; deterrent to birth control, 200–201
Sharp, Lauriston, 185

Sick-well distinction: cultural patterning of, 78, 123–126, 156, 168, 469; deviation and control, 62, 81, 85, 123–126, 474; normality standards, 48, 58–61, 78, 85, 309, 310–311, 318, 469, 474
Simmons, Ozzie G., 103, 325, 348, 470
Simons, H. J., 41
Singh, Rudra Datt, 268
Sitala-Mata (goddess), 128
Smallpox, 16, 108, 156, 168, 252; attributed to a deity, 128, 252
Smith, Carleton Sprague, 376
Smith, T. Lynn, 376
Smithsonian Institution of Washington, 354
Snake-bite: curing, 113, 126–129, 257–258
Social class, 65, 66, 75–76, 77, 79, 82, 138, 192, 193, 194, 223, 224, 275, 289–291, 301, 328, 356, 427; in relation to health and health programs, 57, 66, 93–97, 102, 202, 339–340; of health personnel, 95–96, 98, 102, 206, 337, 339, 346
Social science, iii–iv, 3–4, 206, 457
Social Science Research Council, 242n
Social system (society), 460–464; classroom as, 299–300, 309, clinical team as, 325, 346–347
Social workers, 56, 206; as team members, 299, 326, 404, 438; community service function, 452; duties on staff of Human Relations Service, 299, 308, 311
Sociologists, 464; on project staff, 48, 299
Soil erosion, 35–38, 406
Sorcery. See Witchcraft
Spain, Spanish, 75, 216, 382, 406
Spanish-Americans: historical and cultural background, 381–384, 393–396; perception of health needs, 391–392; response to medical cooperative, 387–390; unfamiliarity with Anglo organizational methods, 393–397
Spoehr, Alexander, 235
Sri Krishna (Hindu temple), 110
Stanton, Alfred H., 321
Star, Shirley, 56, 69
Steed, Gitel P., 242n
Stein, Stanley J., 376
Sterilization (of women), 196, 197, 198, 200; and politics, 204; reason for popularity of, in Puerto Rico, 202–204
Stycos, J. Mayone, 189, 192n, 210, 326
Subercaseaux, Benjamin, 348
Sudsaneh, Saowanni, 155
Sujarupa, India, 112–132 passim; village, 110–111
Surgery, 202, 437; attitudes toward, 134, 170, 340, 437
Synarchism (in Mexico), 417, 425